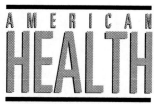

AMERICAN
HEALTH

Demographics and Spending of Health Care Consumers

AMERICAN

HEALTH

Demographics and Spending of Health Care Consumers

BY THE EDITORS OF NEW STRATEGIST PUBLICATIONS

New Strategist Publications, Inc.

Ithaca, New York

New Strategist Publications, Inc.
P.O. Box 242, Ithaca, New York 14851
800/848-0842; 607/273-0913
www.newstrategist.com

ISBN 1-885070-74-8

Printed in the United States of America

Table of Contents

List of Tables

Chapter 5. Births

Chapter 6. Health Care Coverage and Cost

Chapter 7. Deaths

List of Illustrations

Chapter 12. Mental Health

Chapter 13. Sexual Attitudes and Behavior

Chapter 14. Weight and Exercise

American Health: Demographics and Spending of Health Care Consumers

The consumers of health care drive one of the nation's largest and most important industries. Understanding who those consumers are, what they want, and how their wants and needs are changing is vital to health insurance companies, hospitals, doctors, pharmaceutical companies, government policy makers, and every business that provides its employees with health insurance. Fortunately, there are enough statistics collected and published about health care consumers to answer almost any question. The problem is not whether the numbers exist, but how to find and make sense of them.

American Health: Demographics of Health Care Consumers brings together in one volume data on health care consumers from many sources, providing a comprehensive look at the demand for health care. With more than 300 tables, *American Health* includes twice as many tables as the federal government's annual health care reference book, *Health, United States*. It provides a comprehensive look at the demographics of health care consumers and the services they use, ranging from cosmetic surgery to prayer as alternative medicine, from doctor visits to contraception. It includes detailed health care spending data from the federal government's highly respected Consumer Expenditure Survey and the less well-known Medical Expenditure Panel Survey. It presents the latest data on health care coverage and the reasons people do not have health insurance. It has the latest information on the growing girth of the population, in pounds and percentages. It examines teen attitudes toward sex and teen and adult use of contraception.

How to use this book

American Health is divided into 14 chapters, each exploring a different facet of health care. The topics are Addictions, Aging, Alternative Medicine, Attitudes toward Health Care, Births, Coverage and Costs, Deaths, Disability, Diseases and Conditions, Health Care Visits, Hospital Care, Mental Health, Sexual Attitudes and Behavior, and Weight and Exercise. Each chapter includes tables showing the demographics of health care consumers as well as explanatory text and charts revealing the most important trends.

Most of the tables in *American Health* are based on data collected by the federal government, in particular the National Center for Health Statistics. The federal government continues to be the best source of up-to-date, reliable information on the changing characteristics of Americans. Despite the volume of data produced by the federal government, finding relevant health care information and compiling it in a meaningful way is time consuming—and often frustrating—because the government publishes its health care information in a wide array of reports and on numerous web sites. The National Center for Health Statistics attempts to collate its information in the annual publication *Health, United States*. Because the purpose of *Health, United States* is to provide an overview of health care, it focuses only briefly on health care consumers. *American Health* goes further, giving readers a comprehensive look at health care from the public's perspective.

To explore the attitudes of Americans toward health care, *American Health* presents data from the General Social Survey of the University of Chicago's National Opinion Research Center. Other attitudinal data included in the book are from the Medical Expenditure Panel Survey, Pew Internet & American Life Project, the Gallup Organization, and the Kaiser Family Foundation.

While the federal government collected most of the data in *American Health*, the majority of tables published here are not just reprints of the government's tabulations. Instead, most were individually compiled and created by New Strategist's editors to reveal the trends—the story behind the statistics. If you need more information than the tables provide, explore the data source cited at the bottom of each table.

American Health includes a list of tables to help you locate the information you need. For a more detailed search, use the index at the back of the book. Also at the back of the book are a complete bibliography of data sources and a comprehensive glossary defining the terms used in tables and text.

With *American Health* in hand, you will discover the change that lies ahead not just for the health care industry, but also for the nation. Because health care is one of the largest industries in the United States, the ever-changing demands of its customers will shape the future of every American alive today—and those yet to be born.

1

Addictions

■ **More than one in five Americans smokes cigarettes.**

Forty-six million adults smoke cigarettes, and another 46 million have quit smoking.

■ **Two-thirds of high school seniors have tried cigarettes.**

Twenty-six percent have smoked a cigarette in the past 30 days.

■ **Nearly half of adults are regular drinkers.**

The proportion is highest among college graduates and those with household incomes of $75,000 or more.

■ **Forty-five percent of high school students have had a drink in the past month.**

Among high school seniors, more than one-third had five or more drinks on one occasion in the past 30 days.

■ **Marijuana is the most commonly used illicit drug.**

Twenty-one percent of 12-to-17-year-olds and 54 percent of 18-to-25-year-olds have used marijuana.

■ **Twenty-two million needed drug or alcohol treatment during the past year.**

Fewer than 2 million Americans received treatment at a facility specializing in drug and alcohol problems.

Men Are More Likely than Women to Smoke

Most women say they have never smoked.

There are 46 million adults in the U.S. who have quit smoking, and nearly 46 million who still smoke—22 percent of people aged 18 or older. Sixty percent of women have never smoked compared with slightly fewer than half of men. About one-quarter of adult men currently smoke at least occasionally compared with one in five women.

There are differences in smoking rates based on a variety of demographic characteristics, including age, race and Hispanic origin, education, and household income. Perhaps not surprisingly, the share of people who currently smoke falls with age, from 26 percent of those aged 18 to 44 to only 6 percent of those aged 75 or older. One reason for the decline is the health problems caused by smoking, which are more likely to appear at older ages. As smokers get older, many either are forced by health problems to quit or die from a smoking-related illness.

■ In spite of the considerable effort to educate teenagers about the dangers of cigarettes, most still give them a try and many take up the habit.

Most teens have smoked by age 18

(percent of people aged 12 to 17 who have ever smoked, 2003)

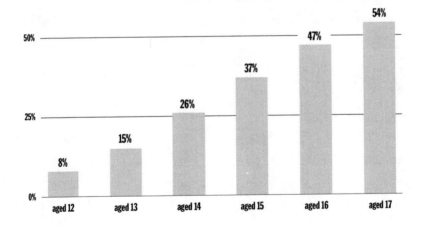

Table 1.1 Cigarette Smoking Status of People Aged 18 or Older by Selected Characteristics, 2002

(number of people aged 18 or older by selected characteristics and cigarette smoking status, 2002; numbers in thousands)

	total	all current smokers	every-day smokers	some-day smokers	former smokers	nonsmokers
Total	**205,825**	**45,821**	**37,495**	**8,327**	**46,019**	**111,817**
Sex						
Men	98,749	24,624	20,023	4,602	25,784	47,201
Women	107,076	21,197	17,472	3,725	20,235	64,616
Age						
Aged 18 to 44	108,114	28,252	22,453	5,799	14,018	64,765
Aged 45 to 64	64,650	14,542	12,386	2,156	18,790	30,643
Aged 65 to 74	17,809	2,088	1,815	273	7,412	8,090
Aged 75 or older	15,252	940	841	98	5,800	8,318
Race and Hispanic origin						
Asian	7,270	951	798	153	848	5,352
Black	23,499	5,152	4,015	1,137	3,578	14,371
Hispanic	22,691	3,749	2,444	1,304	3,374	15,391
Non-Hispanic white	149,584	34,930	29,443	5,487	37,568	75,625
Education						
Less than high school	28,248	7,743	6,619	1,125	6,855	13,436
High school graduate	52,556	14,281	12,252	2,029	13,117	24,622
Some college	48,091	10,765	8,940	1,825	12,526	24,473
College graduate	47,197	4,862	3,458	1,405	11,216	30,790
Household income						
Less than $20,000	37,369	10,827	8,815	2,012	7,077	19,159
$20,000 to $34,999	29,671	8,100	6,743	1,357	6,639	14,802
$35,000 to $54,999	31,814	8,290	6,787	1,503	7,401	15,978
$55,000 to $74,999	23,984	5,424	4,586	838	5,483	12,987
$75,000 or more	41,572	5,740	4,457	1,283	10,255	25,376

Note: Current smokers have smoked at least 100 cigarettes in lifetime and still smoke; every-day smokers are current smokers who smoke every day; some-day smokers are current smokers who smoke on some days; former smokers: have smoked at least 100 cigarettes in lifetime but currently do not smoke; nonsmokers have not smoked at least 100 cigarettes in lifetime. Numbers may not add to total because not all races are shown and Hispanics may be of any race.
Source: National Center for Health Statistics, Summary Health Statistics for U.S. Adults: National Health Interview Survey, 2002, *Series 10, No. 222, 2004*

Table 1.2 Percent Distribution of People Aged 18 or Older by Cigarette Smoking Status, 2002

(percent distribution of people aged 18 or older by cigarette smoking status and selected characteristics, 2002)

	total	all current smokers	every-day smokers	some-day smokers	former smokers	nonsmokers
Total	100.0%	22.3%	18.2%	4.0%	22.4%	54.3%
Sex						
Men	100.0	24.9	20.3	4.7	26.1	47.8
Women	100.0	19.8	16.3	3.5	18.9	60.3
Age						
Aged 18 to 44	100.0	26.1	20.8	5.4	13.0	59.9
Aged 45 to 64	100.0	22.5	19.2	3.3	29.1	47.4
Aged 65 to 74	100.0	11.7	10.2	1.5	41.6	45.4
Aged 75 or older	100.0	6.2	5.5	0.6	38.0	54.5
Race and Hispanic origin						
Asian	100.0	13.1	11.0	2.1	11.7	73.6
Black	100.0	21.9	17.1	4.8	15.2	61.2
Hispanic	100.0	16.5	10.8	5.7	14.9	67.8
Non-Hispanic white	100.0	23.4	19.7	3.7	25.1	50.6
Education						
Less than high school	100.0	27.4	23.4	4.0	24.3	47.6
High school graduate	100.0	27.2	23.3	3.9	25.0	46.8
Some college	100.0	22.4	18.6	3.8	26.0	50.9
College graduate	100.0	10.3	7.3	3.0	23.8	65.2
Household income						
Less than $20,000	100.0	29.0	23.6	5.4	18.9	51.3
$20,000 to $34,999	100.0	27.3	22.7	4.6	22.4	49.9
$35,000 to $54,999	100.0	26.1	21.3	4.7	23.3	50.2
$55,000 to $74,999	100.0	22.6	19.1	3.5	22.9	54.1
$75,000 or more	100.0	13.8	10.7	3.1	24.7	61.0

Note: Current smokers have smoked at least 100 cigarettes in lifetime and still smoke; every-day smokers are current smokers who smoke every day; some-day smokers are current smokers who smoke on some days; former smokers: have smoked at least 100 cigarettes in lifetime but currently do not smoke; nonsmokers have not smoked at least 100 cigarettes in lifetime. Numbers may not add to total because not all races are shown and Hispanics may be of any race.
Source: National Center for Health Statistics, Summary Health Statistics for U.S. Adults: National Health Interview Survey, 2002, *Series 10, No. 222, 2004*

Table 1.3 Current Cigarette Smokers by Selected Characteristics, 2003

(percent of people aged 18 or older who currently smoke cigarettes, by selected characteristics, 2003)

	percent
Total people	**22.0%**
Sex	
Men	24.7
Women	20.2
Age	
Aged 18 to 24	29.5
Aged 25 to 34	25.2
Aged 35 to 44	25.6
Aged 45 to 54	24.1
Aged 55 to 64	19.8
Aged 65 or older	9.5
Race and Hispanic origin	
Black	24.1
Hispanic	21.6
White	21.9
Multiracial	32.7
Other	26.7
Household income	
Under $15,000	30.5
$15,000 to $24,999	29.6
$25,000 to $34,999	25.9
$35,000 to $49,999	23.6
$50,000 or more	16.6
Education	
Not a high school graduate	33.6
High school graduate	28.2
Some college	23.2
College graduate	11.9

Source: Centers for Disease Control and Prevention, Behavioral Risk Factor Surveillance System, Prevalence Data, Internet site http://apps.nccd.cdc.gov/brfss

Table 1.4 Cigarette Smoking by People Aged 12 or Older, 2003

(percent of people aged 12 or older reporting any, past year, or past month use of cigarettes, 2003)

	ever used	used in past year	used in past month
Total people	**68.7%**	**29.4%**	**25.4%**
Aged 12	7.8	3.5	1.7
Aged 13	15.3	7.5	3.3
Aged 14	25.6	14.9	8.4
Aged 15	37.2	22.5	13.6
Aged 16	46.7	30.4	20.1
Aged 17	54.2	35.4	26.4
Aged 18	60.0	42.8	33.7
Aged 19	67.8	45.4	37.2
Aged 20	71.2	51.2	44.1
Aged 21	70.7	48.2	42.0
Aged 22	75.6	50.8	43.5
Aged 23	73.1	48.9	41.6
Aged 24	73.4	49.0	42.1
Aged 25	71.7	45.2	38.6
Aged 26 to 29	73.1	42.7	36.8
Aged 30 to 34	71.7	35.4	30.9
Aged 35 to 39	74.2	32.9	29.0
Aged 40 to 44	75.6	34.0	31.1
Aged 45 to 49	76.8	31.7	28.9
Aged 50 to 54	75.9	27.4	25.0
Aged 55 to 59	77.2	23.5	21.8
Aged 60 to 64	77.4	18.3	16.5
Aged 65 or older	67.2	11.8	10.0

Source: SAMHSA, Office of Applied Studies, National Survey on Drug Use and Health, 2003; Internet site http://oas.samhsa. gov/NHSDA/2k3NSDUH/appg.htm#tabg.I

Health Professionals Are Advising Smokers to Quit

Some smokers are more likely to receive this advice than others, however.

Decades ago, it was common for physicians and other health care workers to smoke, and few advised their patients to give up the habit. Although some health professionals still do not address the issue, the majority of smokers who had a routine health check-up in the past year report that a physician or other health professional told them to quit smoking.

Not all smokers were advised to quit smoking. Women are more likely than men to say their doctor told them to give up cigarettes at their last physical. People aged 45 to 64 were more likely than older or younger adults to say they had been given this advice.

As would be expected, people who characterize their health status as poor were most likely to say they were advised to quit smoking.

■ Health care providers need to do more than admonish their patients. They need to provide guidance on how to quit smoking before their advice can be adopted.

Health status determines smoking advice

(percent of smokers aged 18 or older who had a routine health check-up in the past year and were advised to quit smoking, by self-assessed health status, 2001)

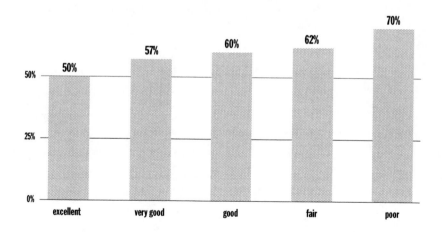

Table 1.5 Advised to Quit Smoking during Routine Health Check-Up, 2001

(number of current smokers aged 18 or older who had a routine health check-up in the previous year, and percent distribution by whether they were advised to quit smoking, 2001; numbers in thousands)

	total	told to quit	not told to quit
Total people	**23,129**	**58.4%**	**37.5%**
Age			
Aged 18 to 44	11,323	54.8	42.1
Aged 45 to 64	8,929	62.1	33.6
Aged 65 or older	2,877	60.9	31.3
Sex			
Male	10,978	53.6	42.0
Female	12,151	62.7	33.4
Race and Hispanic origin			
Black	3,252	54.4	40.9
Hispanic	1,657	54.9	41.3
White and other	18,221	59.4	36.5
Income status			
Poor	3,124	61.7	33.3
Near poor	1,221	54.2	43.4
Low income	3,165	56.0	38.7
Middle income	7,832	55.2	39.7
High income	7,788	61.8	35.5
Self-reported health status			
Excellent	3,502	49.7	46.1
Very good	7,096	56.7	39.8
Good	7,717	59.9	36.6
Fair	3,357	62.3	30.8
Poor	1,457	70.4	25.9

Note: Poor refers to incomes below poverty level. Near poor is incomes from poverty level through 125 percent of poverty level. Low income is more than 125 percent of poverty level through 200 percent of poverty level. Middle income is more than 200 percent of poverty level through 400 percent of poverty level. High income is more than 400 percent of poverty level. Percentages will not sum to 100 because no response is not shown.
Source: Center for Financing, Access and Cost Trends, Agency for Healthcare Research and Quality: Medical Expenditure Panel Survey, 2001; Internet site http://www.meps.ahrq.gov/CompendiumTables/TC_TOC.htm

By 12th Grade, Most Teens Have Tried Cigarettes

Boys are more likely than girls to be tobacco users.

During the teen years, experimentation is common, including trying cigarettes. By the time they reach their senior year, almost two-thirds of students have tried smoking. Most do not continue to smoke, but more than one-quarter are current smokers, a habit they may find difficult to kick.

Similar shares of boys and girls have tried cigarettes or other forms of tobacco, such as cigars and chewing tobacco. But while young women generally stick to cigarettes, young men try a wider variety of tobacco products. As a result, among high school seniors, boys are more likely than girls to be current tobacco users.

Most students in 8th, 10th, and 12th grade disapprove or strongly disapprove of people who smoke one or more packs of cigarettes a day. Disapproval is slightly greater than it was a decade ago. Smaller percentages view cigarettes as a serious health risk, although the share is higher than in 1993. Antismoking efforts seem to have an effect eventually. The share of teens who think smoking poses a great physical risk rises from 53 percent among 8th graders to 70 percent among high school seniors.

■ Attitudes about smoking clearly influence smoking rates. To the degree that teens "disapprove" of smokers, it can discourage them from taking up the habit.

Teens are more likely to think cigarette smoking is risky

(percent of 8th, 10th, and 12th graders who think smoking one or more packs of cigarettes per day presents a "great" physical risk, 1993 and 2003)

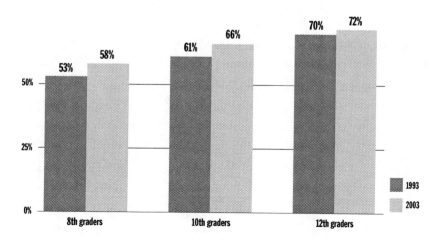

Table 1.6 Tobacco Use among 9th to 12th Graders by Sex, 2003

(percent of 9th to 12th graders by tobacco use status, by sex and grade, 2003)

	total	9th grade	10th grade	11th grade	12th grade
Total					
Lifetime cigarette use (ever tried a cigarette)	58.4%	52.0%	58.3%	60.0%	65.4%
Lifetime daily cigarette use (ever smoked cigarettes every day for 30 days)	15.8	11.5	15.0	18.1	19.8
Current cigarette use (smoked cigarettes in the past 30 days)	21.9	17.4	21.8	23.6	26.2
Current frequent cigarette use (smoked cigarettes on 20 of the past 30 days)	9.7	6.3	9.2	11.2	13.1
Smoked 10 or more cigarettes a day on the days they smoked in the past 30 days	3.1	1.9	2.4	3.3	4.8
Purchased cigarettes at a store or gas station during the past 30 days	18.9	12.0	13.6	27.9	26.1
Used chewing tobacco, snuff, or dip during the past 30 days	6.7	6.6	5.4	7.8	7.1
Smoked cigars, cigarillos, or little cigars in the past 30 days	14.8	11.9	13.2	16.3	19.1
Used tobacco of any kind in the past 30 days	27.5	22.0	26.4	30.4	33.0
Females					
Lifetime cigarette use (ever tried a cigarette)	58.1	50.9	57.7	59.8	65.9
Lifetime daily cigarette use (ever smoked cigarettes every day for 30 days)	15.8	11.6	15.8	18.4	18.3
Current cigarette use (smoked cigarettes in the past 30 days)	21.9	18.9	21.9	24.0	23.3
Current frequent cigarette use (smoked cigarettes on 20 of the past 30 days)	9.7	6.9	9.0	11.8	11.4
Smoked 10 or more cigarettes a day on the days they smoked in the past 30 days	2.4	1.3	2.4	3.1	2.6
Purchased cigarettes at a store or gas station during the past 30 days	13.8	10.4	7.8	21.2	18.9
Used chewing tobacco, snuff, or dip during the past 30 days	2.2	3.8	1.0	2.0	1.3
Smoked cigars, cigarillos, or little cigars in the past 30 days	9.4	10.0	9.3	10.0	7.8
Used tobacco of any kind in the past 30 days	24.6	22.4	23.6	27.0	25.7
Males					
Lifetime cigarette use (ever tried a cigarette)	58.7	53.0	59.0	60.1	64.7
Lifetime daily cigarette use (ever smoked cigarettes every day for 30 days)	15.7	11.4	14.3	17.8	21.0
Current cigarette use (smoked cigarettes in the past 30 days)	21.8	16.0	21.7	23.2	29.0
Current frequent cigarette use (smoked cigarettes on 20 of the past 30 days)	9.6	5.7	9.5	10.5	14.5
Smoked 10 or more cigarettes a day on the days they smoked in the past 30 days	3.6	2.4	2.4	3.5	6.8
Purchased cigarettes at a store or gas station during the past 30 days	24.2	13.8	19.3	34.5	33.6
Used chewing tobacco, snuff, or dip during the past 30 days	11.0	9.1	9.6	13.3	12.7
Smoked cigars, cigarillos, or little cigars in the past 30 days	19.9	13.6	17.0	22.2	29.8
Used tobacco of any kind in the past 30 days	30.3	21.5	29.2	33.7	40.3

Source: Centers for Disease Control and Prevention, Youth Risk Behavior Surveillance–United States, 2003, Mortality and Morbidity Weekly Report, Surveillance Summaries, Vol. 53/SS02, May 21, 2004

Table 1.7 Attitudes toward Cigarette Smoking by 8th, 10th, and 12th Graders, 1993 and 2003

(percent of 8th, 10th, and 12th graders who think smoking one or more packs of cigarettes per day presents a great physical risk, and percent who disapprove or strongly disapprove of those who smoke one or more packs of cigarettes per day, 1993 and 2003; percentage point change, 1993–2003)

	2003	1993	percentage point change
Great risk			
8th graders	57.7%	52.7%	5.0
10th graders	65.7	60.7	5.0
12th graders	72.1	69.5	2.6
Disapprove			
8th graders	84.6	80.6	4.0
10th graders	81.4	76.5	4.9
12th graders	74.8	70.6	4.2

Source: Institute for Social Research, University of Michigan, Monitoring the Future Survey, 2003; Internet site http://monitoringthefuture.org/data/03data.html; calculations by New Strategist

Drinking Varies by Demographics

The affluent are most likely to be regular drinkers.

There are distinct demographic differences in the likelihood of being a regular drinker. Men are more likely to drink regularly, as are non-Hispanic whites, college graduates, and people with household incomes of $75,000 or more.

The percentage of people who drink regularly falls with age. The oldest Americans are more likely to be lifetime abstainers, but opportunities to drink regularly—such as parties with friends—also become less common with age. Metabolic changes related to aging can also make alcohol consumption less appealing.

By law, the sale of alcoholic beverages is restricted to people aged 21 or older. It is clear, however, that people under age 21 have access to alcohol. More than half of 19- and 20-year-olds have consumed alcoholic beverages in the past month. Even among 15-year-olds drinking is not rare—21 percent have drunk alcohol in the past month. More disturbing is the rate of binge drinking among people under age 21. One-quarter of 17-year-olds have had five or more drinks on at least one occasion in the past month. The shares are even higher among those aged 18 to 20, although the highest rate of binge drinking is found among people aged 22 to 23, with nearly half admitting they had done so.

■ News about the health benefits of moderate alcohol consumption may increase the percentage of middle-aged and older adults who drink regularly.

Regular drinking rises with income

(percent of people aged 18 or older who are regular drinkers, by household income, 2002)

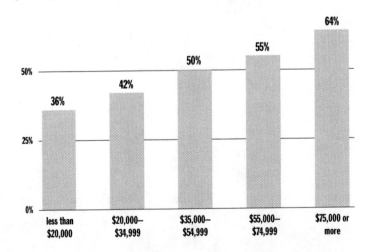

Table 1.8 Alcohol Drinking Status of People Aged 18 or Older by Selected Characteristics, 2002

(number of people aged 18 or older by selected characteristics and alcohol drinking status, 2002; numbers in thousands)

	total	lifetime abstainer	former infrequent	former regular	current infrequent	current regular
Total	**205,825**	**44,478**	**16,756**	**13,537**	**26,678**	**97,791**
Sex						
Men	98,749	14,234	6,919	7,706	9,369	56,955
Women	107,076	30,244	9,837	5,830	17,308	40,835
Age						
Aged 18 to 44	108,114	22,587	5,738	4,186	13,871	58,243
Aged 45 to 64	64,650	11,867	6,300	5,211	9,323	29,946
Aged 65 to 74	17,809	4,780	2,553	2,133	1,997	5,777
Aged 75 or older	15,252	5,244	2,164	2,007	1,486	3,825
Race and Hispanic origin						
Asian	7,270	2,935	345	137	862	2,657
Black	23,499	7,542	2,539	1,494	3,041	7,948
Hispanic	22,691	8,030	1,421	1,045	2,749	8,718
Non-Hispanic white	149,584	25,512	12,190	10,565	19,635	77,135
Education						
Less than high school	28,248	9,462	3,564	3,033	2,931	8,397
High school graduate	52,556	11,591	5,363	4,158	7,747	21,875
Some college	48,091	7,988	4,316	3,181	7,569	23,823
College graduate	47,197	6,526	2,629	2,426	5,622	29,124
Household income						
Less than $20,000	37,369	11,736	3,914	3,348	4,051	13,260
$20,000 to $34,999	29,671	7,430	2,804	2,318	4,098	12,419
$35,000 to $54,999	31,814	5,913	2,920	1,832	4,690	15,890
$55,000 to $74,999	23,984	3,781	1,889	1,369	3,474	13,094
$75,000 or more	41,572	5,265	1,972	2,125	5,155	26,455

Note: Lifetime abstainer had fewer than 12 drinks in lifetime; former drinker had more than 12 drinks in lifetime, but no drinks in past year; current drinker had more than 12 drinks in lifetime, and had drinks in past year; infrequent drinker had fewer than 12 drinks in one year; regular drinker had more than 12 drinks in one year. Numbers by race and Hispanic origin will not sum to total because not all races are shown and Hispanics may be of any race. Numbers may not add to total because unknown is not shown.
Source: National Center for Health Statistics, Summary Health Statistics for U.S. Adults: National Health Interview Survey, 2002, *Series 10, No. 222, 2004*

Table 1.9 Percent Distribution of People Aged 18 or Older by Alcohol Drinking Status, 2002

(percent distribution of people aged 18 or older by alcohol drinking status and selected characteristics, 2002)

	total	lifetime abstainer	former infrequent	former regular	current infrequent	current regular
Total	**100.0%**	**21.6%**	**8.1%**	**6.6%**	**13.0%**	**47.5%**
Sex						
Men	100.0	14.4	7.0	7.8	9.5	57.7
Women	100.0	28.2	9.2	5.4	16.2	38.1
Age						
Aged 18 to 44	100.0	20.9	5.3	3.9	12.8	53.9
Aged 45 to 64	100.0	18.4	9.7	8.1	14.4	46.3
Aged 65 to 74	100.0	26.8	14.3	12.0	11.2	32.4
Aged 75 or older	100.0	34.4	14.2	13.2	9.7	25.1
Race and Hispanic origin						
Asian	100.0	40.4	4.7	1.9	11.9	36.5
Black	100.0	32.1	10.8	6.4	12.9	33.8
Hispanic	100.0	35.4	6.3	4.6	12.1	38.4
Non-Hispanic white	100.0	17.1	8.1	7.1	13.1	51.6
Education						
Less than high school	100.0	33.5	12.6	10.7	10.4	29.7
High school graduate	100.0	22.1	10.2	7.9	14.7	41.6
Some college	100.0	16.6	9.0	6.6	15.7	49.5
College graduate	100.0	13.8	5.6	5.1	11.9	61.7
Household income						
Less than $20,000	100.0	31.4	10.5	9.0	10.8	35.5
$20,000 to $34,999	100.0	25.0	9.5	7.8	13.8	41.9
$35,000 to $54,999	100.0	18.6	9.2	5.8	14.7	49.9
$55,000 to $74,999	100.0	15.8	7.9	5.7	14.5	54.6
$75,000 or more	100.0	12.7	4.7	5.1	12.4	63.6

Note: Lifetime abstainer had fewer than 12 drinks in lifetime; former drinker had more than 12 drinks in lifetime, but no drinks in past year; current drinker had more than 12 drinks in lifetime, and had drinks in past year; infrequent drinker had fewer than 12 drinks in one year; regular drinker had more than 12 drinks in one year. Percentages by race and Hispanic origin will not sum to total because not all races are shown and Hispanics may be of any race. Percentages may not add to total because unknown is not shown.
Source: National Center for Health Statistics, Summary Health Statistics for U.S. Adults: National Health Interview Survey, 2002, *Series 10, No. 222, 2004*

Table 1.10   Alcohol Use by Selected Characteristics, 2003

(percent of people aged 18 or older who have had at least one drink of alcohol in the past thirty days, by selected characteristics, 2003)

	percent
Total people	**58.8%**
Sex	
Men	66.2
Women	50.4
Age	
Aged 18 to 24	60.2
Aged 25 to 34	64.0
Aged 35 to 44	63.2
Aged 45 to 54	60.4
Aged 55 to 64	54.7
Aged 65 or older	41.6
Race and Hispanic origin	
Black	46.6
Hispanic	51.1
White	62.4
Multiracial	55.7
Other	49.1
Household income	
Under $15,000	41.9
$15,000 to $24,999	48.1
$25,000 to $34,999	54.4
$35,000 to $49,999	59.3
$50,000 or more	70.7
Education	
Not a high school graduate	38.3
High school graduate	52.6
Some college	60.5
College graduate	68.8

Source: Centers for Disease Control and Prevention, Behavioral Risk Factor Surveillance System, Prevalence Data, Internet site http://apps.nccd.cdc.gov/brfss

Table 1.11 Alcohol Use by People Aged 12 or Older, 2003

(percent of people aged 12 or older who drank alcoholic beverages during the past month, by level of alcohol use, 2003)

	any	binge	heavy
Total people	**50.1%**	**22.6%**	**6.8%**
Aged 12	2.9	0.9	0.1
Aged 13	6.1	2.2	0.2
Aged 14	13.1	7.1	1.3
Aged 15	20.9	11.7	3.1
Aged 16	28.5	18.0	4.3
Aged 17	35.3	24.5	6.8
Aged 18	43.7	31.5	10.1
Aged 19	52.4	36.3	13.8
Aged 20	59.6	41.4	16.1
Aged 21	69.7	47.8	18.7
Aged 22	69.8	47.0	17.4
Aged 23	67.4	46.1	16.5
Aged 24	65.5	44.0	15.3
Aged 25	66.1	40.0	13.6
Aged 26 to 29	61.7	38.0	11.4
Aged 30 to 34	59.2	29.1	7.9
Aged 35 to 39	59.5	28.1	7.9
Aged 40 to 44	58.6	25.7	7.9
Aged 45 to 49	57.7	23.2	6.8
Aged 50 to 54	54.0	17.9	4.9
Aged 55 to 59	52.9	15.5	4.2
Aged 60 to 64	46.2	11.9	2.5
Aged 65 or older	34.4	7.2	1.8

Note: Binge drinking is defined as having five or more drinks on the same occasion on at least one day in the thirty days prior to the survey. Heavy drinking is having five or more drinks on the same occasion on each of five or more days in the thirty days prior to the survey.
Source: SAMHSA, Office of Applied Studies, National Survey on Drug Use and Health, 2003; Internet site http://oas.samhsa.gov/NHSDA/2k3NSDUH/appg.htm#tabg.1

Most High School Students Have Tried Alcohol

Heavy drinking is common among some teens.

High school students do not find it difficult to get alcoholic beverages. Three-quarters have consumed one or more alcoholic drinks in their lifetime. The share rises with age, from 65 percent among 9th graders to 83 percent among 12th graders. Of greater concern is the number of high school students who have engaged in "episodic heavy drinking," defined as consuming five or more alcoholic beverage on one occasion. Twenty percent of 9th graders reported doing so, as did 37 percent of high school seniors.

Most students do not believe there is a great physical risk in consuming one or two drinks every day. This is precisely the message that has come out of research linking moderate alcohol consumption with health benefits. However, what is good for adults may not be good for teenagers who are still physically developing. Students are also less likely in 2003 than in 1993 to disapprove of people who consume one or two drinks nearly every day, which may reflect greater awareness of the health benefits of moderate drinking. But the majority still disapproves.

■ In spite of efforts to keep alcoholic beverages out of the hands of teenagers, they continue to find ways to get drinks.

Many teens drink heavily

(percent of high school students who have engaged in episodic heavy drinking in the past thirty days, by grade, 2003)

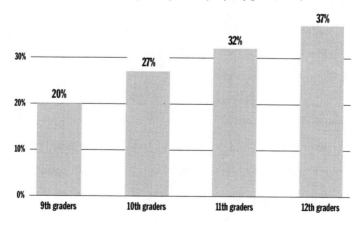

Table 1.12 Alcohol Use by 9th to 12th Graders by Sex, 2003

(percent of 9th to 12th graders who have ever used or currently use alcohol, and percent who have drunk heavily in past 30 days, by grade and sex, 2003)

	lifetime use (ever had a drink)	current use (one or more drinks in past 30 days)	episodic heavy drinking (drank 5 or more drinks in a row in the past 30 days)
Total in 9th to 12th grade	**74.9%**	**44.9%**	**28.3%**
Female	76.1	45.8	27.5
Male	73.7	43.8	29.0
Total 9th graders	**65.0**	**36.2**	**19.8**
Female	66.2	38.5	20.9
Male	64.0	33.9	18.8
Total 10th graders	**76.7**	**43.5**	**27.4**
Female	76.5	44.9	27.2
Male	74.9	42.2	27.7
Total 11th graders	**78.6**	**47.0**	**31.8**
Female	80.9	46.8	29.4
Male	76.4	47.3	34.1
Total 12th graders	**83.0**	**55.9**	**37.2**
Female	83.3	55.5	34.5
Male	82.6	56.0	39.5

Source: Centers for Disease Control and Prevention, Youth Risk Behavior Surveillance–United States, 2003, Mortality and Morbidity Weekly Report, Surveillance Summaries, Vol. 53/SS02, May 21, 2004

Table 1.13 Attitudes toward Drinking by 8th, 10th, and 12th Graders, 1993 and 2003

(percent of 8th, 10th, and 12th graders who think taking one or two drinks of alcohol nearly every day is a great physical risk, and percent who disapprove or strongly disapprove of those who drink one or two drinks of alcohol nearly every day, 1993 and 2003; percentage point change, 1993–2003)

	2003	1993	percentage point change
Great risk			
8th graders	29.9%	32.6%	−2.7
10th graders	30.9	35.9	−5.0
12th graders	20.1	28.2	−8.1
Disapprove			
8th graders	77.1	79.6	−2.5
10th graders	74.2	78.6	−4.4
12th graders	68.9	77.8	−8.9

Source: Institute for Social Research, University of Michigan, Monitoring the Future Survey, 2003; Internet site http://monitoringthefuture.org/data/03data.html; calculations by New Strategist

Marijuana Is the Most Commonly Used Illicit Drug

Forty-one percent of people aged 12 or older have tried it.

A remarkable 46 percent of people aged 12 or older have used illicit drugs at least once in their lifetime. The rate is relatively high primarily because of drug use by baby boomers and younger generations. Only about 10 percent of people aged 65 or older admit to ever using an illicit drug compared with the majority of those aged 18 to 54.

Although many people have given illicit drugs a try, relatively few have used them in the past year (15 percent) and a much smaller 8 percent have used them in the past month. But the share of current (past month) users is much higher among young adults, with 20 percent of those aged 18 to 25 falling into this category.

The most commonly used illicit drug is marijuana. The popularity of marijuana is the primary reason for the relatively high proportion of lifetime drug users in the population. When marijuana is factored out, a smaller 30 percent of people aged 12 or older have ever tried illicit drugs. Other than marijuana, prescribed psychotherapeutic drugs are the most commonly used illicit drug.

■ Recent efforts in some states to soften harsh penalties for drug possession, as well as the movement to allow the medicinal use of marijuana, suggest that public perceptions of drug use—and the best way to deal with it—are changing.

Psychotherapeutics are the second most commonly used illicit drug

(percent of people aged 12 or older using selected illicit drugs in their lifetime, by type of drug, 2003)

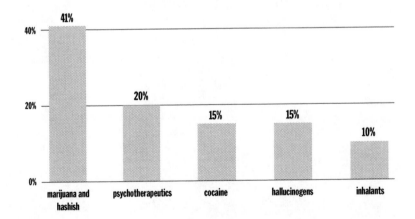

Table 1.14 Illicit Drug Use by People Aged 12 or Older, 2003

(percent of people aged 12 or older who ever used any illicit drug, who used an illicit drug in the past year, and who used an illicit drug in the past month, by age, 2003)

	ever used	used in past year	used in past month
Total people	**46.4%**	**14.7%**	**8.2%**
Aged 12	12.2	6.2	2.7
Aged 13	18.7	11.9	4.9
Aged 14	26.3	18.7	8.5
Aged 15	34.2	25.2	13.3
Aged 16	43.8	33.2	18.6
Aged 17	48.4	36.1	19.7
Aged 18	53.5	38.2	22.6
Aged 19	58.3	39.9	23.5
Aged 20	62.0	40.3	24.0
Aged 21	61.6	35.0	20.7
Aged 22	64.0	33.5	19.6
Aged 23	63.4	32.2	18.0
Aged 24	62.3	30.1	17.2
Aged 25	60.1	25.9	15.7
Aged 26 to 29	57.9	23.6	13.4
Aged 30 to 34	56.8	16.6	8.8
Aged 35 to 39	61.7	15.0	8.4
Aged 40 to 44	65.3	14.0	8.1
Aged 45 to 49	62.3	12.6	6.8
Aged 50 to 54	52.0	7.4	3.9
Aged 55 to 59	38.3	4.4	2.0
Aged 60 to 64	23.8	2.9	1.1
Aged 65 or older	9.9	0.7	0.6

Note: Illicit drugs include marijuana/hashish, cocaine (including crack), heroin, hallucinogens, inhalants, and any prescription-type psychotherapeutic used nonmedically.
Source: SAMHSA, Office of Applied Studies, National Survey on Drug Use and Health, 2003; Internet site http://oas.samhsa. gov/NHSDA/2k3NSDUH/appg.htm#tabg.1

Table 1.15 Illicit Drug Use by Type of Drug and Age, 2003

(percent of people aged 12 or older using selected illicit drugs in their lifetime, during the past year, or during the past month, by age, 2003)

	total	12 to 17	18 to 25	26 or older
LIFETIME				
Any illicit drug	**46.4%**	**30.5%**	**60.5%**	**46.1%**
Marijuana oe hashish	40.6	19.6	53.9	41.2
Cocaine	14.7	2.6	15.0	16.3
Crack	3.3	0.6	3.8	3.6
Heroin	1.6	0.3	1.6	1.7
Hallucinogens	14.5	5.0	23.3	14.2
LSD	10.3	1.6	14.0	10.8
PCP	3.0	0.8	3.0	3.3
Ecstasy	4.6	2.4	14.8	3.1
Inhalants	9.7	10.7	14.9	8.6
Nonmedical use of any psychotherapeutic	20.1	13.4	29.0	19.5
Pain relievers	13.1	11.2	23.7	11.5
Tranquilizers	8.5	3.5	12.3	8.5
Stimulants	8.8	4.0	10.8	9.0
Methamphetamine	5.2	1.3	5.2	5.7
Sedatives	4.0	1.0	1.8	4.8
Any illicit drug other than marijuana	29.9	21.3	40.2	29.3
PAST YEAR				
Any illicit drug	**14.7**	**21.8**	**34.6**	**10.3**
Marijuana or hashish	10.6	15.0	28.5	6.9
Cocaine	2.5	1.8	6.6	1.9
Crack	0.6	0.4	0.9	0.6
Heroin	0.1	0.1	0.3	0.1
Hallucinogens	1.7	3.1	6.7	0.6
LSD	0.2	0.6	1.1	–
PCP	0.1	0.4	0.4	–
Ecstasy	0.9	1.3	3.7	0.3
Inhalants	0.9	4.5	2.1	0.2
Nonmedical use of any psychotherapeutic	6.3	9.2	14.5	4.5
Pain relievers	4.9	7.7	12.0	3.3
Tranquilizers	2.1	2.3	5.3	1.5
Stimulants	1.2	2.3	3.5	0.6
Methamphetamine	0.6	0.7	1.6	0.4
Sedatives	0.3	0.5	0.5	0.3
Any illicit drug other than marijuana	8.5	13.4	19.7	5.9

(continued)

PAST MONTH	total	12 to 17	18 to 25	26 or older
Any illicit drug	**8.2%**	**11.2%**	**20.3%**	**5.6%**
Marijuana and hashish	6.2	7.9	17.0	4.0
Cocaine	1.0	0.6	2.2	0.8
Crack	0.3	0.1	0.2	0.3
Heroin	0.1	0.1	0.1	–
Hallucinogens	0.4	1.0	1.7	0.1
LSD	0.1	0.2	0.2	–
PCP	–	0.1	0.1	–
Ecstasy	0.2	0.4	0.7	0.1
Inhalants	0.2	1.3	0.4	0.1
Nonmedical use of any psychotherapeutic	2.7	4.0	6.0	1.9
Pain relievers	2.0	3.2	4.7	1.3
Tranquilizers	0.8	0.9	1.7	0.6
Stimulants	0.5	0.9	1.3	0.3
Methamphetamine	0.3	0.3	0.6	0.2
Sedatives	0.1	0.2	0.2	0.1
Any illicit drug other than marijuana	3.7	5.7	8.4	2.6

Note: Illicit drugs include marijuana/hashish, cocaine (including crack), heroin, hallucinogens, inhalants, or any prescription-type psychotherapeutic used nonmedically. (–) means percentage is less than 0.05 or sample is too small to make a reliable estimate. Source: SAMHSA, Office of Applied Studies, National Survey on Drug Use and Health, 2003; Internet site http://oas.samhsa. gov/NHSDA/2k3NSDUH/appg.htm#tabg.1

Twenty Percent of High School Students Have Smoked Pot

More than half of people aged 18 to 25 have used marijuana.

Marijuana is the most commonly used illicit drug and is readily available to most teenagers and young adults. In 2002, more than half of 18-to-25-year-olds had ever smoked pot.

In 1965, few young adults had ever smoked marijuana. Use of the drug exploded in the 1970s, rising from 22 percent among people aged 18 to 25 in 1970 to more than 50 percent in 1979. The percentage of those who have experimented with marijuana at least once has hovered around the 50 percent mark ever since.

Overall, 40 percent of students in grades 9 through 12 have tried marijuana, and 22 percent have used it in the past month. The share of high schoolers who have smoked pot rises with age, from 31 percent of 9th graders to 49 percent of high school seniors.

■ The widespread use of marijuana among teenagers and young adults signals a high degree of acceptance of the drug's use. This attitude portends continued division in the nation about marijuana laws and the use of pot for medicinal purposes.

Marijuana use is commonplace among teens and young adults

(percent of people aged 12 to 25 who have ever used marijuana, selected years 1965–2002)

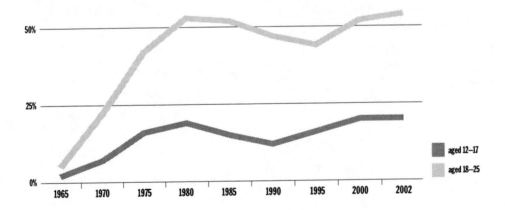

aged 12–17
aged 18–25

Table 1.16 Lifetime Marijuana Use by People Aged 12 to 25, 1965 to 2002

(percent of people aged 12 to 25 who have ever used marijuana, 1965 to 2002)

	12 to 17	18 to 25
2002	20.6%	53.8%
2001	21.9	53.0
2000	20.4	51.8
1999	19.7	50.3
1998	19.9	47.0
1997	18.6	45.7
1996	17.9	44.3
1995	16.4	44.1
1994	13.9	43.5
1993	12.4	43.4
1992	11.8	44.5
1991	11.5	45.1
1990	11.9	46.6
1989	12.5	47.3
1988	13.2	48.8
1987	14.9	49.7
1986	15.2	50.4
1985	15.4	51.5
1984	15.6	53.2
1983	16.0	53.8
1982	16.9	54.4
1981	17.6	54.3
1980	19.4	53.0
1979	19.6	52.1
1978	18.0	51.0
1977	18.7	48.6
1976	17.9	44.9
1975	15.8	41.6
1974	14.8	39.3
1973	13.2	34.5
1972	11.0	30.8
1971	9.4	27.1
1970	7.4	22.0
1969	5.9	16.0
1968	4.9	10.6
1967	2.8	7.7
1966	1.8	6.1
1965	1.8	5.1

Source: SAMHSA, Office of Applied Studies, National Survey on Drug Use and Health, 2002; Internet site http://www.samhsa. gov/

Table 1.17 Marijuana Use by 9th to 12th Graders by Sex, 2003

(percent of 9th to 12th graders who have ever used marijuana or who have used marijuana in the past thirty days, by grade and sex, 2003)

	lifetime	past month
Total in 9th to 12th grade	**40.2%**	**22.4%**
Female	37.6	19.3
Male	42.7	25.1
Total 9th graders	**30.7**	**18.5**
Female	28.1	17.2
Male	33.1	19.6
Total 10th graders	**40.4**	**22.0**
Female	36.4	18.2
Male	44.2	25.7
Total 11th graders	**44.5**	**24.1**
Female	43.5	20.9
Male	45.4	27.3
Total 12th graders	**48.5**	**25.8**
Female	44.9	21.3
Male	51.7	30.0

Source: Centers for Disease Control and Prevention, Youth Risk Behavior Surveillance–United States, 2003, Mortality and Morbidity Weekly Report, *Surveillance Summaries, Vol. 53/SS02, May 21, 2004*

Teen Drug Use Increased in the Past Decade

Fewer students think casual drug use poses a great risk to health.

Between 1993 and 2003, the percentage of high school students using a variety of illicit drugs increased. The largest increase was in the use of marijuana, with the share of 10th graders who had smoked pot in the past thirty days rising from 11 percent to 17 percent. Among high school seniors, drug use rose from 16 percent to 21 percent. Small declines occurred in the use of some drugs, however, particularly inhalants.

The rise in the share of teens using drugs is likely tied to changing attitudes about drug use. Among high school seniors in 1993, 73 percent believed smoking marijuana regularly posed a great physical risk. By 2003, the share was a much smaller 55 percent. The percentages of students who believe that LSD, cocaine, and steroids pose a significant health risk also declined. Teenagers may be somewhat correct in assuming that trying a drug once or twice is unlikely to put their health at risk, but there has been a more troubling decline in the percentage of teens who believe that regular use of drugs is risky.

■ The ambivalence of boomer parents about their own drug use may be one reason for the more casual attitude toward drug use among today's teens.

Twelfth graders are less likely to think drug use is risky

(percent of 12th graders who think selected drug use behavior poses a great physical risk, 1993 and 2003)

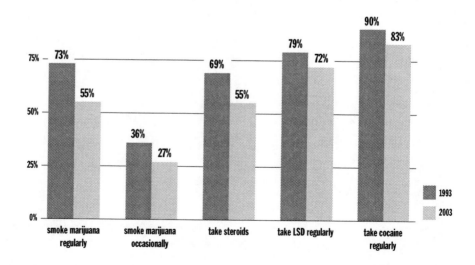

Table 1.18 Drug Use by 8th, 10th, and 12th Graders, 1993 and 2003

(percent of 8th, 10th, and 12th graders who have ever used illicit drugs and who have used illicit drugs in the past 30 days, by type of drug, 1993 and 2003; percentage point change, 1993–2003)

	ever used			used in past thirty days		
	2003	1993	percentage point change	2003	1993	percentage point change
8TH GRADERS						
Any illicit drug	**22.8%**	**22.5%**	**0.3**	**9.7%**	**8.4%**	**1.3**
Any illicit drug other than marijuana	13.6	16.8	−3.2	4.7	5.3	−0.6
Marijuana	17.5	12.6	4.9	7.5	5.1	2.4
Inhalants	15.8	19.4	−3.6	4.1	5.4	−1.3
Hallucinogens	4.0	3.9	0.1	1.2	1.2	0.0
Cocaine	3.6	2.9	0.7	0.9	0.7	0.2
Heroin	1.6	1.4	0.2	0.4	0.4	0.0
Amphetamines	8.4	11.8	−3.4	2.7	3.6	−0.9
Steroids	2.5	1.6	0.9	0.7	0.5	0.2
10TH GRADERS						
Any illicit drug	**41.4**	**32.8**	**8.6**	**19.5**	**14.0**	**5.5**
Any illicit drug other than marijuana	19.7	20.9	−1.2	6.9	6.5	0.4
Marijuana	36.4	24.4	12.0	17.0	10.9	6.1
Inhalants	12.7	17.5	−4.8	2.2	3.3	−1.1
Hallucinogens	6.9	6.8	0.1	1.5	1.9	−0.4
Cocaine	5.1	3.6	1.5	1.3	0.9	0.4
Heroin	1.5	1.3	0.2	0.3	0.3	0.0
Amphetamines	13.1	14.9	−1.8	4.3	4.3	0.0
Steroids	3.0	1.7	1.3	0.8	0.5	0.3
12TH GRADERS						
Any illicit drug	**51.1**	**42.9**	**8.2**	**24.1**	**18.3**	**5.8**
Any illicit drug other than marijuana	27.7	26.7	1.0	10.4	7.9	2.5
Marijuana	46.1	35.3	10.8	21.2	15.5	5.7
Inhalants	11.2	17.4	−6.2	1.5	2.5	−1.0
Hallucinogens	10.6	10.9	−0.3	1.8	2.7	−0.9
Cocaine	7.7	6.1	1.6	2.1	1.3	0.8
Heroin	1.5	1.1	0.4	0.4	0.2	0.2
Amphetamines	14.4	15.1	−0.7	5.0	3.7	1.3
Steroids	3.5	2.0	1.5	1.3	0.7	0.6

Source: Institute for Social Research, University of Michigan, Monitoring the Future Survey, 2003; Internet site http://monitoringthefuture.org/data/03data.html

Table 1.19 Attitudes toward Drug Use by 12th Graders, 1993 and 2003

(percentage of 12th graders who think the use of illicit drugs is a great physical risk and percent who disapprove or strongly disapprove of those aged 18 or older who use illicit drugs, by type of drug, 1993 and 2003; percentage point change, 1993–2003)

	2003	1993	percentage point change
Great risk			
Try marijuana once or twice	16.1%	21.9%	–5.8
Smoke marijuana occasionally	26.6	35.6	–9.0
Smoke marijuana regularly	54.9	72.5	–17.6
Try LSD once or twice	36.2	39.5	–3.3
Take LSD regularly	72.3	79.4	–7.1
Try PCP once or twice	45.2	50.8	–5.6
Try MDMA (Ecstasy) once or twice	56.3	–	–
Try cocaine once or twice	51.0	57.6	–6.6
Take cocaine occasionally	69.1	73.3	–4.2
Take cocaine regularly	83.0	90.1	–7.1
Take steroids	55.0	69.1	–14.1
Disapprove			
Try marijuana once or twice	53.4	63.3	–9.9
Smoke marijuana occasionally	64.2	75.5	–11.3
Smoke marijuana regularly	78.7	87.6	–8.9
Try LSD once or twice	85.5	85.9	–0.4
Take LSD regularly	94.4	95.8	–1.4
Try MDMA (Ecstasy) once or twice	84.7	–	–
Try cocaine once or twice	89.3	92.7	–3.4
Take cocaine regularly	95.8	97.5	–1.7
Take steroids	86.0	92.1	–6.1

Note: (–) means data not available.
Source: Institute for Social Research, University of Michigan, Monitoring the Future Survey, 2003; Internet site http://monitoringthefuture.org/data/03data.html; calculations by New Strategist

Most Addicts Do Not Get the Treatment They Need

Those that get treatment most commonly do so on an outpatient basis.

Although some people who have drug or alcohol problems are able to resolve them on their own, most need some type of assistance. Support groups such as Alcoholics or Narcotics Anonymous can be effective for highly motivated individuals, but many people, particularly those who are heavy users of drugs or alcohol, need more intensive treatment at a specialized facility. Most, however, do not get the needed treatment. Of 22 million people identified as needing specialized treatment for drug or alcohol problems, only 8 percent received treatment at a specialized facility.

The majority of those getting specialized treatment received it on an outpatient basis, and most turned to private, nonprofit institutions for their treatment. Only 10 percent received treatment in a residential facility, although those types of facilities often have better success than outpatient programs. Limited or nonexistent health insurance coverage for residential treatment programs keeps many people from participating.

■ Although lack of financial resources keeps many people from receiving needed drug or alcohol treatment, lack of motivation is also often a factor. More research and trial programs are needed to find ways to encourage addicts to get help.

Few drug or alcohol abusers get help through residential programs

(percent distribution of clients in drug or alcohol treatment facilities by type of care received, 2003)

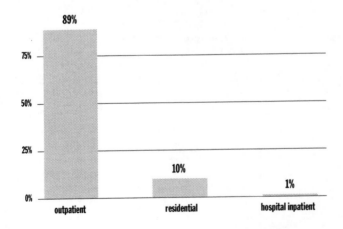

Table 1.20 Treatment for Drug or Alcohol Problems in Past Year, 2003

(number and percent of people aged 12 or older needing treatment for drug or alcohol problems in past year, number and percent receiving treatment at a specialty facility, and percent needing treatment who received treatment at a specialty facility, 2003; numbers in thousands)

	total needing treatment		received treatment at specialty facility		percent of those needing treatment who received treatment at specialty facility
	number	percent of population	number	percent of population	
Total	**22,165**	**9.3%**	**1,874**	**0.8%**	**8.5%**
Age					
Aged 12 to 17	2,253	9.0	168	0.7	7.4
Aged 18 to 25	6,824	21.5	486	1.5	7.1
Aged 26 or older	13,088	7.2	1,221	0.7	9.3
Sex					
Female	7,775	6.3	612	0.5	7.9
Male	14,390	12.5	1,263	1.1	8.8
Race and Hispanic origin					
Not Hispanic	19,182	9.2	1,683	0.8	8.8
American Indian	228	18.2	43	3.4	–
Asian	616	6.3	11	0.1	1.9
Black	2,328	8.5	305	1.1	13.1
White	15,647	9.4	1,286	0.8	8.2
Hispanic	2,983	10.0	191	0.6	6.4

Note: Respondents were classified as needing treatment if they met at least one of three criteria during the past year: (1) dependent on any illicit drug or alcohol; (2) abuse of any illicit drug or alcohol; or (3) received treatment for any illicit drug or alcohol problem at a specialty facility. Specialty facility is defined as drug or alcohol rehabilitation facilities (inpatient or outpatient), hospitals (inpatient only), and mental health centers. Illicit drugs are defined as marijuana/hashish, cocaine (including crack), heroin, hallucinogens, inhalants, or any prescription-type psychotherapeutic used nonmedically. (–) means sample is too small to make a reliable estimate.

Source: SAMHSA, Office of Applied Studies, National Survey on Drug Use and Health, 2003; Internet site http://oas.samhsa.gov/NHSDA/2k3NSDUH/appg.htm#tabg.1

Table 1.21 Clients in Drug or Alcohol Treatment Facilities by Type of Care Received, 2003

(number and percent distribution of clients in drug or alcohol treatment facilities by type of care received and facility operation, March 31, 2003)

	total	private nonprofit	private for profit	local, county, or community government	state government	federal government total	Department of Vet. Affairs	Department of Defense	Indian Health Service	other	tribal government
Total clients	**1,092,546**	**615,410**	**282,161**	**101,826**	**45,649**	**37,155**	**28,386**	**6,020**	**2,331**	**418**	**10,345**
Outpatient	968,719	523,778	265,324	97,665	38,207	33,963	25,468	5,889	2,222	384	9,782
Regular	587,975	331,430	131,147	70,907	24,919	22,217	15,866	4,758	1,422	171	7,355
Intensive	128,127	78,301	29,568	9,567	4,505	4,362	2,737	755	757	113	1,824
Day treatment or partial hospitalization	27,728	17,456	3,869	2,964	1,115	1,983	1,598	344	41	0	341
Detox	11,770	4,216	5,397	461	409	1,138	1,004	32	2	100	149
Methadone or LAAM maintenance	213,119	92,375	95,343	13,766	7,259	4,263	4,263	0	0	0	113
Residential	108,592	84,088	13,019	3,422	4,810	2,727	2,509	107	95	16	526
Short-term	22,926	13,737	4,324	804	2,583	1,342	1,209	105	28	0	136
Long-term	76,605	63,033	7,816	2,063	2,018	1,314	1,233	0	65	16	361
Detox	9,061	7,318	879	555	209	71	67	2	2	0	29
Hospital inpatient	15,235	7,544	3,818	739	2,632	465	409	24	14	18	37
Treatment	8,168	3,136	2,276	386	2,158	192	152	21	12	7	20
Detox	7,067	4,408	1,542	353	474	273	257	3	2	11	17

(continued)

Percent distribution by type of treatment	total	private nonprofit	private for profit	local, county, or community government	state government	federal government					
						total	Department of Vet. Affairs	Department of Defense	Indian Health Service	other	tribal government
Total clients	100.0%	100.0%	100.0%	100.0%	100.0%	100.0%	100.0%	100.0%	100.0%	100.0%	100.0%
Outpatient	88.7	85.1	94.0	95.9	83.7	91.4	89.7	97.8	95.3	91.9	94.6
Regular	53.8	53.9	46.5	69.6	54.6	59.8	55.9	79.0	61.0	40.9	71.1
Intensive	11.7	12.7	10.5	9.4	9.9	11.7	9.6	12.5	32.5	27.0	17.6
Day treatment or partial hospitalization	2.5	2.8	1.4	2.9	2.4	5.3	5.6	5.7	1.8	0.0	3.3
Detox	1.1	0.7	1.9	0.5	0.9	3.1	3.5	0.5	0.1	23.9	1.4
Methadone or LAAM maintenance	19.5	15.0	33.8	13.5	15.9	11.5	15.0	0.0	0.0	0.0	1.1
Residential	9.9	13.7	4.6	3.4	10.5	7.3	8.8	1.8	4.1	3.8	5.1
Short-term	2.1	2.2	1.5	0.8	5.7	3.6	4.3	1.7	1.2	0.0	1.3
Long-term	7.0	10.2	2.8	2.0	4.4	3.5	4.3	0.0	2.8	3.8	3.5
Detox	0.8	1.2	0.3	0.5	0.5	0.2	0.2	0.0	0.1	0.0	0.3
Hospital inpatient	1.4	1.2	1.4	0.7	5.8	1.3	1.4	0.4	0.6	4.3	0.4
Treatment	0.7	0.5	0.8	0.4	4.7	0.5	0.5	0.3	0.5	1.7	0.2
Detox	0.6	0.7	0.5	0.3	1.0	0.7	0.9	0.0	0.1	2.6	0.2

(continued)

Percent distribution by facility operation

	total	private nonprofit	private for profit	local, county, or community government	state government	federal government total	Department of Vet. Affairs	Department of Defense	Indian Health Service	other	tribal government
Total clients	100.0%	56.3%	25.8%	9.3%	4.2%	3.4%	2.6%	0.6%	0.2%	0.0%	0.9%
Outpatient	100.0	54.1	27.4	10.1	3.9	3.5	2.6	0.6	0.2	0.0	1.0
Regular	100.0	56.4	22.3	12.1	4.2	3.8	2.7	0.8	0.2	0.0	1.3
Intensive	100.0	61.1	23.1	7.5	3.5	3.4	2.1	0.6	0.6	0.1	1.4
Day treatment or partial hospitalization	100.0	63.0	14.0	10.7	4.0	7.2	5.8	1.2	0.1	0.0	1.2
Detox	100.0	35.8	45.9	3.9	3.5	9.7	8.5	0.3	0.0	0.8	1.3
Methadone or LAAM maintenance	100.0	43.3	44.7	6.5	3.4	2.0	2.0	0.0	0.0	0.0	0.1
Residential	100.0	77.4	12.0	3.2	4.4	2.5	2.3	0.1	0.1	0.0	0.5
Short-term	100.0	59.9	18.9	3.5	11.3	5.9	5.3	0.5	0.1	0.0	0.6
Long-term	100.0	82.3	10.2	2.7	2.6	1.7	1.6	0.0	0.1	0.0	0.5
Detox	100.0	80.8	9.7	6.1	2.3	0.8	0.7	0.0	0.0	0.0	0.3
Hospital inpatient	100.0	49.5	25.1	4.9	17.3	3.1	2.7	0.2	0.1	0.1	0.2
Treatment	100.0	38.4	27.9	4.7	26.4	2.4	1.9	0.3	0.1	0.1	0.2
Detox	100.0	62.4	21.8	5.0	6.7	3.9	3.6	0.0	0.0	0.2	0.2

Source: Office of Applied Studies, Substance Abuse and Mental Health Services Administration, National Survey of Substance Abuse Treatment Services (N-SSATS), 2003; Internet site http://wwwdasis.samhsa.gov/03nssats/index.htm; calculations by New Strategist

2

Aging

■ **More than 8 million cosmetic procedures were performed in 2003.**

Sixty-nine percent of cosmetic procedures were performed on people aged 35 to 64.

■ **One in five adults is a caregiver.**

Most caregivers are women, their average age is 46, and three-quarters are caring for someone aged 50 or older.

■ **The nation's assisted-living facilities were home to 800,000 Americans in 2000.**

Most assisted-living facilities provide meals, housework, and help with medications, money management, and shopping.

■ **More than 1 million Americans aged 65 or older live in a nursing home.**

The majority of elderly nursing home residents are women. Most need help moving about and most are incontinent.

Women Are More Likely to Get Nipped and Tucked

Young adults account for a large share of some cosmetic procedures.

In 2003, there were more than 8 million cosmetic procedures performed on Americans. The great majority (6 million) were nonsurgical procedures. The most common of these was also one of the most recently developed: botox injections. Of the 2 million surgical procedures performed, the most common was liposuction.

Women are far more likely than men to turn to cosmetic procedures to undo what nature and time have wrought. Women accounted for 87 percent of all cosmetic procedures in 2003. Men account for the majority of those receiving calf augmentations and hair transplants. Nearly all lip augmentations (other than by injectable materials) and upper arm lifts are performed on women.

People aged 35 to 50 account for the largest share of cosmetic procedures. This age group is made up primarily of the large baby-boom generation. But it is not just their numbers that make them such good customers for cosmetic surgeons. This generation is also determined to remain youthful, in appearance as well as spirit. Younger generations are showing signs of following in the boomers' footsteps. Nearly one-quarter of cosmetic procedures in 2003 were performed on people aged 19 to 34. Older adults are more interested in damage control than enhancements. The majority of face lifts are performed on people aged 51 or older.

■ As new procedures carry reduced risks, more people—including men—are likely to turn to cosmetic surgeons to improve their appearance.

People aged 35 to 50 account for the largest share of patients.

(percent distribution of cosmetic surgery and procedures by age, 2003)

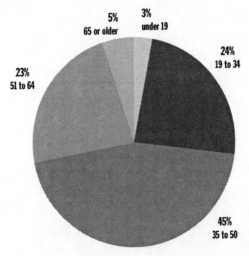

5%
65 or older

3%
under 19

24%
19 to 34

23%
51 to 64

45%
35 to 50

Table 2.1 Cosmetic Surgery by Sex, 2003

(number and percent distribution of cosmetic surgery procedures by sex, 2003)

	total	females		males	
		number	percent	number	percent
TOTAL PROCEDURES	8,251,994	7,177,918	87.0%	1,074,087	13.0%
Total surgical procedures	1,819,485	1,559,367	85.7	260,129	14.3
Abdominoplasty (tummy tuck)	117,693	112,713	95.8	4,975	4.2
Blepharoplasty (cosmetic eyelid surgery)	267,627	216,829	81.0	50,798	19.0
Breast augmentation	280,401	280,401	100.0	NA	NA
Breast lift	76,943	76,943	100.0	NA	NA
Breast nipple enlargement (cosmetic only)	529	529	100.0	0	0.0
Breast nipple reduction (not with breast reduction)	1,591	1,467	92.2	127	8.0
Breast reduction (women)	147,173	147,173	100.0	NA	NA
Buttock augmentation	3,885	2,804	72.2	1,081	27.8
Buttock lift	3,565	3,450	96.8	115	3.2
Calf augmentation	1,170	331	28.3	837	71.5
Cheek implants	8,287	6,926	83.6	1,361	16.4
Chin augmentation	27,999	21,118	75.4	6,881	24.6
Face lift	125,581	112,025	89.2	13,558	10.8
Forehead lift	76,696	65,412	85.3	11,290	14.7
Gynecomastia, treatment of (male breast reduction)	22,049	NA	NA	22,049	100.0
Hair transplantation	16,638	1,748	10.5	14,891	89.5
Lip augmentation (other than by injectable materials)	23,164	22,722	98.1	445	1.9
Lipoplasty (liposuction)	384,626	322,975	84.0	61,646	16.0
Lower body lift	10,964	9,107	83.1	1,861	17.0
Otoplasty (cosmetic ear surgery)	27,814	15,298	55.0	12,515	45.0
Pectoral (male chest) augmentation	1,734	NA	NA	1,734	100.0
Rhinoplasty (nose reshaping)	172,420	119,047	69.0	53,376	31.0
Thigh lift	8,806	8,563	97.2	243	2.8
Umbilicoplasty (not with abdominoplasty)	1,534	1,426	93.0	112	7.3
Upper arm lift	10,595	10,361	97.8	235	2.2
Total nonsurgical procedures	6,432,509	5,618,551	87.3	813,958	12.7
Botox injection	2,272,080	1,963,012	86.4	309,063	13.6
Cellulite treatment (mechanical roller massage therapy)	27,919	26,558	95.1	1,365	4.9
Chemical peel	722,248	640,081	88.6	82,174	11.4
Dermabrasion (not including microdermabrasion)	27,584	22,775	82.6	4,812	17.4
Laser hair removal	923,200	695,210	75.3	227,990	24.7
Laser skin resurfacing	127,470	116,467	91.4	11,010	8.6
Laser treatment of leg veins	170,358	163,149	95.8	7,208	4.2
Microdermabrasion	858,312	774,261	90.2	84,049	9.8
Sclerotherapy	444,416	431,257	97.0	13,168	3.0
Soft tissue fillers: autologous fat	90,321	83,295	92.2	7,017	7.8
Soft tissue fillers: calcium hydroxylapatite (radiance)	31,913	29,013	90.9	2,894	9.1
Soft tissue fillers: collagen	620,476	568,797	91.7	51,674	8.3
Soft tissue fillers: hyaluronic acid (Hylaform, Restylane)	116,211	104,678	90.1	11,534	9.9

Note: NA means does not apply.
Source: The American Society for Aesthetic Plastic Surgery, Internet site http://www.surgery.org

Table 2.2   Cosmetic Surgery by Age, 2003

(total number of cosmetic surgery procedures and percent distribution by age of patient and type of procedure, 2003)

	total number	total percent	under 19	19 to 34	35 to 50	51 to 64	65 or older
TOTAL PROCEDURES	**8,251,994**	**100.0%**	**2.7%**	**23.8%**	**45.4%**	**23.4%**	**4.7%**
Total surgical procedures	**1,819,485**	**100.0**	**3.6**	**30.8**	**41.2**	**20.0**	**4.3**
Abdominoplasty (tummy tuck)	117,693	100.0	0.1	20.7	61.8	16.4	1.2
Blepharoplasty (cosmetic eyelid surgery)	267,627	100.0	0.3	9.1	38.7	39.2	12.7
Breast augmentation	280,401	100.0	4.0	53.6	37.2	4.8	0.4
Breast lift	76,943	100.0	0.5	24.2	58.4	15.3	1.5
Breast nipple enlargement (cosmetic only)	529	100.0	0.0	87.3	9.3	3.2	0.0
Breast nipple reduction (not with breast reduction)	1,591	100.0	0.0	44.5	52.4	3.1	0.0
Breast reduction (women)	147,173	100.0	3.4	35.5	42.1	16.1	2.8
Buttock augmentation	3,885	100.0	0.0	37.6	53.1	8.2	1.0
Buttock lift	3,565	100.0	0.0	31.5	51.9	15.1	1.4
Calf augmentation	1,170	100.0	0.0	58.5	40.3	1.1	0.0
Cheek implants	8,287	100.0	0.0	22.5	48.0	23.3	6.1
Chin augmentation	27,999	100.0	1.8	41.5	38.4	15.8	2.6
Face lift	125,581	100.0	0.0	0.5	30.4	55.4	13.8
Forehead lift	76,696	100.0	0.2	3.2	36.0	49.1	11.4
Gynecomastia, treatment of (male breast reduction)	22,049	100.0	17.2	50.7	25.5	5.1	1.4
Hair transplantation	16,638	100.0	2.3	12.3	63.2	18.1	4.2
Lip augmentation (other than by injectable materials)	23,164	100.0	0.7	31.0	44.0	19.4	4.9
Lipoplasty (liposuction)	384,626	100.0	1.0	38.9	46.7	12.5	0.9
Lower body lift	10,964	100.0	0.0	33.8	57.1	7.8	1.4
Otoplasty (cosmetic ear surgery)	27,814	100.0	58.5	24.7	12.5	3.2	1.2
Pectoral (male chest) augmentation	1,734	100.0	0.2	32.5	60.4	7.0	0.0
Rhinoplasty (nose reshaping)	172,420	100.0	13.3	48.6	28.5	8.4	1.3
Thigh lift	8,806	100.0	0.0	30.8	53.0	15.4	0.8
Umbilicoplasty (not with abdominoplasty)	1,534	100.0	8.5	40.7	47.7	2.4	0.7
Upper arm lift	10,595	100.0	0.7	21.4	50.9	23.0	4.1
Total nonsurgical procedures	**6,432,509**	**100.0**	**2.4**	**21.9**	**46.6**	**24.3**	**4.8**
Botox injection	2,272,080	100.0	0.2	14.1	54.5	26.5	4.6
Cellulite treatment (mechanical roller massage therapy)	27,919	100.0	0.0	37.1	53.2	9.5	0.2
Chemical peel	722,248	100.0	7.2	24.9	39.4	23.3	5.2
Dermabrasion (not including microdermabrasion)	27,584	100.0	3.7	20.3	38.2	28.8	9.0
Laser hair removal	923,200	100.0	5.4	36.0	36.8	18.3	3.5
Laser skin resurfacing	127,470	100.0	0.9	8.0	57.5	25.7	7.9
Laser treatment of leg veins	170,358	100.0	0.4	16.5	50.5	28.6	4.0
Microdermabrasion	858,312	100.0	4.7	31.0	40.5	20.2	3.6
Sclerotherapy	444,416	100.0	1.0	19.2	47.7	27.5	4.7
Soft tissue fillers: autologous fat	90,321	100.0	0.5	21.9	45.6	25.9	6.1
Soft tissue fillers: calcium hydroxylapatite (radiance)	31,913	100.0	0.2	15.9	42.9	31.1	9.9
Soft tissue fillers: collagen	620,476	100.0	0.4	19.0	43.6	29.0	7.9
Soft tissue fillers: hyaluronic acid (Hylaform, Restylane)	116,211	100.0	0.0	20.0	52.4	21.1	6.6

Source: The American Society for Aesthetic Plastic Surgery, Internet site http://www.surgery.org

Twenty-One Percent of Adults Are Caregivers

Many are caring for an aging parent.

More than 44 million people in the United States provide care (without pay) to someone aged 18 or older, according to a 2003 study by the National Alliance for Caregiving and the AARP. This represents more than one out of every five adults. Three quarters of caregivers are assisting someone aged 50 or older, usually a parent or grandparent. The majority of caregivers are women, and their average age is 46. Most have household incomes below $50,000 a year.

The most common types of assistance provided by caregivers are with transportation, grocery shopping, housework, and other instrumental activities of daily living. Among those receiving care, 15 percent need assistance because of aging-related conditions such as mobility impairments. Among people aged 18 to 49 who need the assistance of a caregiver, the largest share (23 percent) have a mental illness.

■ The growing number of elderly in the U.S. population means more Americans will become caregivers.

Most caregivers are aged 35 to 64

(percent distributuion of caregivers by age, 2003)

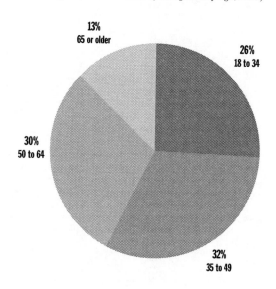

13%
65 or older

26%
18 to 34

30%
50 to 64

32%
35 to 49

Table 2.3 Caregivers by Demographic Characteristic, 2003

(number of caregivers by age of care recipient and percent distribution of caregivers by selected demographic characteristic, 2003)

	total	care recipient aged 18 to 49	care recipient aged 50 or older
Number of caregivers	**44,443,800**	**10,581,900**	**33,861,900**
Percent of population	**21%**	**5%**	**16%**
Total caregivers	**100%**	**100%**	**100%**
Sex			
Female	61	56	63
Male	39	44	37
Age of caregiver			
Aged 18 to 34	26	42	22
Aged 35 to 49	32	30	33
Aged 50 to 64	30	19	32
Aged 65 or older	13	9	13
Average age (years)	46	41	47
Race and Hispanic origin of caregiver			
African American	12	16	11
Asian American	4	4	4
Hispanic	10	11	10
White	73	69	74
Marital status of caregiver			
Married/living with partner	62	53	63
Single, never married	18	22	17
Separated/divorced	14	17	14
Widowed	6	7	6
Educational attainment of caregiver			
High school or less	34	41	33
Some college	27	3	26
Technical school	3	2	3
College graduate	22	18	23
Graduate school or more	13	8	14
Employment status of caregiver			
Employed full-time	48	54	47
Employed part-time	11	12	10
Not employed	41	33	43
Household income of caregiver			
Under $30,000	25	32	22
$30,000 to $49,999	26	27	25
$50,000 to $74,999	18	19	18
$75,000 to $99,999	9	9	9
$100,000 or more	15	7	17

Source: National Alliance for Caregiving and AARP, Caregiving in the U.S., *2004; Internet site http://research.aarp.org/il/us_caregiving.html*

Table 2.4 Assistance Provided by Caregivers, 2003

(percent of caregivers providing assistance by type, 2003)

	percent
TOTAL CAREGIVERS	**100%**
Instrumental activities of daily living (IADL)	
Transportation	82
Grocery shopping	75
Housework	69
Managing finances	64
Preparing meals	59
Giving medicines	41
Arranging services	30
Three or more IADLs	80
Activities of daily living (ADL)	
In/out of bed and chairs	36
Dressing	29
Bathing	26
Toileting	23
Feeding	18
Continence/diapers	16
Three or more ADLs	26
None of these ADLs	50

Note: Caregivers were defined as those providing at least one IADL to another person. Therefore, all caregivers provided at least one IADL.

Source: National Alliance for Caregiving and AARP, Caregiving in the U.S., 2004; *Internet site http://research.aarp.org/il/us_caregiving.html*

Table 2.5   Caregivers by Recipient's Relationship to Them, 2003

(percent distribution of caregivers by relationship and age of care recipient, 2003)

	total	recipients aged 18 to 49	recipients aged 50 or older
Total recipients	**100%**	**100%**	**100%**
Relative	83	74	85
Mother	28	7	34
Grandmother	9	–	11
Father	8	3	10
Mother-in-law	7	1	8
Spouse	6	6	6
Sibling	5	20	4
Daughter/son	6	27	1
Nonrelative	17	25	14

Note: (–) means less than .05 percent.
Source: National Alliance for Caregiving and AARP, Caregiving in the U.S., 2004; *Internet site http://research.aarp.org/il/us_caregiving.html*

Table 2.6 Caregivers by Main Problem with Care Recipient, 2003

(percent distribution of caregivers by main problem with and age of care recipient, 2003)

	total	recipients aged 18 to 49	recipients aged 50 or older
Total caregivers	**100%**	**100%**	**100%**
Old age	12	–	15
Cancer	8	4	9
Diabetes	8	4	9
Mental illness	7	23	3
Heart disease	7	1	9
Alzheimer's	6	–	8
Stroke	5	3	6
Mobility	5	3	6
Arthritis	4	–	5
Blindness/vision	3	2	3

Note: Numbers will not add to 100 because not all problems are shown. (–) means less than .05 percent.
Source: National Alliance for Caregiving and AARP, Caregiving in the U.S., 2004; *Internet site http://research.aarp.org/il/us_caregiving.html*

Demand for Assisted-Living Facilities Is Likely to Grow

These facilities can help older adults maintain some independence.

Assisted-living facilities provide care to people who need help with one or more activities of daily living, such as bathing and dressing, but are not in need of the full-time nursing care provided by nursing homes. By providing an intermediate level of care, these facilities can help older adults maintain a degree of independence without having to rely on family members.

There were about 33,000 assisted-living facilities in the United States in 2000. About 800,000 people live in these types of facilities, most of them older women. Most assisted-living facilities provide some prepared meals and help residents with cleaning and other housework. Most also provide local transportation and assist with shopping.

Most residents of assisted-living facilities have some type of physical problem, such as heart disease or diabetes. About one-quarter have been diagnosed with depression, and a similar share have a mild form of dementia. Few have more serious forms of dementia, such as Alzheimer's disease, because assisted-living facilities do not provide the level of care usually required by these individuals.

■ The demand for high-quality assisted-living facilities will grow along with the number of older adults. But the cost of these facilities will place a significant financial burden on the elderly and their families, leading some to seek lower-cost alternatives.

Meals and housework help are provided to nearly all assisted-living facility residents

(percent of assisted-living facility residents who receive help with selected activities, 2000)

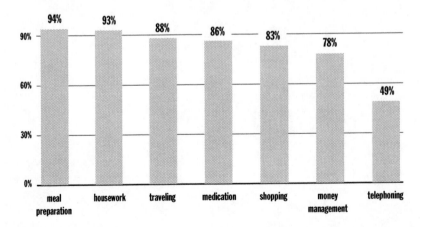

Table 2.7 Assisted Living Facilities and Residents, 2000

(characteristics of assisted living facilities and residents, 2000)

Total facilities	**33,000**
Average number of beds per facility	30
Average monthly fee	$1,873
Total residents	**800,000**
Average age of resident (years)	80
Percent female	69%
Percent male	31
Percent who need help with at least one activity of daily living (ADL)	81
Average number of ADLs for which help is needed	2.25
Percent needing at least some help with ADL:	
Bathing	72%
Dressing	57
Toileting	41
Transferring	36
Eating	23
Percent who receive help with:	
Meal preparation	94
Housework	93
Traveling	88
Medication	86
Shopping	83
Money management	78
Telephoning	49
Percent using mobility aid:	
Walker	30
Wheelchair	15
Cane	11
Percent with medical condition:	
Bladder incontinence	33
Heart disease	28
Bowel incontinence	18
Osteoporosis	16
Diabetes	13
Stroke	11
Parkinson's	5
Cancer	4
Multiple sclerosis	1
Pressure ulcers	1

(continued)

Percent with mental condition:

Alzheimer's, early stage	11%
Alzheimer's, mid-stage	8
Alzheimer's, late stage	4
Other dementia, mild	25
Other dementia, severe	4
Depression	24
Mental retardation/ developmental disability	10

Assisted-living residents came from:

Home	46
Another assisted-living residence	20
Hospitals	14
Nursing facility	10

Assisted-living residents moved to:

Nursing facility	33
Deceased	28
Another assisted-living facility	14
Home	12
Hospital	11

Source: National Center for Assisted Living, 2001 Facts and Trends: The Assisted Living Sourcebook; *Internet site http://www. ahca.org/research/index.html*

Most Nursing Home Residents Are Older Women

Men are more likely than women to need nursing home care before age 65.

Among women in nursing homes, only 7 percent are under age 65. More than half are aged 85 or older. Men, on the other hand, are more likely to enter a nursing home at a younger age. Although most men in nursing homes are aged 65 or older, a substantial 17 percent are under age 65. Similarly, blacks are more likely than whites to need nursing home care before they reach age 65.

The types of health conditions that are common among nursing home residents point at the reasons they are not being cared for at home. The great majority have mobility problems and require assistance to move around or feed themselves. Family caregivers often have difficulty providing this level of care 24 hours a day.

■ As the large baby-boom generation reaches its senior years, the number of people needing nursing home care will certainly rise.

Most women in nursing homes are aged 85 or older

(percent of nursing home residents who are aged 85 or older, by sex, 1999)

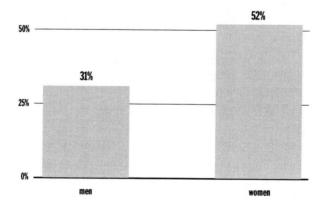

Table 2.8 Nursing Home Residents by Sex and Race, 1999

(number and percent distribution of current nursing home residents by age, sex, and race, 1999)

	total	sex		race	
		female	male	black	white
Total residents	**1,628,300**	**1,170,400**	**457,900**	**178,700**	**1,397,000**
Under age 65	158,700	78,700	80,000	32,800	115,800
Aged 65 or older	1,469,500	1,091,700	377,800	145,900	1,281,200
Aged 65 to 74	194,800	110,700	84,100	30,300	157,300
Aged 75 to 84	517,600	368,100	149,500	58,700	441,600
Aged 85 or older	757,100	612,900	144,200	56,900	682,400
Percent distribution by age					
Total residents	**100.0%**	**100.0%**	**100.0%**	**100.0%**	**100.0%**
Under age 65	9.8	6.7	17.5	18.4	8.3
Aged 65 or older	90.3	93.3	82.5	81.7	91.7
Aged 65 to 74	12.0	9.5	18.4	17.0	11.3
Aged 75 to 84	31.8	31.5	32.7	32.8	31.6
Aged 85 or older	46.5	52.4	31.5	31.8	48.9
Percent distribution by sex and race					
Total residents	**100.0%**	**71.9%**	**28.1%**	**11.0%**	**85.8%**
Under age 65	100.0	49.6	50.4	20.7	73.0
Aged 65 or older	100.0	74.3	25.7	9.9	87.2
Aged 65 to 74	100.0	56.8	43.2	15.6	80.7
Aged 75 to 84	100.0	71.1	28.9	11.3	85.3
Aged 85 or older	100.0	81.0	19.0	7.5	90.1

Note: Figures by race do not add to total because not all races are shown.
Source: National Center for Health Statistics, 1999 National Nursing Home Survey; Internet site http://www.cdc.gov/nchs/about/ major/nnhsd/nnhsd.htm; calculations by New Strategist

Table 2.9 Nursing Home Residents by Functional Status, 1999

(percent distribution of nursing home residents aged 65 or older by age, sex, race, and functional status, 1999)

	total residents	dependent mobility	incontinent	dependent eating	dependent mobility, eating, and incontinent
Total aged 65 or older	**100.0%**	**80.4%**	**65.7%**	**47.4%**	**37.0%**
Aged 65 to 74	100.0	73.9	58.5	43.1	31.7
Aged 75 to 84	100.0	77.8	64.2	46.6	35.4
Aged 85 or older	100.0	83.8	68.6	49.0	39.4
Female residents	**100.0**	**81.9**	**65.6**	**8.1**	**37.7**
Aged 65 to 74	100.0	76.4	57.7	41.6	29.3
Aged 75 to 84	100.0	78.2	62.2	47.7	35.6
Aged 85 or older	100.0	85.2	69.0	49.7	40.4
Male residents	**100.0**	**75.9**	**66.0**	**45.1**	**35.0**
Aged 65 to 74	100.0	70.5	59.6	45.0	34.8
Aged 75 to 84	100.0	76.9	68.9	44.7	35.2
Aged 85 or older	100.0	78.1	66.8	45.7	34.9
Black residents	**100.0**	**81.5**	**70.6**	**54.9**	**45.7**
Aged 65 to 74	100.0	78.7	64.6	53.3	42.6
Aged 75 to 84	100.0	80.1	67.5	49.7	41.0
Aged 85 or older	100.0	84.5	77.0	61.0	52.1
White residents	**100.0**	**80.2**	**65.1**	**46.2**	**35.8**
Aged 65 to 74	100.0	72.6	57.1	40.7	28.8
Aged 75 to 84	100.0	77.5	63.8	45.8	34.8
Aged 85 or older	100.0	83.6	67.8	47.7	38.1

Note: Nursing home residents who are dependent in mobility and eating require the assistance of a person or special equipment. Nursing home residents who are incontinent have difficulty in controlling bowels and/or bladder or have an ostomy or indwelling catheter.

Source: National Center for Health Statistics, 1999 National Nursing Home Survey; Internet site http://www.cdc.gov/nchs/about/ major/nnhsd/nnhsd.htm; calculations by New Strategist

3

Alternative Medicine

■ **Sixty-two percent of adults have used alternative medicine in the past year.**

Women are more likely than men to use alternative medicine, and the likelihood of use rises with age.

■ **Forty-five percent of adults have used prayer as an alternative therapy in the past year.**

Most of those using prayer are praying for their own health, but many are praying for the health of others.

■ **Back pain is the condition for which alternative therapy is most frequently used.**

Seventeen percent of the users of alternative medicine sought treatment for back pain.

■ **Half of users tried alternative therapy because they thought it would be interesting.**

The 55 percent majority used alternative medicine in combination with conventional therapy.

Most Americans Have Used Some Type of Alternative Therapy

The most commonly used alternative therapy is prayer.

The majority of adults (62 percent) had used some type of therapy that could be considered alternative (or complementary) medicine in the past year, according to a 2002 survey. Women are more likely than men to have used alternative therapies, and the likelihood of use increases with age. Included within the category of alternative therapies, however, are prayer and the use of large doses of vitamins. When these two approaches are excluded, a much smaller 35 percent of respondents say they have used some type of alternative therapy.

Among people under age 65, those without health insurance are less likely than those with health insurance to use alternative therapies. People who had been hospitalized in the past year were much more likely than those who had not been hospitalized to use alternative therapies.

Overall, 75 percent of adults have tried some type of alternative therapy at some point in their lives. One-quarter have used some type of "biologically based" therapy (other than vitamins and minerals). Generally, these are herbal remedies, such as Echinacea, which is used to prevent the onset of colds. Twenty percent of adults have used chiropractic care, and 10 percent have tried meditation. The largest share (55 percent) have turned to prayer, usually to improve their own health, although many have also prayed for the health of others.

■ The use of alternative therapies has become widely accepted by Americans and is even encouraged by some medical doctors.

Many people turn to herbal remedies to solve their medical problems

(percent of adults using biologically based therapies, excluding megavitamins, in the past twelve months, by age, 2002)

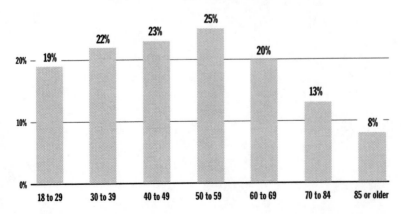

Table 3.1 Users of Alternative and Complementary Medicine by Sex, 2002

(percent of people aged 18 or older who used selected complementary and alternative medicine categories during the past twelve months by sex, 2002; numbers in thousands)

	total	female	male
Any, including megavitamin therapy and prayer	62.1%	69.3%	54.1%
Biologically based therapies, including megavitamins	21.9	24.1	19.6
Mind-body therapies including prayer	52.6	61.1	43.4
Any, excluding megavitamin therapy and prayer	35.1	39.7	30.2
Biologically based therapies excluding megavitamins	20.6	22.9	18.2
Mind-body therapies excluding prayer	16.9	21.1	12.5
Alternative medical systems	2.7	3.2	2.2
Energy therapies	0.5	0.7	0.3
Manipulative and body-based therapies	10.9	12.2	9.5

Source: National Center for Health Statistics, Complementary and Alternative Medicine Use among Adults: United States, 2002, *Advance Data, No. 343, 2004; Internet site http://www.cdc.gov/nchs/pressroom/04news/adultsmedicine.htm*

Table 3.2 Users of Alternative and Complementary Medicine by Age, 2002

(percent of people aged 18 or older who used selected complementary and alternative medicine categories during the past twelve months by age, 2002; numbers in thousands)

	total	18 to 29	30 to 39	40 to 49	50 to 59	60 to 69	70 to 84	85 or older
Any, incl. megavitamin therapy and prayer	62.1%	53.5%	60.7%	64.1%	66.1%	64.8%	68.6%	70.3%
Biologically based therapies, including megavitamins	21.9	19.6	23.2	24.7	26.2	21.3	15.3	9.1
Mind-body therapies including prayer	52.6	44.2	49.8	53.3	56.1	56.3	63.3	66.0
Any, excl. megavitamin therapy and prayer	35.1	32.9	37.8	39.4	39.6	32.6	25.1	14.9
Biologically based therapies excluding megavitamins	20.6	18.8	22.1	23.3	24.7	19.6	13.3	8.4
Mind-body therapies excluding prayer	16.9	17.7	18.3	18.9	19.6	14.4	9.4	6.4
Alternative medical systems	2.7	2.3	3.3	3.2	3.3	2.1	1.4	–
Energy therapies	0.5	0.4	0.6	0.7	0.8	–	–	–
Manipulative and body-based therapies	10.9	9.5	12.8	13.0	11.3	9.8	7.7	2.1

Note: (–) means sample too small to make a reliable estimate.
Source: National Center for Health Statistics, Complementary and Alternative Medicine Use among Adults: United States, 2002, *Advance Data, No. 343, 2004; Internet site http://www.cdc.gov/nchs/pressroom/04news/adultsmedicine.htm*

Table 3.3 Users of Alternative and Complementary Medicine by Race and Hispanic Origin, 2002

(percent of people aged 18 or older who used selected complementary and alternative medicine categories during the past twelve months by race and Hispanic origin, 2002; numbers in thousands)

	total	race			Hispanic origin	
		Asian	black	white	Hispanic	non-Hispanic
Any, including megavitamin therapy and prayer	62.1%	61.7%	71.3%	60.4%	61.4%	62.3%
Biologically based therapies, incl. megavitamins	21.9	29.5	16.5	22.3	20.6	22.3
Mind-body therapies including prayer	52.6	48.1	68.3	50.1	55.1	52.4
Any, excluding megavitamin therapy and prayer	35.1	43.1	26.2	35.9	28.3	36.1
Biologically based therapies excl. megavitamins	20.6	28.9	15.2	20.9	19.8	20.9
Mind-body therapies excluding prayer	16.9	20.9	14.7	17.0	10.9	17.7
Alternative medical systems	2.7	4.5	1.4	2.8	2.4	2.8
Energy therapies	0.5	–	–	0.5	–	0.6
Manipulative and body-based therapies	10.9	7.2	4.4	12.0	5.8	11.6

Note: (–) means sample too small to make a reliable estimate.
Source: National Center for Health Statistics, Complementary and Alternative Medicine Use among Adults: United States, 2002, *Advance Data, No. 343, 2004; Internet site http://www.cdc.gov/nchs/pressroom/04news/adultsmedicine.htm*

Table 3.4 Users of Alternative and Complementary Medicine by Education, 2002

(percent of people aged 18 or older who used selected complementary and alternative medicine categories during the past twelve months by education, 2002; numbers in thousands)

	total	less than high school	high school graduate	some college, no degree	associate's degree	bachelor's degree	graduate degree
Any, incl. megavitamin therapy, prayer	62.1%	57.4%	58.3%	64.7%	64.1%	66.7%	65.5%
Biologically based therapies, including megavitamins	21.9	12.5	17.8	24.1	24.6	29.8	31.5
Mind-body therapies including prayer	52.6	52.0	49.6	54.8	53.8	54.9	52.7
Any, excluding megavitamin therapy and prayer	35.1	20.8	29.5	38.8	39.8	45.9	48.8
Biologically based therapies excluding megavitamins	20.6	11.7	16.8	22.6	23.1	27.7	29.8
Mind-body therapies excluding prayer	16.9	8.0	12.4	19.1	20.2	25.0	26.5
Alternative medical systems	2.7	1.3	1.6	2.7	3.0	4.6	5.2
Energy therapies	0.5	–	0.3	0.7	–	0.9	–
Manipulative and body-based therapies	10.9	5.1	9.4	12.5	12.6	15.3	12.8

Note: (–) means sample too small to make a reliable estimate.
Source: National Center for Health Statistics, Complementary and Alternative Medicine Use among Adults: United States, 2002, *Advance Data, No. 343, 2004; Internet site http://www.cdc.gov/nchs/pressroom/04news/adultsmedicine.htm*

Table 3.5 Users of Alternative and Complementary Medicine by Household Income, 2002

(percent of people aged 18 or older who used selected complementary and alternative medicine categories during the past twelve months by household income, 2002; numbers in thousands)

	total	less than $20,000	$20,000 to $34,999	$35,000 to $54,999	$55,000 to $74,999	$75,000 or more
Any, including megavitamin therapy and prayer	62.1%	64.9%	63.5%	62.8%	60.9%	61.9%
Biologically based therapies, incl. megavitamins	21.9	18.9	21.1	22.6	22.7	27.1
Mind-body therapies including prayer	52.6	58.8	55.3	52.8	50.1	48.7
Any, excluding megavitamin therapy and prayer	35.1	29.6	34.1	36.6	37.4	43.3
Biologically based therapies excl. megavitamins	20.6	18.0	19.9	21.2	21.2	25.6
Mind-body therapies excluding prayer	16.9	14.8	16.9	17.9	18.2	20.7
Alternative medical systems	2.7	2.4	2.0	2.9	2.4	4.0
Energy therapies	0.5	0.4	0.5	0.6	0.4	0.7
Manipulative and body-based therapies	10.9	6.7	10.0	11.8	11.0	15.2

Source: National Center for Health Statistics, Complementary and Alternative Medicine Use among Adults: United States, 2002, *Advance Data, No. 343, 2004; Internet site http://www.cdc.gov/nchs/pressroom/04news/adultsmedicine.htm*

Table 3.6 Users of Alternative and Complementary Medicine by Region, 2002

(percent of people aged 18 or older who used selected complementary and alternative medicine categories during the past twelve months by region, 2002; numbers in thousands)

	total	Northeast	Midwest	South	West total	West Pacific states
Any, including megavitamin therapy and prayer	62.1%	57.9%	61.4%	64.6%	62.1%	64.0%
Biologically based therapies, incl. megavitamins	21.9	22.6	20.9	19.3	27.7	27.7
Mind-body therapies including prayer	52.6	46.9	52.0	57.2	50.3	52.4
Any, excluding megavitamin therapy and prayer	35.1	35.7	37.0	29.9	42.2	43.0
Biologically based therapies excl. megavitamins	20.6	21.1	19.7	18.0	26.4	26.4
Mind-body therapies excluding prayer	16.9	16.9	18.2	14.0	21.1	22.4
Alternative medical systems	2.7	3.1	2.2	1.9	4.6	4.8
Energy therapies	0.5	0.7	0.5	0.3	0.8	0.8
Manipulative and body-based therapies	10.9	10.9	13.2	7.9	13.8	13.3

Source: National Center for Health Statistics, Complementary and Alternative Medicine Use among Adults: United States, 2002, *Advance Data, No. 343, 2004; Internet site http://www.cdc.gov/nchs/pressroom/04news/adultsmedicine.htm*

Table 3.7 Users of Alternative and Complementary Medicine by Health Insurance Status, 2002

(percent of people aged 18 or older who used selected complementary and alternative medicine categories during the past twelve months by health insurance status, 2002; numbers in thousands)

	total	under age 65			aged 65 or older		
		private insurance	public insurance	uninsured	private insurance	public insurance	uninsured
Any, including megavitamin therapy and prayer	62.1%	61.4%	65.1%	57.7%	68.2%	65.9%	74.4%
Biologically based therapies, including megavitamins	21.9	24.6	17.9	21.1	16.0	14.6	18.2
Mind-body therapies including prayer	52.6	50.0	59.8	49.5	61.9	61.1	73.2
Any, excluding megavitamin therapy and prayer	35.1	39.4	31.1	31.2	27.2	21.3	19.7
Biologically based therapies excluding megavitamins	20.6	23.2	16.5	20.4	14.0	13.4	18.2
Mind-body therapies excluding prayer	16.9	19.3	18.0	14.7	10.6	8.4	–
Alternative medical systems	2.7	3.0	2.3	3.1	1.4	1.3	–
Energy therapies	0.5	0.6	–	0.7	–	–	–
Manipulative and body-based therapies	10.9	13.1	7.3	8.0	9.4	4.5	–

Note: (–) means sample too small to make a reliable estimate.
Source: National Center for Health Statistics, Complementary and Alternative Medicine Use among Adults: United States, 2002, *Advance Data, No. 343, 2004; Internet site http://www.cdc.gov/nchs/pressroom/04news/adultsmedicine.htm*

Table 3.8 Users of Alternative and Complementary Medicine by Drinking and Smoking Status, 2002

(percent of people aged 18 or older who used selected complementary and alternative medicine categories during the past twelve months by drinking and smoking status, 2002; numbers in thousands)

	total	lifetime drinking status				lifetime cigarette smoking status		
		abstainer	former drinker	infrequent or light drinker	moderate or heavy drinker	never	former	current
Any, including megavitamin therapy and prayer	62.1%	61.6%	69.2%	62.2%	57.0%	62.8%	66.6%	57.2%
Biologically based therapies, including megavitamins	21.9	14.9	20.5	24.3	25.5	21.2	27.0	19.7
Mind-body therapies including prayer	52.6	56.9	62.3	51.6	43.5	54.3	55.6	47.6
Any, excl. megavitamin therapy and prayer	35.1	24.3	33.4	39.7	38.5	34.1	41.9	32.9
Biologically based therapies excluding megavitamins	20.6	14.0	19.0	23.0	24.0	20.0	25.3	18.7
Mind-body therapies excluding prayer	16.9	10.8	16.6	19.6	18.4	16.1	21.1	16.8
Alternative medical systems	2.7	1.5	2.3	3.1	3.4	2.6	4.0	2.0
Energy therapies	0.5	–	0.5	0.7	0.6	0.5	0.8	0.5
Manipulative and body-based therapies	10.9	6.1	9.4	13.3	12.1	10.7	13.6	9.2

Note: (–) means sample too small to make a reliable estimate.
Source: National Center for Health Statistics, Complementary and Alternative Medicine Use among Adults: United States, 2002, *Advance Data, No. 343, 2004; Internet site http://www.cdc.gov/nchs/pressroom/04news/adultsmedicine.htm*

Table 3.9 Users of Alternative and Complementary Medicine by Hospitalization Status, 2002

(percent of people aged 18 or older who used selected complementary and alternative medicine categories during the past twelve months by whether respondent had been hospitalized, 2002; numbers in thousands)

	total	hospitalized in past year	
		yes	no
Any, including megavitamin therapy and prayer	62.1%	75.9%	60.6%
Biologically based therapies, including megavitamins	21.9	22.1	22.0
Mind-body therapies including prayer	52.6	70.4	50.8
Any, excluding megavitamin therapy and prayer	35.1	37.4	34.9
Biologically based therapies excluding megavitamins	20.6	20.5	20.7
Mind-body therapies excluding prayer	16.9	19.5	16.7
Alternative medical systems	2.7	3.1	2.7
Energy therapies	0.5	–	0.5
Manipulative and body-based therapies	10.9	11.2	10.9

Note: (–) means sample too small to make a reliable estimate.
Source: National Center for Health Statistics, Complementary and Alternative Medicine Use among Adults: United States, 2002, *Advance Data, No. 343, 2004; Internet site http://www.cdc.gov/nchs/pressroom/04news/adultsmedicine.htm*

Table 3.10   Use of Alternative and Complementary Medicine by Type of Therapy, 2002

(number and percent of people aged 18 or older ever using and using in the past twelve months complementary and alternative medicine, by type of therapy, 2002; numbers in thousands)

	ever used		used during past 12 months	
	number	percent	number	percent
Any complementary or alternative medicine	**149,271**	**74.6%**	**123,606**	**62.1%**
Alternative medical systems				
Acupuncture	8,188	4.0	2,136	1.1
Ayurveda	751	0.4	154	0.1
Homeopathic treatment	7,379	3.6	3,433	1.7
Naturopathy	1,795	0.9	498	0.2
Biologically based therapies				
Chelation therapy	270	0.1	66	–
Folk medicine	1,393	0.7	233	0.1
Nonvitamin, nonmineral, natural products	50,613	25.0	38,183	18.9
Diet-based therapies	13,799	6.8	7,099	3.5
Vegetarian diet	5,324	2.6	3,184	1.6
Macrobiotic diet	1,368	0.7	317	0.2
Atkins diet	7,312	3.6	3,417	1.7
Pritikin diet	580	0.3	137	0.1
Ornish diet	290	0.1	76	–
Zone diet	1,062	0.5	430	0.2
Megavitamin therapy	7,935	3.9	5,739	2.8
Manipulative and body-based therapies				
Chiropractic care	40,242	19.9	15,226	7.5
Massage	18,899	9.3	10,052	5.0
Mind-body therapies				
Biofeedback	1,986	1.0	278	0.1
Meditation	20,698	10.2	15,336	7.6
Guided imagery	6,067	3.0	4,194	2.1
Progressive relaxation	8,518	4.2	6,185	3.0
Deep breathing exercises	29,658	14.6	23,457	11.6
Hypnosis	3,733	1.8	505	0.2
Yoga	15,232	7.5	10,386	5.1
Tai chi	5,056	2.5	2,565	1.3
Qi gong	950	0.5	527	0.3
Prayer for health reasons	110,012	55.3	89,624	45.2
Prayed for own health	103,662	52.1	85,432	43.0
Others ever prayed for your health	62,348	31.3	48,467	24.4
Participate in prayer group	25,167	23.0	18,984	9.6
Healing ritual for own health	9,230	4.6	4,045	2.0
Energy healing therapy/Reiki	2,264	1.1	1,080	0.5

Note: (–) means sample is too small to make a reliable estimate.
Source: National Center for Health Statistics, Complementary and Alternative Medicine Use among Adults: United States, 2002, *Advance Data, No. 343, 2004; Internet site http://www.cdc.gov/nchs/pressroom/04news/adultsmedicine.htm*

Alternative Therapies Are Most Commonly Used for Back Problems

The lack of effective conventional treatment encourages experimentation.

Among people who have used alternative therapies other than megavitamins or prayer in the past twelve months, back pain was the most common condition for which relief was sought. Neck problems were also among the most commonly cited conditions, as was joint pain. These problems are often not fully relieved by conventional medicine, making it understandable that sufferers would seek other treatments. Notably, people did not turn to alternative therapies to treat the most serious and life-threatening conditions, such as cancer or heart disease.

Most people who have ever used alternative medicine did so because they felt it would be beneficial when combined with conventional medical treatment. Half said they thought it would be interesting to try an alternative therapy. One-quarter said that a medical professional had suggested they give alternative treatments a try.

Echinacea, generally used to ward off colds, was the most commonly used herbal supplement in the past twelve months. Forty percent of those using natural products had used Echinacea, while 24 percent had used ginseng, and 21 percent had used Gingkobiloba.

■ Most people who use alternative therapies do so in combination with conventional treatment, making it important for physicians to know what else their patients are doing to solve their medical problem.

Colds are commonly treated with alternative therapies

(percent of alternative medicine users by condition being treated, 2002)

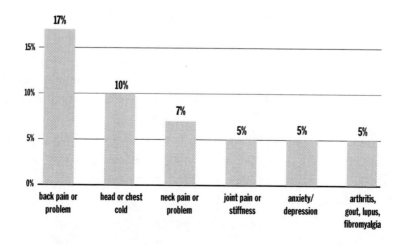

Table 3.11 Alternative Medicine Use by Disease or Condition, 2002

(number and percent of people aged 18 or older who used complementary and alternative medicine, excluding megavitamin therapy and prayer, during the past twelve months by disease or condition for which it was used, 2002; numbers in thousands)

	number	percent
Back pain or problem	11,965	16.8%
Head or chest cold	6,924	9.5
Neck pain or problem	4,756	6.6
Joint pain or stiffness	3,420	4.9
Anxiety/depression	3,249	4.5
Arthritis, gout, lupus, or fibromyalgia	3,216	4.9
Stomach or intestinal illness	2,656	3.7
Severe headache or migraine	2,307	3.1
Recurring pain	1,762	2.4
Insomnia or trouble sleeping	1,595	2.2
Sinusitis	900	1.2
Cholesterol	797	1.1
Asthma	788	1.1
Hypertension	714	1.0
Menopause	657	0.8

Source: National Center for Health Statistics, Complementary and Alternative Medicine Use among Adults: United States, 2002, *Advance Data, No. 343, 2004; Internet site http://www.cdc.gov/nchs/pressroom/04news/adultsmedicine.htm*

Table 3.12 Reason for Use of Complementary and Alternative Medicine, 2002

(percent of people aged 18 or older ever having used complementary and alternative medicine by type of therapy and reason for use, 2002; numbers in thousands)

	conventional medical treatments would not help	conventional medical treatments were too expensive	therapy combined with conventional medical treatments would help	suggested by a conventional medical professional	thought it would be interesting to try
Any complementary or alternative medicine use	**27.7%**	**13.2%**	**54.9%**	**25.8%**	**50.1%**
Alternative medical systems					
Acupuncture	44.2	7.4	56.2	24.8	51.6
Ayurveda	60.6	–	–	–	100.0
Homeopathic treatment	36.7	19.4	43.1	14.2	45.8
Naturopathy	53.1	28.3	62.4	16.5	43.9
Biologically based therapies					
Chelation therapy	28.5	–	84.6	76.4	–
Folk medicine	43.1	47.6	53.5	–	49.3
Nonvitamin, nonmineral, natural products	19.2	14.4	47.5	15.3	51.7
Diet-based therapies	22.4	11.3	38.1	26.3	52.6
Megavitamin therapy	27.5	13.5	55.0	38.3	37.7
Manipulative and body-based therapies					
Chiropractic care	39.6	9.5	52.9	20.2	31.8
Massage	33.9	12.6	59.6	33.4	44.1
Mind-body therapies					
Biofeedback	–	–	61.0	62.7	45.5
Relaxation techniques	20.6	12.5	56.1	36.3	54.5
Hypnosis	30.0	–	22.9	21.1	65.2
Yoga, tai chi, qi gong	30.9	14.4	52.3	21.0	59.2
Healing ritual for own health	19.1	13.6	66.9	8.4	34.1
Energy healing therapy/Reiki	46.5	22.9	60.6	18.0	50.4

Note: (–) means sample too small to make a reliable estimate.
Source: National Center for Health Statistics, Complementary and Alternative Medicine Use among Adults: United States, 2002, *Advance Data, No. 343, 2004; Internet site http://www.cdc.gov/nchs/pressroom/04news/adultsmedicine.htm*

Table 3.13 Use of Natural Products by Type, 2002

(number and percent of people aged 18 or older who used nonvitamin, nonmineral, natural products during the past twelve months for health reasons, 2002; numbers in thousands)

	number	percent
Echinacea	14,665	40.3%
Ginseng	8,777	24.1
Ginkgobiloba	7,679	21.1
Garlic supplements	7,096	19.9
Glucosamine with or without chondroitin	5,249	14.9
St. John's wort	4,390	12.0
Peppermint	4,308	11.8
Fish oils/omega fatty acids	4,253	11.7
Ginger supplements	3,768	10.5
Soy supplements	3,480	9.4
Ragweed/chamomile	3,111	8.6
Bee pollen or royal jelly	2,755	7.4
Kava kava	2,441	6.6
Valerian	2,131	5.9
Saw palmetto	2,054	5.8

Source: National Center for Health Statistics, Complementary and Alternative Medicine Use among Adults: United States, 2002, *Advance Data, No. 343, 2004; Internet site http://www.cdc.gov/nchs/pressroom/04news/adultsmedicine.htm*

4

Attitudes toward Health Care

■ **Few have much confidence in the medical community.**

Only 37 percent say they have a "great deal" of confidence in the medical community, down from 54 percent in 1973.

■ **Sixty-seven percent of Americans say their health is "excellent" or "very good."**

Fifty-six percent of parents say their children's health is excellent and another 28 percent say their children's health is very good.

■ **Eleven percent of families had problems getting health care in the past year.**

The 57 percent majority of those having problems said inability to pay was the reason.

■ **Many people do not get enough time with their health care provider.**

Only 43 percent say they "always" get enough time with their provider, while 15 percent say they only "sometimes" or "never" do.

■ **Young adults are more critical of the health care they receive.**

People aged 65 or older are most likely to rate the health care they receive at 9 or higher on a scale of 1 to 10.

■ **Health care is one of Americans' biggest concerns.**

The 52 percent majority of the public is "very" or "somewhat" concerned about a substantial increase in insurance premiums.

Fewer Americans Have Confidence in the Medical Community

The medical community's reputation is eroding as problems with the health care system persist.

The percentage of people saying they have a "great deal" of confidence in the leaders of the medical community is at the lowest level since the question was first asked in the 1973 General Social Survey. In that year, the 54 percent majority of respondents had a great deal of confidence in the medical community, but in 2002 only 37 percent felt that way. Eleven percent have "hardly any" confidence, and 51 percent have "only some" confidence in the medical community.

One reason for declining confidence in the medical community is the sense that the nation is not doing enough to protect and improve the public's health. Seventy-four percent of adults say we are spending too little on health issues, up from 61 percent in 1973.

In 1975, 36 percent of adults believed it was primarily the government's responsibility to make sure people could pay their medical bills. The share fell in the 1980s and 1990s, and was as low as 25 percent in 1998. Since then, however, the percentage who believe government should take responsibility has been rising, reaching 32 percent in 2002. The percentage who believe there should be no government assistance dropped by a sizable margin between 1975 and 2002. A growing share of Americans take the middle position—both individuals and the government should share responsibility for medical bills.

■ As the percentage of people without health insurance increases and those with insurance face sharply rising costs, more Americans are becoming frustrated with the current health care system.

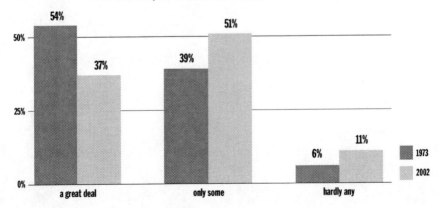

The majority has "only some" confidence in the medical community

(percent distribution of people aged 18 or older by degree of confidence in the leaders of the medical community, 1973 and 2002)

Table 4.1 Confidence in Leaders of the Medical Community, 1973 to 2002

As far as the people running these institutions are concerned, would you say you have a great deal of confidence, only some, or hardly any confidence at all in the medical community?

(number of respondents aged 18 or older, and percent distribution by response, 1973–2002)

	number of respondents	total	a great deal	only some	hardly any	don't know
2002	912	100.0%	37.0%	51.3%	11.2%	0.5%
2000	1,887	100.0	43.7	45.4	9.5	1.4
1998	1,905	100.0	44.3	45.4	8.8	1.6
1996	1,924	100.0	44.5	45.3	8.9	1.3
1994	2,003	100.0	41.5	48.0	9.8	0.7
1993	1,052	100.0	39.1	51.2	8.5	1.2
1991	1,013	100.0	47.5	43.6	7.6	1.3
1990	898	100.0	45.7	46.5	6.8	1.0
1989	1,030	100.0	46.3	45.4	6.8	1.5
1988	993	100.0	51.3	41.9	5.9	0.9
1987	1,813	100.0	51.7	41.9	5.2	1.2
1986	1,466	100.0	45.9	45.3	7.5	1.3
1984	977	100.0	51.1	41.7	6.3	0.9
1983	1,596	100.0	51.6	41.0	6.0	1.4
1982	1,854	100.0	45.3	46.4	7.3	1.1
1980	1,467	100.0	52.4	38.7	7.4	1.5
1978	1,527	100.0	46.0	44.0	9.2	0.8
1977	1,526	100.0	51.5	41.2	6.2	1.1
1976	1,492	100.0	54.1	35.3	9.2	1.3
1975	1,487	100.0	50.5	40.1	7.9	1.5
1974	1,482	100.0	60.4	33.7	4.5	1.5
1973	1,496	100.0	54.1	39.2	5.7	0.9

Source: General Social Surveys, National Opinion Research Center, University of Chicago; calculations by New Strategist

Table 4.2 Spending on Improving the Nation's Health, 1973 to 2002

We are faced with many problems in this country, none of which can be solved easily or inexpensively. Are we spending too much, too little money, or about the right amount on improving and protecting the nation's health?

(number of respondents aged 18 or older, and percent distribution by response, 1973–2002)

	number of respondents	total	too little	about right	too much	don't know
2002	1,357	100.0%	73.7%	20.9%	3.8%	1.5%
2000	1,406	100.0	71.8	22.7	3.6	1.9
1998	1,379	100.0	66.9	25.0	5.7	2.5
1996	1,436	100.0	66.2	23.1	7.9	2.9
1994	1,502	100.0	64.2	23.2	8.5	4.1
1993	794	100.0	71.9	17.3	7.6	3.3
1991	749	100.0	69.2	25.5	2.7	2.7
1990	670	100.0	72.2	22.5	2.7	2.5
1989	766	100.0	68.0	25.3	3.0	3.7
1988	714	100.0	66.0	27.7	3.2	3.1
1987	594	100.0	68.9	25.1	4.0	2.0
1986	726	100.0	58.7	34.0	4.0	3.3
1985	749	100.0	57.7	33.1	6.3	2.9
1984	486	100.0	57.6	31.5	6.6	4.3
1983	1,591	100.0	57.4	33.7	5.2	3.8
1982	1,855	100.0	56.0	32.3	6.5	5.1
1980	1,467	100.0	54.7	33.5	7.6	4.1
1978	1,532	100.0	55.4	33.7	6.9	4.0
1977	1,526	100.0	55.8	32.6	6.9	4.7
1976	1,491	100.0	60.5	31.2	5.0	3.4
1975	1,485	100.0	62.6	28.4	5.1	4.0
1974	1,477	100.0	63.9	28.1	4.5	3.5
1973	1,497	100.0	60.8	31.1	4.7	3.5

Source: General Social Surveys, National Opinion Research Center, University of Chicago; calculations by New Strategist

Table 4.3 Should Government Help the Sick, 1975 to 2002

In general, some people think that it is the responsibility of the government in Washington to see to it that people have help in paying for doctors and hospital bills. Others think that these matters are not the responsibility of the federal government and that people should take care of these things themselves. Where would you place yourself on this scale?

(number of respondents aged 18 or older, and percent distribution by response, 1975–2002)

	number of respondents	total	1 government should help	2	3 agree with both	4	5 people should help themselves	don't know
2002	911	100.0%	31.5%	19.2%	33.8%	7.1%	6.9%	1.4%
2000	1,887	100.0	28.6	21.3	31.1	10.3	5.8	3.0
1998	1,905	100.0	24.8	22.2	32.0	9.7	8.3	2.9
1996	1,918	100.0	27.0	21.0	32.4	10.3	6.6	2.7
1994	1,998	100.0	25.2	21.0	31.0	10.9	9.3	2.7
1993	1,049	100.0	28.3	22.3	31.6	9.3	6.2	2.2
1991	1,013	100.0	31.7	24.7	26.8	9.2	5.7	2.0
1990	897	100.0	29.7	25.5	30.1	7.5	4.3	2.9
1989	1,031	100.0	30.5	22.4	30.1	7.6	7.5	2.0
1988	993	100.0	26.6	21.6	34.7	8.6	6.4	2.1
1987	1,813	100.0	26.4	20.1	35.2	8.4	7.6	2.2
1986	1,463	100.0	28.4	20.0	31.6	11.2	6.4	2.5
1984	1,449	100.0	23.9	18.6	34.9	12.1	7.7	2.8
1983	1,593	100.0	25.9	18.8	31.6	10.2	10.1	3.3
1975	1,484	100.0	35.8	12.7	28.5	7.7	13.1	2.1

Source: General Social Surveys, National Opinion Research Center, University of Chicago; calculations by New Strategist

Most People Say Their Health Is Good or Excellent

But the percentage declines with age.

Between 1972 and 2002, the plurality of respondents to the General Social Survey reported that their health was good. The next largest share said they were in excellent health. As might be expected, the share of people saying their health is good or excellent declines with age. There is also a strong correlation between self-reported health status and income, with the percentage saying their health is excellent increasing with income. People with private health insurance are more likely than the uninsured and those on public insurance to say they are in excellent health. Often the living conditions of people with low incomes contribute to health problems, and health problems, in turn, can make it difficult to earn a decent income and obtain good health insurance.

The percentage of people reporting one or more days of poor physical health in the past month rises with age, from a low of less than 2 percent among those aged 18 to 24 to a high of 12 percent among those aged 65 or older. Interestingly, however, the oldest adults are least likely to report being in poor mental health. Although physical health can certainly influence one's mental status, for most older adults this does seem to be the case.

■ Boomers and younger generations have high expectations for medical science. They may complain about health problems more than today's older generations as they age.

The middle aged are most likely to report poor mental health

(percent of people aged 18 or older reporting one or more days of poor physical or mental health in past 30 days, by age, 2001)

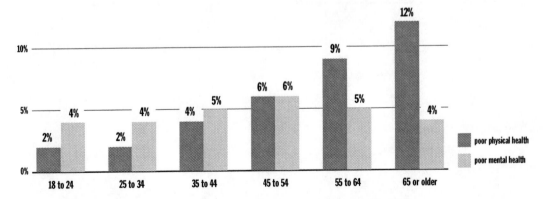

Table 4.4 Health Status, 1972 to 2002

Would you say your own health, in general, is excellent, good, fair, or poor?

(number of respondents aged 18 or older, and percent distribution by self-reported health status, 1972–2002)

	number of respondents	total	excellent	good	fair	poor	don't know
2002	1,851	100.0%	30.7%	46.1%	17.4%	5.6%	0.2%
2000	2,326	100.0	30.2	47.4	16.9	5.4	0.1
1998	2,823	100.0	31.0	47.6	16.5	4.8	0.1
1996	2,421	100.0	30.9	49.0	16.0	3.9	0.1
1994	1,994	100.0	31.4	46.7	17.3	4.6	0.0
1993	1,072	100.0	31.6	45.4	16.6	6.3	0.1
1991	988	100.0	31.3	44.5	19.8	4.4	0.0
1990	916	100.0	31.1	45.7	17.7	5.2	0.2
1989	1,032	100.0	33.1	44.6	17.7	4.3	0.3
1988	976	100.0	30.7	45.1	17.8	6.4	0.0
1987	1,817	100.0	34.0	42.8	18.0	5.2	0.1
1985	1,531	100.0	33.5	42.3	17.6	6.6	0.1
1984	1,462	100.0	29.9	47.7	17.6	4.7	0.1
1982	1,859	100.0	31.8	42.0	18.9	7.3	0.0
1980	1,466	100.0	31.8	42.0	19.6	6.5	0.0
1977	1,527	100.0	31.8	40.9	20.5	6.9	0.0
1976	1,499	100.0	31.3	42.0	19.7	6.9	0.1
1975	1,489	100.0	32.4	39.8	21.4	6.4	0.0
1974	1,480	100.0	32.8	39.8	21.2	6.1	0.0
1973	1,501	100.0	31.9	39.9	21.0	7.1	0.1
1972	1,612	100.0	30.0	44.8	19.9	5.3	0.0

Source: General Social Surveys, National Opinion Research Center, University of Chicago; calculations by New Strategist

Table 4.5 Health Status by Selected Characteristics, 2002

(total number of people, and percent distribution by self-reported health status, by selected characteristics, 2002; numbers in thousands)

	total number	total percent	excellent	very good	good	fair	poor
Total people	278,789	100.0%	36.7%	30.5%	23.1%	6.9%	2.3%
Sex							
Female	142,731	100.0	35.4	30.3	23.9	7.4	2.5
Male	136,058	100.0	38.1	30.8	22.2	6.3	2.0
Age							
Under age 12	48,356	100.0	56.5	27.3	14.2	1.5	0.3
Aged 12 to 17	24,612	100.0	51.6	29.2	16.5	2.0	0.2
Aged 18 to 44	108,111	100.0	38.5	34.2	21.4	4.5	1.0
Aged 45 to 64	64,650	100.0	25.4	30.7	28.6	10.6	4.0
Aged 65 to 74	17,752	100.0	15.5	26.1	35.7	16.2	5.8
Aged 75 or older	15,308	100.0	10.4	21.5	36.2	21.8	9.4
Race and Hispanic origin							
Asian	10,740	100.0	39.2	31.7	23.0	4.2	0.9
Black	34,037	100.0	30.9	29.4	27.2	9.0	2.9
Hispanic	35,254	100.0	34.8	29.3	26.0	7.5	2.1
Non-Hispanic white	193,860	100.0	37.9	30.9	21.9	6.6	2.2
Household income							
Under $20,000	46,934	100.0	25.2	26.2	28.8	13.8	5.7
$20,000 to $34,999	36,568	100.0	30.3	29.4	28.1	9.0	3.1
$35,000 to $54,999	40,451	100.0	37.1	33.1	22.7	5.8	1.2
$55,000 to $74,999	31,344	100.0	42.1	34.1	19.2	3.7	0.9
$75,000 or more	55,653	100.0	50.9	31.1	14.9	2.5	0.5
Education							
Not a high school graduate	27,467	100.0	15.1	22.7	33.4	19.5	9.0
High school graduate	52,064	100.0	22.8	31.2	31.1	11.2	3.5
Some college	46,703	100.0	30.0	34.2	25.5	7.9	2.2
College graduate	45,541	100.0	42.9	34.3	18.1	3.7	1.0
Health insurance coverage among people under age 65							
Private	169,418	100.0	43.8	32.7	18.8	3.7	0.7
Medicaid	27,538	100.0	32.2	25.7	26.7	10.2	4.8
Other	5,883	100.0	30.1	21.1	23.6	15.0	9.8
Uninsured	40,127	100.0	31.0	31.8	27.7	7.0	1.7

Note: Numbers by race and Hispanic origin will not sum to total because not all races are shown and Hispanics may be of any race.
Source: National Center for Health Statistics, Summary Health Statistics for the U.S. Population: National Health Interview Survey, 2002, Vital and Health Statistics, Series 10, No. 220, 2004; Internet site http://www.cdc.gov/nchs/nhis.htm

Table 4.6 Health Status of Children by Selected Characteristics, 2002

(number of people under age 18, and percent distribution by parent-reported health status, by selected characteristics, 2002; numbers in thousands)

	total		excellent	very good	good	fair/poor
	number	percent				
Total children	**72,970**	**100.0%**	**55.7%**	**27.9%**	**14.3%**	**2.1%**
Sex						
Female	35,659	100.0	57.1	27.3	13.5	2.0
Male	37,311	100.0	54.4	28.5	15.0	2.1
Age						
Aged 0 to 4	19,827	100.0	58.9	27.7	11.7	1.6
Aged 5 to 11	28,780	100.0	55.3	27.7	14.5	2.4
Aged 12 to 17	24,363	100.0	53.5	28.5	16.0	2.0
Race and Hispanic origin						
Asian	2,554	100.0	55.5	28.6	14.7	1.2
Black	10,578	100.0	45.8	29.7	20.8	3.7
Hispanic	12,563	100.0	45.9	29.8	21.1	3.1
Non-Hispanic white	45,253	100.0	60.4	27.1	10.9	1.5
Family structure						
Mother and father	52,588	100.0	59.4	27.2	11.9	1.5
Mother, no father	16,175	100.0	46.0	29.7	20.4	3.8
Father, no mother	2,124	100.0	53.3	32.4	12.5	1.6
Neither mother nor father	2,081	100.0	40.4	28.0	27.7	3.8
Parent's education						
Less than high school diploma	9,438	100.0	41.5	28.1	25.3	5.0
High school diploma	16,411	100.0	46.8	31.1	19.2	2.9
More than high school	44,560	100.0	63.0	26.5	9.5	1.0
Household income						
Less than $20,000	12,299	100.0	43.3	29.2	22.1	5.3
$20,000 to $34,999	10,174	100.0	48.0	29.4	20.3	2.2
$35,000 to $54,999	11,667	100.0	56.4	29.4	12.7	1.5
$55,000 to $74,999	9,565	100.0	59.7	29.1	10.2	0.9
$75,000 or more	16,223	100.0	68.5	23.5	7.3	0.6
Health insurance coverage						
Private	46,640	100.0	62.1	26.7	10.1	1.1
Medicaid/other public	17,243	100.0	41.1	30.2	23.9	4.7
Other	1,464	100.0	63.7	25.3	9.8	1.2
Uninsured	7,378	100.0	47.7	31.2	18.8	2.2

Note: Mother and father can include biological, adoptive, step, in-law, or foster relationships. Legal guardians are classified as neither mother nor father. Parent's education is the education level of the parent with the higher level of education.
Source: National Center for Health Statistics, Summary Health Statistics for U.S. Children: National Health Interview Survey, *2002, Series 10, No. 221, 2004; Internet site http://www.cdc.gov/nchs/nhis.htm*

Table 4.7 Health Problems in Past 30 Days by Age, 2001

(percent of people aged 18 or older reporting one or more days of poor physical or mental health during the past 30 days or activity limitations due to poor health, by age, 2001)

	poor physical health	poor mental health	activity limitations due to poor health
Total people	**5.9%**	**4.7%**	**3.2%**
Aged 18 to 24	1.5	4.4	0.8
Aged 25 to 34	2.4	4.1	1.3
Aged 35 to 44	4.0	4.9	2.4
Aged 45 to 54	6.2	5.7	3.8
Aged 55 to 64	9.0	4.9	5.3
Aged 65 or older	12.2	3.8	5.4

Source: Centers for Disease Control and Prevention, Behavioral Risk Factor Surveillance System Online Prevalence Data, 2001; Internet site http://apps.nccd.cdc.gov/brfss/

Inability to Pay for Health Care Is a Problem for Many

For the uninsured, this is a serious issue.

In 2001, 13.6 million families—almost 12 percent of all families—had problems receiving health care for at least one family member. The ability to pay for health care is the most commonly cited reason for having difficulty getting health care, with more half of those having problems (57 percent) giving this reason. Another 19 percent had problems related to their insurance coverage. The remainder (24 percent) cited other reasons, which includes such things as transportation difficulties or problems getting time off work.

The impact of the Medicare program, which covers nearly everyone aged 65 or older, can be seen in these statistics. People aged 65 or older are much less likely than younger adults to have problems receiving health care. Among those with problems, only 38 percent said the problem was due to an inability to pay. In contrast, fully 89 of people under age 65 without health insurance who had problems receiving health care said inability to pay was the reason.

Among people with incomes below poverty level who had problems getting care, 69 percent said it was because they could not afford it. The near poor were even more likely to cite financial problems (74 percent). The difference is likely due to the fact that poverty-level families are eligible for Medicaid while the "working poor" are not.

■ As health costs rise, affordability is keeping many Americans from getting care.

Older Americans are least likely to experience problems paying for care

(among families who had problems receiving health care, percent who had problems because of ability to pay, by age and health insurance status, 2001)

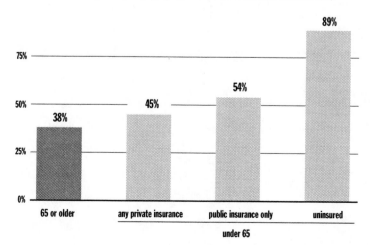

Table 4.8 Families with Problems Receiving Health Care by Reason, 2001

(total number of families, number reporting at least one family member having problems receiving health care in past 12 months, and percent distribution of families with problems by reason, 2001; families in thousands)

	total families	total with problems number	total with problems percent	could not afford	insurance related	other reasons
Total families	**118,796**	**13,635**	**100.0%**	**57.2%**	**18.7%**	**24.0%**
Age						
Aged 18 to 44	56,213	7,645	100.0	62.5	15.8	21.8
Aged 45 to 64	38,796	4,632	100.0	53.8	22.1	23.8
Aged 65 or older	23,631	1,326	100.0	38.2	24.6	37.2
Sex						
Female	57,370	7,338	100.0	60.9	17.8	21.3
Male	61,425	6,297	100.0	52.7	19.9	27.2
Race and Hispanic origin						
Black	13,966	1,451	100.0	56.2	15.0	28.8
Hispanic	12,117	1,638	100.0	71.2	7.8	20.9
White and other	92,713	10,546	100.0	55.1	20.9	23.9
Health insurance status of people under age 65						
Any private insurance	72,666	6,890	100.0	44.8	24.6	30.4
Public insurance only	8,245	1,775	100.0	53.6	22.0	24.4
Uninsured	14,252	3,644	100.0	89.1	3.8	7.0
Income status						
Poor	15,806	2,950	100.0	69.2	12.1	18.7
Near poor	5,586	925	100.0	73.8	8.1	18.2
Low income	16,743	2,802	100.0	69.3	16.8	14.0
Middle income	36,649	4,001	100.0	56.2	20.7	23.0
High income	44,012	2,957	100.0	29.7	27.8	42.1

Note: Uninsured refers to people uninsured for the entire year. Poor refers to incomes below poverty level. Near poor is incomes from poverty level through 125 percent of poverty level. Low income is more than 125 percent of poverty level through 200 percent of poverty level. Middle income is more than 200 percent of poverty level through 400 percent of poverty level. High income is more than 400 percent of poverty level.
Source: Center for Financing, Access and Cost Trends, Agency for Healthcare Research and Quality: Medical Expenditure Panel Survey, 2001; Internet site http://www.meps.ahrq.gov/CompendiumTables/TC_TOC.htm

Many Patients Want More Time with Health Care Providers

Younger people are most likely to feel they have been hurried.

Among people who have made appointments for routine health care in the past 12 months, the largest share (42 percent) say they always get an appointment as soon as they want and 34 percent say they usually do. They have better luck getting appointments for their children, with two-thirds saying they always get in as soon they want.

Fewer than half (43 percent) of adults who visited a physician or health care clinic in the past 12 months say their health care provider always spent enough time with them. Forty percent say they usually got enough time with their provider, but 15 percent say they only sometimes or never get enough time. There are striking differences by age in responses to this question. Only 38 percent of people aged 18 to 44 say their provider always spends enough time with them. Among people aged 65 or older, the 52 percent majority says providers give them enough time.

■ Older adults have more—and more complex—health problems, requiring health care providers to spend more time with them.

Older people are most satisfied with time provider spends with them

(percent of people aged 18 or older who saw a health care provider in the past 12 months who say their provider "always" spent enough time with them, by age, 2001)

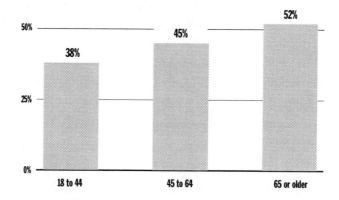

Table 4.9 Attitude toward Scheduling of Routine Health Care Appointments for Adults, 2001

(total number of people aged 18 or older, number who made appointments for routine health care in past 12 months, and percent distribution by how often they got appointment as soon as wanted, 2001; people in thousands)

	total	total with appointments number	total with appointments percent	always	usually	sometimes/ never
Total adults	**208,272**	**138,643**	**100.0%**	**41.7%**	**34.3%**	**19.2%**
Age						
Aged 18 to 44	107,916	60,851	100.0	36.2	33.7	26.5
Aged 45 to 64	65,740	48,429	100.0	42.1	36.4	16.7
Aged 65 or older	34,616	29,363	100.0	52.3	31.9	8.5
Sex						
Female	108,448	81,702	100.0	40.9	34.5	19.5
Male	99,824	56,941	100.0	42.8	34.0	18.9
Race and Hispanic origin						
Black	23,305	14,415	100.0	44.7	27.4	22.1
Hispanic	24,431	12,249	100.0	39.2	28.1	27.4
White and other	160,536	111,979	100.0	41.6	35.8	18.0
Health insurance status						
Under age 65						
Any private insurance	134,689	90,262	100.0	38.8	36.3	21.2
Public insurance only	13,041	9,230	100.0	41.4	29.2	22.9
Uninsured	25,926	9,787	100.0	36.8	27.3	30.6
Aged 65 or older						
Medicare only	10,737	9,132	100.0	51.7	31.0	9.0
Medicare and private	20,251	17,454	100.0	53.2	33.3	7.5
Medicare and other public	3,543	2,754	100.0	49.2	25.8	12.8
Income status						
Poor	20,753	12,629	100.0	42.4	28.7	23.0
Near poor	8,145	4,970	100.0	43.9	30.4	18.8
Low income	27,360	16,731	100.0	45.6	30.6	18.0
Middle income	65,619	42,191	100.0	41.7	33.6	19.9
High income	86,394	62,121	100.0	40.3	37.1	18.4

Note: Uninsured refers to people uninsured for the entire year. Poor refers to incomes below poverty level. Near poor is incomes from poverty level through 125 percent of poverty level. Low income is more than 125 percent of poverty level through 200 percent of poverty level. Middle income is more than 200 percent of poverty level through 400 percent of poverty level. High income is more than 400 percent of poverty level. Percentages will not sum to 100 because no response is not shown.
Source: Center for Financing, Access and Cost Trends, Agency for Healthcare Research and Quality: Medical Expenditure Panel Survey, 2001; Internet site http://www.meps.ahrq.gov/CompendiumTables/TC_TOC.htm

Table 4.10 Attitude toward Scheduling of Routine Health Care Appointments for Children, 2001

(total number of people under age 18, number who had appointments for routine health care in past 12 months, and percent distribution by how often they got appointment as soon as wanted, 2001; people in thousands)

	total	total with appointments number	total with appointments percent	always	usually	sometimes/ never
Total children	**72,936**	**47,346**	**100.0%**	**67.6%**	**20.6%**	**11.6%**
Age						
Under age 6	23,678	18,077	100.0	69.5	19.9	10.5
Aged 6 to 17	49,258	29,268	100.0	66.4	21.1	12.3
Sex						
Female	35,609	23,297	100.0	66.3	21.3	12.2
Male	37,326	24,049	100.0	68.8	20.0	11.0
Race and Hispanic origin						
Black	11,226	7,051	100.0	66.2	21.4	12.0
Hispanic	13,019	7,501	100.0	63.9	20.6	15.3
White and other	48,691	32,794	100.0	68.7	20.5	10.6
Health insurance status						
Any private insurance	49,156	33,339	100.0	68.1	20.8	10.9
Public insurance only	17,525	11,502	100.0	66.0	20.2	13.4
Uninsured	6,254	2,505	100.0	66.9	20.4	12.0
Income status						
Poor	12,167	7,302	100.0	64.4	21.1	14.1
Near poor	3,958	2,245	100.0	63.1	23.5	13.3
Low income	12,005	6,642	100.0	61.7	24.7	13.5
Middle income	23,480	15,005	100.0	66.7	21.6	11.5
High income	21,326	16,153	100.0	72.7	17.5	9.6

Note: Uninsured refers to people uninsured for the entire year. Poor refers to incomes below poverty level. Near poor is incomes from poverty level through 125 percent of poverty level. Low income is more than 125 percent of poverty level through 200 percent of poverty level. Middle income is more than 200 percent of poverty level through 400 percent of poverty level. High income is more than 400 percent of poverty level. Percentages will not sum to 100 because "don't know" and no response is not shown.
Source: Center for Financing, Access and Cost Trends, Agency for Healthcare Research and Quality: Medical Expenditure Panel Survey, 2001; Internet site http://www.meps.ahrq.gov/CompendiumTables/TC_TOC.htm

Table 4.11 Health Care Provider Spent Enough Time with Adult Patient, 2001

(total number of people aged 18 or older, number visiting a doctor or health care clinic in past 12 months, and percent distribution by whether the health care provider spent enough time with them, 2001; people in thousands)

	total	total with health care visit number	total with health care visit percent	always	usually	sometimes/ never
Total adults	**208,272**	**147,562**	**100.0%**	**43.1%**	**39.5%**	**15.4%**
Age						
Aged 18 to 44	107,916	68,662	100.0	38.3	40.9	19.7
Aged 45 to 64	65,740	50,052	100.0	45.0	39.8	13.5
Aged 65 or older	34,616	28,847	100.0	51.6	35.7	8.4
Sex						
Female	108,448	85,176	100.0	42.3	39.4	16.2
Male	99,824	62,385	100.0	44.3	39.6	14.3
Race and Hispanic origin						
Black	23,305	14,834	100.0	48.7	31.8	16.3
Hispanic	24,431	12,967	100.0	41.1	36.5	20.2
White and other	160,536	119,760	100.0	42.7	40.8	14.8
Health insurance status						
Under age 65						
Any private insurance	134,689	97,538	100.0	41.1	41.9	15.9
Public insurance only	13,041	9,918	100.0	43.9	32.9	20.8
Uninsured	25,926	11,258	100.0	39.1	34.4	24.4
Aged 65 or older						
Medicare only	10,737	8,957	100.0	50.1	36.2	9.5
Medicare and private	20,251	17,040	100.0	52.1	36.5	7.3
Medicare and other public	3,543	2,825	100.0	53.3	29.6	11.4
Income status						
Poor	20,753	13,560	100.0	43.1	33.6	20.6
Near poor	8,145	5,399	100.0	48.7	35.0	13.4
Low income	27,360	17,780	100.0	45.6	33.7	18.1
Middle income	65,619	45,121	100.0	41.3	40.8	15.8
High income	86,394	65,701	100.0	43.3	41.8	13.5

Note: Uninsured refers to people uninsured for the entire year. Poor refers to incomes below poverty level. Near poor is incomes from poverty level through 125 percent of poverty level. Low income is more than 125 percent of poverty level through 200 percent of poverty level. Middle income is more than 200 percent of poverty level through 400 percent of poverty level. High income is more than 400 percent of poverty level. Percentages will not sum to 100 because "don't know" and no response is not shown.
Source: Center for Financing, Access and Cost Trends, Agency for Healthcare Research and Quality: Medical Expenditure Panel Survey, 2001; Internet site http://www.meps.ahrq.gov/CompendiumTables/TC_TOC.htm

Table 4.12 Health Care Provider Spent Enough Time with Patients under Age 18 and Their Parents, 2001

(total number of people under age 18, number visiting a doctor or health care clinic in past 12 months, and percent distribution by whether the health care provider spent enough time with them and their parents, 2001; people in thousands)

| | total | total with health care visit | | always | usually | sometimes/ never |
		number	percent			
Total children	**72,936**	**54,448**	**100.0%**	**67.3%**	**22.6%**	**9.6%**
Age						
Under age 6	23,678	19,563	100.0	67.8	21.4	10.7
Aged 6 to 17	49,258	34,885	100.0	67.0	23.2	9.0
Sex						
Female	35,609	26,671	100.0	67.4	22.6	9.5
Male	37,326	27,777	100.0	67.2	22.5	9.7
Race and Hispanic origin						
Black	11,226	7,797	100.0	70.3	19.8	8.8
Hispanic	13,019	8,522	100.0	62.2	24.2	13.1
White and other	48,691	38,129	100.0	67.8	22.8	9.0
Health insurance status						
Any private insurance	49,156	38,286	100.0	68.5	23.2	7.8
Public insurance only	17,525	13,033	100.0	64.0	21.4	14.2
Uninsured	6,254	3,129	100.0	65.8	19.1	12.8
Income status						
Poor	12,167	8,447	100.0	64.6	20.0	15.0
Near poor	3,958	2,592	100.0	64.8	24.4	10.4
Low income	12,005	7,827	100.0	62.2	24.0	13.0
Middle income	23,480	17,604	100.0	65.2	24.2	10.0
High income	21,326	17,977	100.0	73.2	21.3	5.2

Note: Uninsured refers to people uninsured for the entire year. Poor refers to incomes below poverty level. Near poor is incomes from poverty level through 125 percent of poverty level. Low income is more than 125 percent of poverty level through 200 percent of poverty level. Middle income is more than 200 percent of poverty level through 400 percent of poverty level. High income is more than 400 percent of poverty level. Percentages will not sum to 100 because "don't know" and no response is not shown.
Source: Center for Financing, Access and Cost Trends, Agency for Healthcare Research and Quality: Medical Expenditure Panel Survey, 2001; Internet site http://www.meps.ahrq.gov/CompendiumTables/TC_TOC.htm

Most Patients Say Providers Always Explain, Listen, and Show Respect

But the shares could be higher.

More than half (56 percent) of adults who visited a doctor or health care clinic in the past year say their health care provider always explained things clearly to them, while slightly more than one-third said this is usually true. Parents are more likely to say their child's health care provider always explains things clearly to them, with 74 percent saying this is always true. One reason for the difference between parents and adults seeking care may be the fact that it is more difficult to ask enough questions and elicit information as a patient than as an observer.

Fifty-four percent of adults say their health care provider always listens carefully to them. Parents are even more likely to say their children's health care provided listens carefully (72 percent). Fifty-seven percent of adults and 74 percent of parents say their health care provider shows respect for what they had to say.

Older adults are more likely than younger ones to say their providers always explain, listen, and show respect. This may reflect differing expectations and attitudes toward "authority figures." Younger generations may expect more information and may want to participate more in decisions about their care.

■ While explaining things clearly, listening carefully, and showing respect may not always be important to a patient's well-being, they certainly enhance a patient's opinion of the quality of care he or she receives.

Younger adults are least likely to think health care providers listen carefully or show respect

(percent of people aged 18 or older who say their health care provider always explains things clearly, listens carefully, and shows respect for what they had to say, 2001)

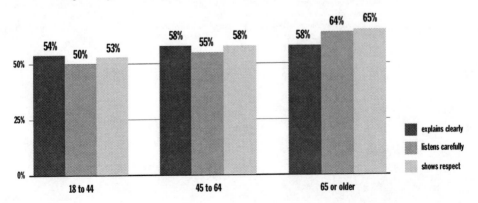

Table 4.13 Health Care Provider Explained Things Clearly to Adult Patient, 2001

(total number of people aged 18 or older, number visiting a doctor or health care clinic in past 12 months, and percent distribution by whether the health care provider explained things clearly to them, 2001; people in thousands)

		total with health care visit				sometimes/
	total	number	percent	always	usually	never
Total adults	**208,272**	**147,562**	**100.0%**	**55.8%**	**34.5%**	**8.7%**
Age						
Aged 18 to 44	107,916	68,662	100.0	53.5	36.0	10.0
Aged 45 to 64	65,740	50,052	100.0	57.8	33.2	8.0
Aged 65 or older	34,616	28,847	100.0	57.6	33.0	6.9
Sex						
Female	108,448	85,176	100.0	56.2	33.9	8.9
Male	99,824	62,385	100.0	55.2	35.2	8.5
Race and Hispanic origin						
Black	23,305	14,834	100.0	61.5	25.6	10.9
Hispanic	24,431	12,967	100.0	57.8	27.4	13.4
White and other	160,536	119,780	100.0	54.8	36.3	7.9
Health insurance status						
Under age 65						
Any private insurance	134,689	97,538	100.0	55.6	36.0	7.9
Public insurance only	13,041	9,918	100.0	55.5	27.7	15.4
Uninsured	25,926	11,258	100.0	52.7	30.8	14.7
Aged 65 or older						
Medicare only	10,737	8,957	100.0	58.4	31.6	7.9
Medicare and private	20,251	17,040	100.0	57.7	34.2	5.4
Medicare and other public	3,543	2,825	100.0	54.9	29.9	12.0
Income status						
Poor	20,753	13,560	100.0	55.2	28.7	14.2
Near poor	8,145	5,399	100.0	56.6	31.9	10.8
Low income	27,360	17,780	100.0	55.4	31.3	11.7
Middle income	65,619	45,121	100.0	54.3	35.6	8.9
High income	86,394	65,701	100.0	57.0	35.9	6.5

Note: Uninsured refers to people uninsured for the entire year. Poor refers to incomes below poverty level. Near poor is incomes from poverty level through 125 percent of poverty level. Low income is more than 125 percent of poverty level through 200 percent of poverty level. Middle income is more than 200 percent of poverty level through 400 percent of poverty level. High income is more than 400 percent of poverty level. Percentages will not sum to 100 because "don't know" and no response is not shown.
Source: Center for Financing, Access and Cost Trends, Agency for Healthcare Research and Quality: Medical Expenditure Panel Survey, 2001; Internet site http://www.meps.ahrq.gov/CompendiumTables/TC_TOC.htm

Table 4.14 Health Care Provider Explained Things Clearly to Parents of Patients under Age 18, 2001

(total number of people under age 18, number visiting a doctor or health care clinic in past 12 months, and percent distribution by whether the health care provider explained things clearly to their parents, 2001; people in thousands)

	total	total with health care visit number	total with health care visit percent	always	usually	sometimes/ never
Total children	**72,936**	**54,448**	**100.0%**	**74.3%**	**19.6%**	**5.6%**
Age						
Under age 6	23,678	19,563	100.0	74.9	18.6	6.4
Aged 6 to 17	49,258	34,885	100.0	73.9	20.1	5.1
Sex						
Female	35,609	26,671	100.0	74.6	19.2	5.6
Male	37,326	27,777	100.0	74.0	19.9	5.5
Race and Hispanic origin						
Black	11,226	7,797	100.0	76.5	16.7	5.8
Hispanic	13,019	8,522	100.0	71.5	19.7	8.3
White and other	48,691	38,129	100.0	74.4	20.1	4.9
Health insurance status						
Any private insurance	49,156	38,286	100.0	75.9	19.6	4.1
Public insurance only	17,525	13,033	100.0	70.1	19.7	9.5
Uninsured	6,254	3,129	100.0	72.5	18.9	6.8
Income status						
Poor	12,167	8,447	100.0	69.4	18.2	11.7
Near poor	3,958	2,592	100.0	71.1	20.0	8.4
Low income	12,005	7,827	100.0	67.1	24.4	7.6
Middle income	23,480	17,604	100.0	75.5	19.3	4.6
High income	21,326	17,977	100.0	79.0	18.4	2.3

Note: Uninsured refers to people uninsured for the entire year. Poor refers to incomes below poverty level. Near poor is incomes from poverty level through 125 percent of poverty level. Low income is more than 125 percent of poverty level through 200 percent of poverty level. Middle income is more than 200 percent of poverty level through 400 percent of poverty level. High income is more than 400 percent of poverty level. Percentages will not sum to 100 because "don't know" and no response is not shown.
Source: Center for Financing, Access and Cost Trends, Agency for Healthcare Research and Quality: Medical Expenditure Panel Survey, 2001; Internet site http://www.meps.ahrq.gov/CompendiumTables/TC_TOC.htm

Table 4.15 Health Care Provider Listened Carefully to Adult Patient, 2001

(total number of people aged 18 or older, number visiting a doctor or health care clinic in past 12 months, and percent distribution by whether the health care provider listened carefully to them, 2001; people in thousands)

| | total | total with health care visit | | always | usually | sometimes/ never |
		number	percent			
Total adults	**208,272**	**147,562**	**100.0%**	**54.4%**	**34.3%**	**10.1%**
Age						
Aged 18 to 44	107,916	68,662	100.0	50.0	36.5	12.9
Aged 45 to 64	65,740	50,052	100.0	55.1	34.7	9.1
Aged 65 or older	34,616	28,847	100.0	63.5	28.5	5.2
Sex						
Female	108,448	85,176	100.0	53.9	34.6	10.3
Male	99,824	62,385	100.0	55.0	34.0	9.8
Race and Hispanic origin						
Black	23,305	14,834	100.0	63.7	23.5	10.7
Hispanic	24,431	12,967	100.0	57.5	27.3	13.7
White and other	160,536	119,780	100.0	52.9	36.4	9.7
Health insurance status						
Under age 65						
Any private insurance	134,689	97,538	100.0	52.0	37.2	10.2
Public insurance only	13,041	9,918	100.0	53.7	28.1	16.5
Uninsured	25,926	11,258	100.0	51.7	30.0	16.4
Aged 65 or older						
Medicare only	10,737	8,957	100.0	61.4	31.4	4.5
Medicare and private	20,251	17,040	100.0	64.4	27.5	5.3
Medicare and other public	3,543	2,825	100.0	64.7	24.8	7.2
Income status						
Poor	20,753	13,560	100.0	55.6	28.4	13.8
Near poor	8,145	5,399	100.0	59.2	28.8	10.3
Low income	27,360	17,780	100.0	55.9	29.7	12.6
Middle income	65,619	45,121	100.0	54.0	33.9	10.7
High income	86,394	65,701	100.0	53.6	37.5	8.2

Note: Uninsured refers to people uninsured for the entire year. Poor refers to incomes below poverty level. Near poor is incomes from poverty level through 125 percent of poverty level. Low income is more than 125 percent of poverty level through 200 percent of poverty level. Middle income is more than 200 percent of poverty level through 400 percent of poverty level. High income is more than 400 percent of poverty level. Percentages will not sum to 100 because "don't know" and no response is not shown.
Source: Center for Financing, Access and Cost Trends, Agency for Healthcare Research and Quality: Medical Expenditure Panel Survey, 2001; Internet site http://www.meps.ahrq.gov/CompendiumTables/TC_TOC.htm

Table 4.16 Health Care Provider Listened Carefully to Parents of Patients under Age 18, 2001

(total number of people under age 18, number visiting a doctor or health care clinic in past 12 months, and percent distribution by whether the health care provider listened carefully to their parents, 2001; people in thousands)

| | total | total with health care visit | | always | usually | sometimes/ never |
		number	percent			
Total children	**72,936**	**54,448**	**100.0%**	**71.5%**	**21.1%**	**6.8%**
Age						
Under age 6	23,678	19,563	100.0	72.0	21.0	6.9
Aged 6 to 17	49,258	34,885	100.0	71.2	21.2	6.8
Sex						
Female	35,609	26,671	100.0	71.3	21.2	7.0
Male	37,326	27,777	100.0	71.7	21.1	6.7
Race and Hispanic origin						
Black	11,226	7,797	100.0	77.5	15.2	6.4
Hispanic	13,019	8,522	100.0	69.7	20.7	9.3
White and other	48,691	38,129	100.0	70.7	22.4	6.4
Health insurance status						
Any private insurance	49,156	38,286	100.0	72.7	21.3	5.5
Public insurance only	17,525	13,033	100.0	67.8	21.5	10.3
Uninsured	6,254	3,129	100.0	72.0	17.3	8.9
Income status						
Poor	12,167	8,447	100.0	68.5	19.1	12.0
Near poor	3,958	2,592	100.0	71.7	21.3	6.6
Low income	12,005	7,827	100.0	66.9	23.2	9.0
Middle income	23,480	17,604	100.0	70.4	22.5	6.5
High income	21,326	17,977	100.0	76.0	19.8	3.9

Note: Uninsured refers to people uninsured for the entire year. Poor refers to incomes below poverty level. Near poor is incomes from poverty level through 125 percent of poverty level. Low income is more than 125 percent of poverty level through 200 percent of poverty level. Middle income is more than 200 percent of poverty level through 400 percent of poverty level. High income is more than 400 percent of poverty level. Percentages will not sum to 100 because "don't know" and no response is not shown.
Source: Center for Financing, Access and Cost Trends, Agency for Healthcare Research and Quality: Medical Expenditure Panel Survey, 2001; Internet site http://www.meps.ahrq.gov/CompendiumTables/TC_TOC.htm

Table 4.17 Health Care Provider Showed Respect for What Adult Patient Had to Say, 2001

(total number of people aged 18 or older, number visiting a doctor or health care clinic in past 12 months, and percent distribution by whether the health care provider showed respect for what they had to say, 2001; people in thousands)

| | | total with health care visit | | | | sometimes/ |
	total	number	percent	always	usually	never
Total adults	**208,272**	**147,562**	**100.0%**	**56.8%**	**32.9%**	**9.2%**
Age						
Aged 18 to 44	107,916	68,662	100.0	52.6	35.6	11.1
Aged 45 to 64	65,740	50,052	100.0	58.1	32.5	8.5
Aged 65 or older	34,616	28,847	100.0	64.6	27.2	5.7
Sex						
Female	108,448	85,176	100.0	56.7	33.2	9.0
Male	99,824	62,385	100.0	56.9	32.6	9.4
Race and Hispanic origin						
Black	23,305	14,834	100.0	65.9	23.7	8.4
Hispanic	24,431	12,967	100.0	61.4	25.8	11.4
White and other	160,536	119,780	100.0	55.2	34.8	9.0
Health insurance status						
Under age 65						
Any private insurance	134,689	97,538	100.0	54.9	35.7	8.8
Public insurance only	13,041	9,918	100.0	56.8	26.1	15.7
Uninsured	25,926	11,258	100.0	53.6	29.3	15.4
Aged 65 or older						
Medicare only	10,737	8,957	100.0	63.8	27.7	6.3
Medicare and private	20,251	17,040	100.0	64.7	27.8	5.0
Medicare and other public	3,543	2,825	100.0	67.0	22.0	8.0
Income status						
Poor	20,753	13,560	100.0	58.6	25.9	13.8
Near poor	8,145	5,399	100.0	61.9	28.0	9.2
Low income	27,360	17,780	100.0	58.4	29.0	10.9
Middle income	65,619	45,121	100.0	55.4	33.0	10.3
High income	86,394	65,701	100.0	56.6	35.8	7.0

Note: Uninsured refers to people uninsured for the entire year. Poor refers to incomes below poverty level. Near poor is incomes from poverty level through 125 percent of poverty level. Low income is more than 125 percent of poverty level through 200 percent of poverty level. Middle income is more than 200 percent of poverty level through 400 percent of poverty level. High income is more than 400 percent of poverty level. Percentages will not sum to 100 because "don't know" and no response is not shown.
Source: Center for Financing, Access and Cost Trends, Agency for Healthcare Research and Quality: Medical Expenditure Panel Survey, 2001; Internet site http://www.meps.ahrq.gov/CompendiumTables/TC_TOC.htm

Table 4.18 Health Care Provider Showed Respect for What Parents of Patients under Age 18 Had to Say, 2001

(total number of people under age 18, number visiting a doctor or health care clinic in past 12 months, and percent distribution by whether the health care provider showed respect for what parents had to say, 2001; people in thousands)

	total	total with health care visit number	total with health care visit percent	always	usually	sometimes/ never
Total children	**72,936**	**54,448**	**100.0%**	**74.0%**	**19.5%**	**6.0%**
Age						
Under age 6	23,678	19,563	100.0	74.3	18.8	6.7
Aged 6 to 17	49,258	34,885	100.0	73.8	19.9	5.6
Sex						
Female	35,609	26,671	100.0	74.1	19.5	5.9
Male	37,326	27,777	100.0	73.9	19.5	6.1
Race and Hispanic origin						
Black	11,226	7,797	100.0	79.1	15.5	4.3
Hispanic	13,019	8,522	100.0	73.1	19.0	7.3
White and other	48,691	38,129	100.0	73.1	20.4	6.0
Health insurance status						
Any private insurance	49,156	38,286	100.0	74.9	20.0	4.6
Public insurance only	17,525	13,033	100.0	71.6	18.5	9.6
Uninsured	6,254	3,129	100.0	72.8	17.8	7.3
Income status						
Poor	12,167	8,447	100.0	71.1	17.4	11.1
Near poor	3,958	2,592	100.0	71.4	20.3	7.9
Low income	12,005	7,827	100.0	67.7	23.7	7.6
Middle income	23,480	17,604	100.0	74.2	19.9	5.4
High income	21,326	17,977	100.0	78.2	18.2	3.1

Note: Uninsured refers to people uninsured for the entire year. Poor refers to incomes below poverty level. Near poor is incomes from poverty level through 125 percent of poverty level. Low income is more than 125 percent of poverty level through 200 percent of poverty level. Middle income is more than 200 percent of poverty level through 400 percent of poverty level. High income is more than 400 percent of poverty level. Percentages will not sum to 100 because "don't know" and no response is not shown.
Source: Center for Financing, Access and Cost Trends, Agency for Healthcare Research and Quality: Medical Expenditure Panel Survey, 2001; Internet site http://www.meps.ahrq.gov/CompendiumTables/TC_TOC.htm

Americans Rate Their Health Care Provider Highly

Parents rate their children's health care provider even more highly than their own.

In 2001, 71 percent of people aged 18 or older visited a doctor or health care clinic. Asked to rate the health care they received on a scale of 0 (worst) to 10 (best), the largest share (45 percent) rated the care a 9 or 10. Another 39 percent rated the care they received at 7 or 8 on the scale. Only 14 percent rated the care they received a 6 or lower.

There were sizable differences in opinions by demographic characteristic. Younger adults are more likely to rate the care they receive a 6 or lower and are more likely to give it a 7 or 8. People aged 65 or older are most likely to rate the care they receive a 9 or higher. Perhaps not surprisingly, people without insurance are more likely than the insured to give the care they receive a rating of 6 or below. The uninsured have fewer health care options than those with insurance and often cannot refuse to return to a health care provider who does not provide the best care.

Parents have a higher opinion of the care their children receive than the care they receive. More than two-thirds rate their child's health care provider a 9 or 10, and only 7 percent rate the provider at a 6 or below. Even among parents without insurance or who use public insurance such as Medicaid, more than 60 percent rate their children's care at a 9 or 10.

■ Although many Americans express dissatisfaction with the health care system in general, most have a fairly high opinion of their own health care providers.

Older Americans are most likely to give their health care provider the highest rating

(percent of people aged 18 or older who rate the health care they receive at a 9 or 10 on a 10-point scale, by age, 2001)

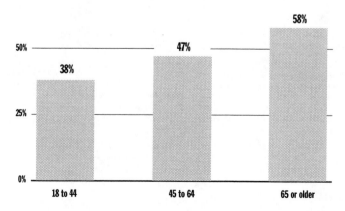

Table 4.19 Adult Patients' Rating of Health Care Received from Doctor's Office or Clinic, 2001

(total number of people aged 18 or older, number visiting a doctor or health care clinic in past 12 months, and percent distribution by rating given for health care received on a scale from 0 (worst) to 10 (best), 2001; people in thousands)

		total with health care visit		rating		
	total	number	percent	0 to 6	7 to 8	9 to 10
Total adults	208,272	147,562	100.0%	14.3%	38.5%	44.7%
Age						
Aged 18 to 44	107,916	68,662	100.0	16.7	44.3	37.5
Aged 45 to 64	65,740	50,052	100.0	13.6	37.0	46.8
Aged 65 or older	34,616	28,847	100.0	10.2	27.2	58.3
Sex						
Female	108,448	85,176	100.0	14.1	38.1	45.2
Male	99,824	62,385	100.0	14.7	38.9	44.2
Race and Hispanic origin						
Black	23,305	14,834	100.0	17.2	33.0	46.0
Hispanic	24,431	12,967	100.0	19.4	33.6	44.1
White and other	160,536	119,780	100.0	13.4	39.7	44.7
Health insurance status						
Under age 65						
Any private insurance	134,689	97,538	100.0	13.5	42.8	42.0
Public insurance only	13,041	9,918	100.0	25.4	31.1	40.5
Uninsured	25,926	11,258	100.0	23.1	35.9	37.1
Aged 65 or older						
Medicare only	10,737	8,957	100.0	13.5	27.1	55.2
Medicare and private	20,251	17,040	100.0	7.4	27.9	60.6
Medicare and other public	3,543	2,825	100.0	16.1	22.5	54.5
Income status						
Poor	20,753	13,560	100.0	21.7	30.3	44.8
Near poor	8,145	5,399	100.0	13.5	34.2	49.9
Low income	27,360	17,780	100.0	19.6	30.6	46.4
Middle income	65,619	45,121	100.0	15.4	38.5	43.4
High income	86,394	65,701	100.0	10.8	42.6	44.8

Note: Uninsured refers to people uninsured for the entire year. Poor refers to incomes below poverty level. Near poor is incomes from poverty level through 125 percent of poverty level. Low income is more than 125 percent of poverty level through 200 percent of poverty level. Middle income is more than 200 percent of poverty level through 400 percent of poverty level. High income is more than 400 percent of poverty level. Percentages will not sum to 100 because "don't know" and no response is not shown.
Source: Center for Financing, Access and Cost Trends, Agency for Healthcare Research and Quality: Medical Expenditure Panel Survey, 2001; Internet site http://www.meps.ahrq.gov/CompendiumTables/TC_TOC.htm

Table 4.20 Parents' Rating of Health Care Received by Children at Doctor's Office or Clinic, 2001

(total number of people under age 18, number visiting a doctor or health care clinic in past 12 months, and percent distribution by rating given by parents for health care received by children on a scale from 0 (worst) to 10 (best), 2001; people in thousands)

		total with health care visit		rating		
	total	number	percent	0 to 6	7 to 8	9 to 10
Total children	**72,936**	**54,448**	**100.0%**	**6.8%**	**29.0%**	**64.0%**
Age						
Under age 6	23,678	19,563	100.0	6.5	28.6	64.7
Aged 6 to 17	49,258	34,885	100.0	6.9	29.2	63.6
Sex						
Female	35,609	26,671	100.0	6.3	28.7	64.7
Male	37,326	27,777	100.0	7.2	29.3	63.3
Race and Hispanic origin						
Black	11,226	7,797	100.0	7.7	28.3	63.5
Hispanic	13,019	8,522	100.0	8.6	28.6	62.7
White and other	48,691	38,129	100.0	6.1	29.3	64.4
Health insurance status						
Any private insurance	49,156	38,286	100.0	5.3	29.0	65.4
Public insurance only	17,525	13,033	100.0	10.5	29.1	60.2
Uninsured	6,254	3,129	100.0	9.0	28.3	62.4
Income status						
Poor	12,167	8,447	100.0	10.7	27.5	61.4
Near poor	3,958	2,592	100.0	8.0	29.4	62.2
Low income	12,005	7,827	100.0	8.8	32.1	59.0
Middle income	23,480	17,604	100.0	6.5	29.3	63.9
High income	21,326	17,977	100.0	4.1	28.0	67.8

Note: Uninsured refers to people uninsured for the entire year. Poor refers to incomes below poverty level. Near poor is incomes from poverty level through 125 percent of poverty level. Low income is more than 125 percent of poverty level through 200 percent of poverty level. Middle income is more than 200 percent of poverty level through 400 percent of poverty level. High income is more than 400 percent of poverty level. Percentages will not sum to 100 because "don't know" and no response is not shown.
Source: Center for Financing, Access and Cost Trends, Agency for Healthcare Research and Quality: Medical Expenditure Panel Survey, 2001; Internet site http://www.meps.ahrq.gov/CompendiumTables/TC_TOC.htm

Most Americans Get Some Health Information Online

But few purchase prescriptions through Internet sources.

One of the primary uses of the Internet is to obtain information about a wide variety of topics, including health. Seventy-five percent of men and 85 percent of women who use the Internet say they have searched online for health-related information. Most commonly, they are seeking information about a specific condition or treatment.

Women search for information about a wider variety of health topics than men. For almost every health topic considered in the Pew survey, women were more likely than men to say they had sought information about it. This may reflect women's traditional role as the family's health-care "point person." Many women may be online seeking health information for other family members, including their husbands.

Although the majority of adults turn to the Internet for health information, most do not shop for prescription drugs online. Only 4 percent of respondents say they have purchased prescription drugs online. The primary reason more people do not do so is suggested by the fact that 62 percent of respondents believe that purchasing drugs over the Internet is not as safe as obtaining them through their local pharmacy.

■ There is a wealth of information about medical issues and medications on the Internet, some of it accurate and some not. Health care providers should discuss with patients the results of their Internet research.

Women are more likely to search for health information online

(percent of Internet users aged 18 or older who have searched for health information online, by sex, 2003)

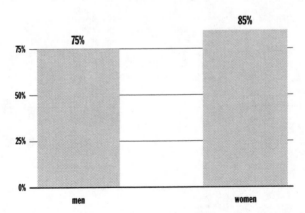

Table 4.21 Searching for Health Information Online, 2003

(percent of Internet users aged 18 or older who have searched for health information online by type of information and sex, 2003)

	total	men	women
Percent who have ever searched for health information online	**80%**	**75%**	**85%**
Specific disease or medical problem	63	54	72
Certain medical treatment or procedure	47	40	54
Diet, nutrition, vitamins, or nutritional supplements	44	39	48
Exercise or fitness	36	34	38
Prescription or over-the-counter drugs	34	29	38
Alternative treatments or medicines	28	23	33
Health insurance	25	22	29
Depression, anxiety, stress, or mental health issues	21	17	25
A particular doctor or hospital	21	17	25
Experimental treatments or medicines	18	16	20
Environmental health hazards	17	16	17
Immunizations or vaccinations	13	11	14
Sexual health information	10	12	9
Medicare or Medicaid	9	8	11
Problems with drugs or alcohol	8	9	8
How to quit smoking	6	7	5

Source: Pew Internet & American Life Project, Internet Health Resources, 2003; *Internet site http://www.pewinternet.org/PPF/ r/95/report_display.asp*

Table 4.22 Online Purchasing of Prescription Drugs, 2004

(percent of people aged 18 or older participating in researching and purchasing prescription drugs online, 2004)

	percent
RESEARCHING PRESCRIPTION DRUGS ONLINE	
Percent who have researched prescription drugs online	**26%**
Age	
Aged 18 to 27	17
Aged 28 to 39	23
Aged 40 to 49	28
Aged 50 to 58	24
Aged 59 to 68	18
Aged 69 or older	8
Education	
High school graduate	15
Some college	23
College graduate	32
Race and Hispanic origin	
Black	12
Hispanic (English-speaking)	14
White	24
ATTITUDE TOWARD PURCHASING PRESCRIPTION DRUGS ONLINE	
Purchasing prescription drugs online is less safe than purchasing at a local pharmacy	62%
Online purchases are as safe as local purchases	20
Don't know or depends	18
Percent who have ever purchased prescription drugs online	**4%**
Percent of Internet users who have ever received unsolicited email advertising a prescription drug	**55%**

Source: Pew Internet & American Life Project, Prescription Drugs Online, 2004; *Internet site http://www.pewinternet.org/PPF/ r/139/report_display.asp*

Americans Have Mixed Feelings about Quality of Health Care Coverage

Only 59 percent think the quality of health care in the nation is good or excellent.

Fully 80 percent of respondents to a Gallup Organization survey on health care said the quality of the health care they personally receive is excellent or good, but a smaller 59 percent have the same opinion of health care nationally. Similarly, while 69 percent rate the quality of their own health insurance coverage as good or excellent, only 30 percent believe this is true nationwide. Fifty-eight percent think the amount they pay for health care is satisfactory, while only 21 percent believe national health care costs are satisfactory.

In a survey by the Kaiser Family Foundation, 82 percent of people aged 18 to 64 said they had some form of health insurance coverage. While basic medical care is covered by nearly all health insurance policies, many types of services and procedures are not covered. Only 76 percent say they have prescription drug coverage, for example, and just over half have coverage for dental, vision, and mental health services. Only 57 percent of respondents think their health insurance provides good protection for their health care needs, while 38 percent feel it is inadequate. Asked to grade their current health insurance plan, the largest share (45 percent) give it a "B" and only 27 percent feel it deserves an "A."

■ Although most Americans are relatively satisfied with the quality of the health care they personally receive, they have a much lower opinion about the quality of care received by everyone else.

Seventy-six percent of working-age Americans have prescription drug coverage

(percent of people aged 18 to 64 with specific types of health insurance coverage, 2003)

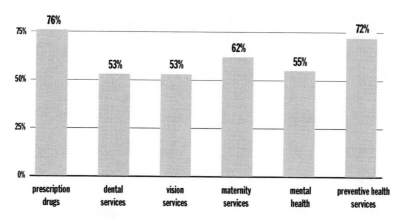

Table 4.23 Attitude toward National and Personal Health Care, 2004

(percent distribution of people aged 18 or older by attitude toward national and personal health care quality and cost, 2004)

	national	personal
Quality of health care		
Excellent/good	59%	80%
Only fair/poor	40	19
Health care coverage		
Excellent/good	30	69
Only fair/poor	70	27
Satisfaction with costs		
Satisfied	21	58
Dissatisfied	78	41

Source: The Gallup Organization, Public: Healthcare Costs and Availability Are Major Concerns; *Internet site http://www.gallup.com/*

Table 4.24   Health Insurance Coverage by Type, 2003

Are you insured? Does your current insurance plan cover...?

(percent distribution of people aged 18 to 64 by response, 2003)

	percent
Total population	**100%**
Total insured	82
Prescription drugs	76
Dental services	53
Vision services	53
Maternity services	62
Mental health	55
Preventive health services	72
Total uninsured	18

Source: "Health Insurance Survey" (#7204), The Henry J. Kaiser Family Foundation, *October 2004; Internet site http://www.kff. org/kaiserpolls/pomr110104pkg.cfm*

Americans Worry about Paying for Health Care Costs

Almost three-quarters are concerned with rising health care costs.

For the 71 percent majority of working-age Americans, the most important function of health insurance is to protect them from high medical bills in case of a severe illness or accident, according to a Kaiser Family Foundation survey of people aged 18 to 64. Only 25 percent think it is most important for health insurance to pay for everyday expenses, such as check-ups and prescriptions.

Substantial numbers of people report having problems with insurance payments. Thirty-five percent say their insurance paid less than expected for medical care, such as physician or hospital bills. And 21 percent say they were surprised to find that care they or a family member received was not covered by their insurance. Many Americans feel insecure about their health care bills. Sixty-five percent are somewhat or very worried that their health care costs will rise substantially.

Most working-age Americans would feel vulnerable to high medical bills if their insurance did not cover hospitalization, even if it offered a wide range of other benefits. Yet many find it difficult to afford even minimal payments toward health insurance. Nearly half of people aged 18 to 64 say premiums would have to be $200 or less per month for them to be able to afford to purchase health insurance on their own. This may be the reason that slightly more than half would accept lower wages in exchange for comprehensive health benefits if they had to choose.

■ Paying for health care is a concern for many Americans. Until some form of health-care security is available to all, uneasiness is likely to grow along with health care costs.

The largest share give their health insurance plan a grade of B

(percent distribution of people aged 18 to 64 by grade given to current main health insurance plan, 2003)

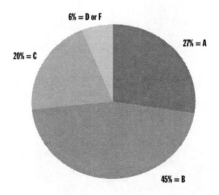

6% = D or F

27% = A

20% = C

45% = B

Table 4.25 Description of Health Insurance Coverage, 2003

Which of the following three statements comes closest to your own view about your current health insurance coverage?

(percent distribution of people aged 18 to 64 with health insurance coverage by response, 2003)

	percent
My health insurance is good and I feel well-protected when it comes to my (family's) health care needs	57%
My health insurance is adequate, but I worry that (I/my family) might have health care needs that it won't pay for	38
My health insurance is inadequate, and I feel very worried about my (family's) health care needs not being paid for	4
Don't know	1

Source: "Health Insurance Survey" (#7204), The Henry J. Kaiser Family Foundation, *October 2004; Internet site http://www.kff. org/kaiserpolls/pomr110104pkg.cfm*

Table 4.26 Letter Grade for Health Insurance Plan, 2003

Based on all your experience with your current main health insurance plan, what letter grade would you give it for its performance: A for excellent, B for good, C for average, D for poor, or F for failing?

(percent distribution of people aged 18 to 64 with health insurance coverage by response, 2003)

	percent
A for excellent	27%
B for good	45
C for average	20
D for poor	4
F for failing	2
Don't know	2

Source: "Health Insurance Survey" (#7204), The Henry J. Kaiser Family Foundation, *October 2004; Internet site http://www.kff. org/kaiserpolls/pomr110104pkg.cfm*

Table 4.27   Out-of-Pocket Health Care Expenses in Past 12 Months, 2003

In the past 12 months, what would you estimate your (and your family's) out-of-pocket health care costs to be? This does not include the amount you pay or have deducted from your paycheck for health insurance premiums.

(percent distribution of people aged 18 to 64 with health insurance coverage by response, 2003)

	percent
Out-of-pocket expenses for the insured	
Less than $50	20%
$50 to less than $100	11
$100 to less than $500	29
$500 to less than $1,000	14
$1,000 to less than $2,000	10
$2,000 or more	9
Don't know	6

In the past 12 months, what would you estimate you (and your family) have paid out of your own pocket for your health care costs?

(percent distribution of people aged 18 to 64 without health insurance coverage by response, 2003)

	percent
Out-of-pocket expenses for the uninsured	
Less than $50	22%
$50 to less than $100	6
$100 to less than $500	22
$500 to less than $1,000	13
$1,000 to less than $2,000	10
$2,000 or more	15
Don't know	11

Source: "Health Insurance Survey" (#7204), The Henry J. Kaiser Family Foundation, *October 2004; Internet site http://www.kff. org/kaiserpolls/pomr110104pkg.cfm*

Table 4.28   Most Important Reason to Have Health Insurance, 2003

Which one of the following do you think is the most
important reason to have health insurance?

(percent distribution of people aged 18 to 64 with health insurance coverage by response, 2003)

	percent
To pay for everyday health care expenses, like check-ups and prescriptions	25%
To protect against high medical bills in case of severe illness or accident	71
Don't know	3

Source: "Health Insurance Survey" (#7204), The Henry J. Kaiser Family Foundation, *October 2004; Internet site http://www.kff. org/kaiserpolls/pomr110104pkg.cfm*

Table 4.29 Problems with Health Insurance, 2003

Have you ever had these problems with your current health insurance plan?

(percent of people aged 18 to 64 with health insurance coverage who had problem, 2003)

	percent
You were surprised to find out that your plan would not pay anything for care you (or your family) received, that you thought was covered	21%
Your plan paid less than you expected for a bill you received from a doctor, hospital, or lab	35
You reached the limit of what your insurance company would pay for treatment of a specific illness or injury	12

Source: "Health Insurance Survey" (#7204), The Henry J. Kaiser Family Foundation, *October 2004; Internet site http://www.kff.org/kaiserpolls/pomr110104pkg.cfm*

Table 4.30 Worries about Health Insurance, 2003

Thinking about the next six months, please tell me how worried
you are that the following might happen to you?

Your (or your spouse's) employer will no longer offer
health insurance to you and other employees?

(percent distribution of people aged 18 to 64 with health insurance coverage through their or their spouse's employer by response 2003)

	percent
Very worried	17%
Somewhat worried	13
Not too worried	20
Not at all worried	50

The benefits under your current health insurance
plan will be cut back substantially?

(percent distribution of people aged 18 to 64 with health insurance coverage by response 2003)

	percent
Very worried	20%
Somewhat worried	26
Not too worried	23
Not at all worried	31

The amount you pay for your health insurance
will increase substantially?

(percent distribution of people aged 18 to 64 with health insurance coverage by response 2003)

	percent
Very worried	23%
Somewhat worried	29
Not too worried	21
Not at all worried	26
Don't know	1

(continued)

The amount you pay for health care services will increase substantially?

(percent distribution of people aged 18 to 64 without health insurance coverage by response 2003)

	percent
Very worried	42%
Somewhat worried	23
Not too worried	16
Not at all worried	16
Don't know	3
Refused	1

You might not be able to get the health care services you think you need because of the cost?

(percent distribution of people aged 18 to 64 without health insurance coverage by response 2003)

	percent
Very worried	24%
Somewhat worried	21
Not too worried	22
Not at all worried	32

Source: "Health Insurance Survey" (#7204), The Henry J. Kaiser Family Foundation, *October 2004; Internet site http://www.kff. org/kaiserpolls/pomr110104pkg.cfm*

Table 4.31 What Is Important in a Health Insurance Plan? 2003

What is important to you (and your family) in a health insurance plan?

(percent of people aged 18 to 64 who answered "very important," 2003)

	percent
Having a wide range of benefits	80%
Having a plan that offers a wide choice of doctors and hospitals	77
Having a low monthly premium	68
Having low co-pays when you visit the doctor or fill a prescription	67
Having a low annual deductible, that is the amount you have to pay in medical expenses yourself before your insurance begins paying	62

Source: "Health Insurance Survey" (#7204), The Henry J. Kaiser Family Foundation, *October 2004; Internet site http://www.kff. org/kaiserpolls/pomr110104pkg.cfm*

Table 4.32 Well Protected by Health Insurance Plan? 2003

If you had a health insurance plan that did not pay for the following items but covered everything else, would you feel well-protected by your health insurance or would you feel vulnerable to high medical bills?

(percent of people aged 18 to 64 with health insurance coverage who would feel vulnerable without coverage for selected items, 2003)

	percent who would feel vulnerable
If health insurance plan did not cover:	
Hospitalizations	93%
Visits to medical specialists	88
Prescription drugs	81
Routine doctor's visits and check-ups	76
Home health care	63
Pregnancy and maternity care	58
Mental health	56

Source: "Health Insurance Survey" (#7204), The Henry J. Kaiser Family Foundation, *October 2004; Internet site http://www.kff. org/kaiserpolls/pomr110104pkg.cfm*

Table 4.33 How Much Would You Pay for Health Insurance? 2003

If you were shopping for a health insurance policy for yourself (and your family), what would be the highest dollar amount you would consider for the monthly premium, that is the amount you pay each month for your health insurance? In other words, anything higher would be unaffordable and you would not consider buying the policy.

(percent distribution of people aged 18 to 64 by response, 2003)

	percent
$50 or less	14%
$51 to $100	16
$101 to $200	19
$201 to $300	11
$301 to $500	10
More than $500	6
Don't know	24

Source: "Health Insurance Survey" (#7204), The Henry J. Kaiser Family Foundation, *October 2004; Internet site http://www.kff. org/kaiserpolls/pomr110104pkg.cfm*

Table 4.34 Health Insurance or Higher Wages? 2003

If you had to choose between having more comprehensive health insurance benefits and lower wages, or less comprehensive health insurance benefits and higher wages, which would you choose?

(percent distribution of people aged 18 to 64 who have health insurance coverage through their or their spouse's employer by response, 2003)

	percent
More comprehensive health insurance benefits and lower wages	52%
Less comprehensive health insurance benefits and higher wages	36
Don't know	11
Refused	1

Source: "Health Insurance Survey" (#7204), The Henry J. Kaiser Family Foundation, *October 2004; Internet site http://www.kff. org/kaiserpolls/pomr110104pkg.cfm*

5

Births

■ **Americans are ambivalent about abortion.**

Only 42 percent support a woman's right to abortion for any reason.

■ **More than one-third of newborns are Hispanic or black.**

Of the 4 million babies born in 2003, only 57 percent were born to non-Hispanic whites.

■ **Most babies are born to women in their twenties.**

More than half of Asian births are to women aged 30 or older, however.

■ **Thirty-four percent of births are to unmarried women.**

The percentage varies from a low of 15 percent among Asians to a high of 68 percent among blacks.

■ **The Caesarean rate rises with age.**

Only 18 percent of teenagers giving birth in 2002 had a Caesarean delivery compared with 40 percent of women aged 40 or older.

■ **Eleven percent of women smoked during their pregnancy.**

Among American Indian women, 20 percent smoked during their pregnancy.

Only 63 Percent of Pregnancies Result in Live Births

Women in their early thirties are most likely to carry their pregnancies to term.

In 2000, there were 6.4 million pregnancies, but only 4.1 million births. Twenty-one percent of pregnancies were terminated by induced abortion, while 16 percent ended as the result of "fetal loss"—miscarriage or stillbirth.

Women aged 30 to 34 are most likely to see their pregnancies through to a live birth. Women under age 20 are most likely to terminate their pregnancy through abortion, while those aged 40 or older were slightly more likely to have a miscarriage than an abortion.

Fewer than half of black women who became pregnant in 2000 gave birth. Of those who did not carry the pregnancy to term, most had induced abortions. Among non-Hispanic whites and Hispanics, about two-thirds of pregnancies ended in a live birth. Among Hispanics who became pregnant but did not give birth, a larger share had induced abortions than fetal losses. The opposite was true for non-Hispanic white women, more of whom lost the fetus than had an abortion.

■ As women delay childbearing until their thirties or forties, the risk of miscarriage rises.

Non-Hispanic white women are least likely to end a pregnancy through abortion

(percent distribution of pregnancies by outcome, race, and Hispanic origin, 2000)

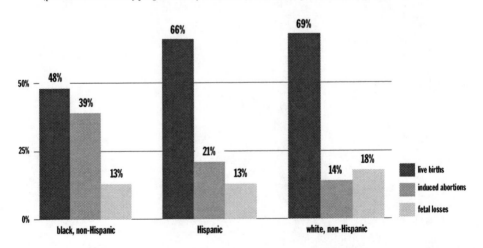

Table 5.1 Pregnancy Outcomes by Age, 2000

(number and percent distribution of pregnancies, live births, induced abortions, and fetal losses by age, 2000; numbers in thousands)

	total	under 20	20 to 24	25 to 29	30 to 34	35 to 39	40 or older
Total pregnancies	**6,401**	**852**	**1,653**	**1,622**	**1,347**	**756**	**172**
Live births	4,059	478	1,018	1,088	929	452	95
Induced abortions	1,313	244	430	303	190	110	37
Fetal losses	1,029	129	206	232	228	194	40
PERCENT DISTRIBUTION							
Total pregnancies	**100.0%**	**100.0%**	**100.0%**	**100.0%**	**100.0%**	**100.0%**	**100.0%**
Live births	63.4	56.1	61.6	67.1	69.0	59.8	55.2
Induced abortions	20.5	28.6	26.0	18.7	14.1	14.6	21.5
Fetal losses	16.1	15.1	12.5	14.3	16.9	25.7	23.3

Source: National Center for Health Statistics, Estimated Pregnancy Rates for the United States, 1990–2000: An Update, *National Vital Statistics Reports, Volume 52, No. 23, 2004*

Table 5.2 Pregnancy Outcomes by Race and Hispanic Origin, 2000

(number and percent distribution of pregnancies, live births, induced abortions, and fetal losses by race and Hispanic origin, 2000; numbers in thousands)

	total	Hispanic	black	non-Hispanic white
Total pregnancies	**6,401**	**1,237**	**1,265**	**3,497**
Live births	4,059	816	607	2,400
Induced abortions	1,313	261	488	479
Fetal losses	1,029	161	170	618
PERCENT DISTRIBUTION				
Total pregnancies	**100.0%**	**100.0%**	**100.0%**	**100.0%**
Live births	63.4	66.0	48.0	68.6
Induced abortions	20.5	21.1	38.6	13.7
Fetal losses	16.1	13.0	13.4	17.7

Source: National Center for Health Statistics, Estimated Pregnancy Rates for the United States, 1990–2000: An Update, *National Vital Statistics Reports, Volume 52, No. 23, 2004*

Many Americans Support Abortion Rights

More favor abortion now than in the 1980s, but abortion rates are down.

The abortion rate declined substantially between 1980 and 2001, from 35.9 to 24.6 abortions per 100 live births. The annual number of abortions dropped from 1.3 million to 853,000 during those years. Women under age 15 are most likely to have an abortion. The rate declines with age before rising again among women aged 35 or older. Unmarried women are far more likely than married women to have an abortion.

Americans are ambivalent about abortion. Forty-two percent of the population believes women should be able to obtain an abortion for any reason, while 56 percent disagree with this notion. A large majority favors the availability of abortion if there is a chance of a serious birth defect, danger to a woman's health, or a woman has been raped, but fewer than half believe that being unmarried, not wanting more children, or not being able to afford more children should be grounds for getting a legal abortion.

■ Most Americans support legal abortion, but only under certain circumstances.

More than 80 percent support abortion if a woman's health is in danger

(percent of people aged 18 or older who support legal abortion, by circumstance, 2002)

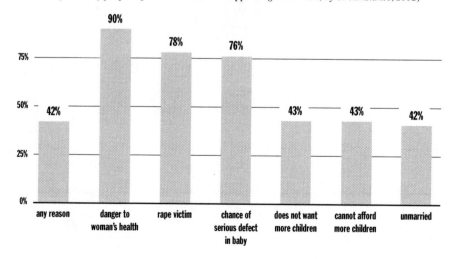

Table 5.3 Abortions, 1980 to 2001

(number of legal abortions and rate per 100 live births by selected characteristics. 1980, 1990, and 2001; number of abortions in thousands)

	2001	1990	1980
Number of abortions	**853**	**1,429**	**1,298**
ABORTIONS PER 100 LIVE BIRTHS			
Total	**24.6**	**34.4**	**35.9**
Age			
Under age 15	74.4	81.8	139.7
Aged 15 to19	36.6	51.1	71.4
Aged 20 to 24	30.4	37.8	39.5
Aged 25 to 29	20.0	21.8	23.7
Aged 30 to 34	14.7	19.0	23.7
Aged 35 to 39	18.0	27.3	41.0
Aged 40 to 44	30.4	50.6	80.7
Race			
Black	49.1	53.7	54.3
White	16.5	25.8	33.2
Hispanic origin			
Hispanic	23.0	–	–
Non-Hispanic	23.2	–	–
Marital status			
Married	6.5	8.7	10.5
Unmarried	57.2	86.3	147.6
Previous live births			
None	26.4	36.0	45.7
One	18.0	22.7	20.2
Two	25.5	31.5	29.5
Three	26.4	30.1	29.7
Four or more	21.9	26.6	24.3

Note: (–) means data unavailable.
Source: National Center for Health Statistics, Health, United States, 2004; Internet site http://www.cdc.gov/nchs/hus.htm

Table 5.4 Abortion for Any Reason, 1977 to 2002

"Do you think it should be possible for a pregnant woman to obtain
a legal abortion if the woman wants it for any reason?"

(number of respondents aged 18 or older, and percent distribution by response, 1977–2002)

	number of respondents	total	yes	no	don't know
2002	923	100.0%	41.9%	55.6%	2.5%
2000	1,855	100.0	38.0	57.3	4.7
1998	1,876	100.0	38.8	56.0	5.2
1996	1,915	100.0	42.8	52.3	4.9
1994	1,990	100.0	45.0	52.2	2.8
1993	1,069	100.0	42.8	51.6	5.5
1991	986	100.0	41.1	55.4	3.5
1990	913	100.0	41.7	54.3	3.9
1989	1,028	100.0	38.8	57.4	3.8
1988	973	100.0	34.7	61.5	3.8
1987	1,807	100.0	38.6	57.2	4.2
1985	1,529	100.0	35.8	61.1	3.1
1984	1,462	100.0	37.5	59.6	2.9
1983	1,565	100.0	33.2	63.6	3.2
1982	1,852	100.0	38.9	56.8	4.3
1980	1,465	100.0	39.5	56.5	4.0
1978	1,527	100.0	32.4	64.8	2.8
1977	1,523	100.0	36.6	60.5	2.9

Source: General Social Surveys, National Opinion Research Center, University of Chicago; calculations by New Strategist

Table 5.5 Abortion if Chance of Serious Defect in Baby, 1972 to 2002

"Do you think it should be possible for a pregnant woman to obtain a legal abortion if there is a strong chance of serious defect in the baby?"

(number of respondents aged 18 or older, and percent distribution by response, 1972–2002)

	number of respondents	total	yes	no	don't know
2002	920	100.0%	76.4%	21.0%	2.6%
2000	1,857	100.0	75.2	20.3	4.5
1998	1,879	100.0	75.3	20.5	4.2
1996	1,916	100.0	79.0	17.5	3.4
1994	1,994	100.0	79.5	17.1	3.4
1993	1,070	100.0	78.5	18.0	3.5
1991	985	100.0	80.0	15.8	4.2
1990	915	100.0	78.1	18.0	3.8
1989	1,029	100.0	78.6	18.1	3.3
1988	975	100.0	76.3	20.5	3.2
1987	1,811	100.0	77.3	19.4	3.3
1985	1,531	100.0	76.2	20.8	2.9
1984	1,465	100.0	77.8	19.2	3.0
1983	1,567	100.0	76.2	20.4	3.4
1982	1,855	100.0	81.6	14.6	3.8
1980	1,467	100.0	80.4	16.4	3.3
1978	1,528	100.0	80.3	17.7	2.0
1977	1,524	100.0	83.4	14.2	2.4
1976	1,495	100.0	81.8	15.7	2.5
1975	1,487	100.0	80.4	16.3	3.3
1974	1,484	100.0	82.6	14.4	3.0
1973	1,500	100.0	82.5	15.1	2.4
1972	1,607	100.0	74.6	20.3	5.0

Source: General Social Surveys, National Opinion Research Center, University of Chicago; calculations by New Strategist

Table 5.6 Abortion if Woman's Health Is Seriously Endangered, 1972 to 2002

"Do you think it should be possible for a pregnant woman to obtain a legal abortion if the woman's own health is seriously endangered by the pregnancy?"

(number of respondents aged 18 or older, and percent distribution by response, 1972–2002)

	number of respondents	total	yes	no	don't know
2002	922	100.0%	89.5%	8.2%	2.3%
2000	1,857	100.0	85.1	11.0	3.9
1998	1,879	100.0	84.0	11.6	4.4
1996	1,915	100.0	88.5	8.1	3.4
1994	1,993	100.0	88.0	9.1	3.0
1993	1,071	100.0	86.2	9.8	4.0
1991	986	100.0	88.6	8.2	3.1
1990	914	100.0	89.1	8.0	3.0
1989	1,027	100.0	88.0	9.6	2.3
1988	974	100.0	85.8	10.9	3.3
1987	1,814	100.0	85.6	11.2	3.3
1985	1,531	100.0	87.0	10.4	2.6
1984	1,462	100.0	87.6	10.3	2.1
1983	1,567	100.0	87.1	10.0	3.0
1982	1,855	100.0	89.2	8.2	2.6
1980	1,466	100.0	87.9	9.6	2.5
1978	1,528	100.0	88.5	9.2	2.4
1977	1,522	100.0	88.5	9.3	2.2
1976	1,492	100.0	89.1	9.1	1.9
1975	1,487	100.0	88.4	9.1	2.6
1974	1,484	100.0	90.4	7.4	2.2
1973	1,502	100.0	90.7	7.6	1.7
1972	1,605	100.0	83.4	12.5	4.1

Source: General Social Surveys, National Opinion Research Center, University of Chicago; calculations by New Strategist

Table 5.7 Abortion in Case of Rape, 1972 to 2002

"Do you think it should be possible for a pregnant woman to obtain a
legal abortion if she became pregnant as a result of rape?"

(number of respondents aged 18 or older, and percent distribution by response, 1972–2002)

	number of respondents	total	yes	no	don't know
2002	924	100.0%	78.0%	19.9%	2.1%
2000	1,855	100.0	76.0	18.3	5.7
1998	1,879	100.0	76.6	19.0	4.4
1996	1,916	100.0	80.9	15.1	4.0
1994	1,994	100.0	81.0	15.9	3.0
1993	1,071	100.0	79.4	16.3	4.3
1991	986	100.0	82.9	13.0	4.2
1990	912	100.0	81.1	14.6	4.3
1989	1,028	100.0	80.3	16.1	3.6
1988	974	100.0	76.9	18.0	5.1
1987	1,811	100.0	77.3	18.6	4.1
1985	1,531	100.0	78.2	18.1	3.7
1984	1,463	100.0	77.2	18.9	3.9
1983	1,567	100.0	79.5	16.5	4.0
1982	1,852	100.0	83.0	12.9	4.1
1980	1,465	100.0	80.3	16.0	3.7
1978	1,526	100.0	80.7	16.3	2.9
1977	1,521	100.0	80.9	15.6	3.4
1976	1,492	100.0	80.8	15.8	3.5
1975	1,487	100.0	80.0	15.6	4.4
1974	1,482	100.0	82.9	13.0	4.2
1973	1,501	100.0	80.7	15.9	3.3
1972	1,604	100.0	74.6	19.7	5.7

Source: General Social Surveys, National Opinion Research Center, University of Chicago; calculations by New Strategist

Table 5.8 Abortion if a Woman Is Unmarried, 1972 to 2002

"Do you think it should be possible for a pregnant woman to obtain a legal abortion if she is not married and does not want to marry the man?"

(number of respondents aged 18 or older, and percent distribution by response, 1972–2002)

	number of respondents	total	yes	no	don't know
2002	922	100.0%	40.8%	56.3%	2.9%
2000	1,855	100.0	37.3	58.0	4.7
1998	1,877	100.0	40.3	55.0	4.6
1996	1,912	100.0	43.0	52.8	4.2
1994	1,990	100.0	46.4	51.0	2.6
1993	1,070	100.0	45.6	49.2	5.2
1991	986	100.0	43.2	53.1	3.7
1990	913	100.0	43.3	52.2	4.5
1989	1,028	100.0	43.5	52.3	4.2
1988	973	100.0	37.7	58.1	4.2
1987	1,812	100.0	40.8	55.6	3.6
1985	1,529	100.0	40.0	57.2	2.8
1984	1,462	100.0	43.0	54.2	2.9
1983	1,566	100.0	37.5	57.8	4.7
1982	1,854	100.0	46.2	49.0	4.7
1980	1,466	100.0	46.4	49.4	4.2
1978	1,528	100.0	39.7	56.7	3.6
1977	1,523	100.0	47.7	48.1	4.2
1976	1,494	100.0	48.4	47.9	3.7
1975	1,485	100.0	45.9	49.3	4.8
1974	1,484	100.0	47.9	47.8	4.3
1973	1,499	100.0	47.5	49.2	3.3
1972	1,605	100.0	40.7	52.8	6.4

Source: General Social Surveys, National Opinion Research Center, University of Chicago; calculations by New Strategist

Table 5.9 Abortion if Married Woman Wants No More Children, 1972 to 2002

"Do you think it should be possible for a pregnant woman to obtain a legal abortion if she is married and does not want any more children?"

(number of respondents aged 18 or older, and percent distribution by response, 1972–2002)

	number of respondents	total	yes	no	don't know
2002	922	100.0%	43.4%	53.5%	3.1%
2000	1,855	100.0	38.8	56.6	4.6
1998	1,877	100.0	40.4	55.0	4.6
1996	1,916	100.0	44.5	50.7	4.8
1994	1,990	100.0	46.7	50.0	3.3
1993	1,070	100.0	44.9	50.4	4.8
1991	986	100.0	43.0	53.3	3.7
1990	912	100.0	43.4	53.0	3.6
1989	1,028	100.0	42.9	53.5	3.6
1988	975	100.0	38.9	58.5	2.7
1987	1,811	100.0	41.1	55.6	3.4
1985	1,529	100.0	39.2	58.1	2.7
1984	1,463	100.0	41.4	55.6	2.9
1983	1,569	100.0	37.7	59.1	3.1
1982	1,855	100.0	45.8	49.4	4.8
1980	1,465	100.0	45.3	50.8	4.0
1978	1,529	100.0	39.1	57.9	3.0
1977	1,523	100.0	44.6	51.3	4.0
1976	1,493	100.0	44.7	52.2	3.1
1975	1,488	100.0	43.8	52.0	4.2
1974	1,484	100.0	44.6	50.5	4.9
1973	1,502	100.0	46.1	50.6	3.3
1972	1,608	100.0	37.7	57.3	5.0

Source: General Social Surveys, National Opinion Research Center, University of Chicago; calculations by New Strategist

Table 5.10 Abortion if Low-Income Woman Cannot Afford More Children, 1972 to 2002

"Do you think it should be possible for a pregnant woman to obtain
a legal abortion if the family has a very low income
and cannot afford any more children?"

(number of respondents aged 18 or older, and percent distribution by response, 1972–2002)

	number of respondents	total	yes	no	don't know
2002	921	100.0%	43.0%	53.9%	3.1%
2000	1,854	100.0	40.4	55.2	4.4
1998	1,878	100.0	42.0	52.9	5.1
1996	1,916	100.0	44.5	51.0	4.5
1994	1,993	100.0	48.7	47.9	3.4
1993	1,070	100.0	47.5	47.8	4.8
1991	985	100.0	46.5	49.4	4.1
1990	912	100.0	45.6	49.2	5.2
1989	1,028	100.0	46.0	50.5	3.5
1988	975	100.0	40.5	56.0	3.5
1987	1,813	100.0	44.3	52.1	3.5
1985	1,530	100.0	42.5	54.8	2.7
1984	1,459	100.0	44.8	52.1	3.1
1983	1,568	100.0	42.0	54.1	3.9
1982	1,852	100.0	48.7	47.2	4.2
1980	1,466	100.0	49.7	46.4	4.0
1978	1,528	100.0	45.6	50.6	3.9
1977	1,522	100.0	51.8	45.3	2.9
1976	1,491	100.0	51.0	45.1	3.8
1975	1,485	100.0	50.7	44.6	4.6
1974	1,482	100.0	52.4	43.3	4.4
1973	1,502	100.0	51.8	45.1	3.1
1972	1,605	100.0	45.8	48.1	6.1

Source: General Social Surveys, National Opinion Research Center, University of Chicago; calculations by New Strategist

More Women Are Childless

Once they reach their forties, many childless women will have fertility problems.

Between 1960 and 2002, the percentage of women aged 15 to 44 who had never had a child grew in every age group. The biggest increase occurred among women aged 25 to 29, with the childless percentage rising from 20 to 41 percent. Most of the increase occurred between 1960 and 1980, however, as boomers reached the age group and decided to delay (or forego) childbearing.

A key reason for not having children is not having a spouse. Women who have never married are far more likely than the married to be childless. But the demographics of childless women also suggest that many are pursuing higher education and careers rather than becoming mothers. While motherhood and career are not wholly incompatible, the time and energy needed to be both a mother and a professional can be overwhelming.

In 2002, the majority of women aged 15 to 29 had not yet had children, while most women aged 30 or older had at least one child. The majority of women aged 15 to 44 have only one or two children. Ten percent of women aged 35 to 44 have had four or more children.

■ Women who delay childbearing often have difficulty having children, creating the booming fertility industry.

Among women aged 25 to 29, the childless percentage has doubled since 1960

(percent of women aged 15 to 44 who have not had a live birth, by age, 1960 to 2002)

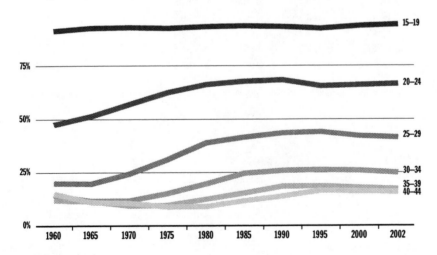

Table 5.11   Childless Women by Age, 1960 to 2002

(percent of women aged 15 to 44 who have not had a live birth, by age, 1960 to 2002)

	15–19	20–24	25–29	30–34	35–39	40–44
2002	94.3%	66.5%	41.3%	24.8%	17.2%	15.8%
2001	94.0	66.5	41.6	25.4	17.6	16.0
2000	93.7	66.0	42.1	25.9	17.9	16.2
1999	93.4	65.5	42.5	26.1	18.1	16.4
1998	93.1	65.1	43.0	26.1	18.2	16.5
1997	92.8	64.9	43.5	26.2	18.4	16.6
1996	92.5	65.0	43.8	26.2	18.5	16.6
1995	92.5	65.5	44.0	26.2	18.6	16.5
1994	92.6	66.1	43.9	26.2	18.7	16.2
1993	92.6	66.7	43.8	26.1	18.8	15.8
1992	92.7	67.3	43.7	26.0	18.8	15.2
1991	93.0	67.9	43.6	26.0	18.7	14.5
1990	93.3	68.3	43.5	25.9	18.5	13.9
1989	93.7	68.4	43.3	25.9	18.2	13.5
1988	93.8	68.4	43.0	25.7	17.7	13.0
1987	93.8	68.2	42.5	25.5	16.9	12.6
1986	93.8	68.0	42.0	25.1	16.1	12.2
1985	93.7	67.7	41.5	24.6	15.4	11.7
1980	93.4	66.2	38.9	19.7	12.5	9.0
1975	92.6	62.5	31.1	15.2	9.6	8.8
1970	93.0	57.0	24.4	11.8	9.4	10.6
1965	92.7	51.4	19.7	11.7	11.4	11.0
1960	91.4	47.5	20.0	14.2	12.0	15.1

Source: National Center for Health Statistics, Health, United States, 2004; *Internet site http://www.cdc.gov/nchs/hus.htm*

Table 5.12 Childless Women Aged 15 to 44 by Selected Characteristics, 2002

(percent of women aged 15 to 44 who have not had children, by selected characteristics and age, 2002)

	total	15 to 24	25 to 34	35 to 44
Total women aged 15 to 44	**43.5%**	**79.1%**	**35.9%**	**19.0%**
Marital status				
Ever married	19.1	39.8	23.9	12.7
Never married	77.2	85.8	62.7	59.2
Race and Hispanic origin				
Asian	50.8	87.4	50.8	20.0
Black	39.0	69.1	27.6	19.4
Hispanic	35.8	70.0	22.7	13.3
Non-Hispanic white	45.6	83.2	39.7	19.9
Education				
Not a high school graduate	58.8	84.3	15.3	13.6
High school graduate	30.7	62.6	24.1	15.3
Some college, no degree	45.9	82.2	31.3	17.7
Associate's degree	33.0	78.0	35.5	17.5
Bachelor's degree	46.6	91.9	55.2	24.9
Graduate or professional degree	44.6	92.0	60.2	30.2
Labor force status				
In labor force	44.0	78.1	20.0	13.9
Not in labor force	42.4	79.8	41.3	20.7
Household income				
Under $10,000	40.0	63.9	24.4	18.0
$10,000 to $19,999	39.9	65.5	26.0	19.9
$20,000 to $24,999	38.2	68.2	26.7	16.9
$25,000 to $29,999	41.9	72.6	34.4	19.6
$30,000 to $34,999	43.7	76.2	36.5	20.4
$35,000 to $49,999	43.0	82.2	35.3	18.3
$50,000 to $74,999	43.6	87.2	37.0	17.1
$75,000 or more	47.2	91.3	46.0	18.6
Region				
Northeast	46.1	84.2	41.3	19.4
Midwest	43.8	80.4	36.1	17.0
South	40.9	75.4	32.9	18.8
West	45.1	79.4	36.3	21.2
Metropolitan status				
In central cities	46.4	76.6	40.5	22.9
Outside central cities	43.8	81.8	37.1	18.9
Nonmetropolitan	37.3	76.3	22.8	13.2
Nativity				
Native born	44.8	80.0	36.5	19.4
Foreign born	35.6	71.5	33.2	17.1

Source: Bureau of the Census, Fertility of American Women: June 2002, *detailed tables, Internet site http://www.census.gov/population/www/socdemo/fertility/cps2002.html*

Table 5.13   Number of Children Born to Women Aged 15 to 44, 2002

(total number of women aged 15 to 44, and percent distribution of women by number of children ever borne, by age, 2002; numbers in thousands)

	total number	number of children							
		percent	none	one	two	three	four	five	six or more
Total women	**61,361**	**100.0%**	**43.5%**	**17.5%**	**22.2%**	**11.2%**	**3.8%**	**1.5%**	**0.3%**
Aged 15 to 19	9,809	100.0	91.2	5.2	2.4	0.8	0.2	0.1	0.0
Aged 20 to 24	9,683	100.0	67.0	19.6	9.3	3.2	0.6	0.3	0.1
Aged 25 to 29	9,221	100.0	45.2	22.2	19.8	9.1	2.7	0.9	0.1
Aged 30 to 34	10,284	100.0	27.6	21.8	29.6	14.1	4.7	1.9	0.2
Aged 35 to 39	10,803	100.0	20.2	18.6	32.4	18.8	6.9	2.6	0.5
Aged 40 to 44	11,561	100.0	17.9	17.4	35.4	18.9	6.8	2.8	0.8

Source: Bureau of the Census, Fertility of American Women: June 2002, *detailed tables, Internet site http://www.census.gov/population/www/socdemo/fertility/cps2002.html*

The Birth Rate Has Risen Since the Late 1990s

Much of the increase stems from births among women aged 30 or older.

Between 1990 and 2003, the birth rate (the number of live births per 1,000 women aged 15 to 44) declined, dropping from 70.9 in 1990 to 66.1 in 2003. But the rate bottomed out in 1997 and has been increasing since then. The rise since 1997 is primarily the result of increased childbearing by women aged 30 or older. The birth rate among women aged 30 to 34 climbed 18 percent between 1990 and 2003, while the rate among women aged 35 to 39 rose 38 percent.

The rising birth rate among women aged 40 or older is in part the result of technological developments enabling them to overcome difficulties in getting pregnant or carrying a pregnancy to term. But the birth rate among older women is still low, largely because most older women no longer want to have children.

Differing socioeconomic and cultural backgrounds are readily apparent in the age at which women begin having children. On average, first-time mothers in the United States are about 25 years old. But women of Chinese or Japanese descent have their first child at age 30 or 31. In contrast, American Indians have their first child at age 22.

■ Women who have their first child at a younger age tend to have more children than those who start later.

The birth rate is higher today than it was in 1997

(number of births per 1,000 women aged 15 to 44, 1990 to 2003)

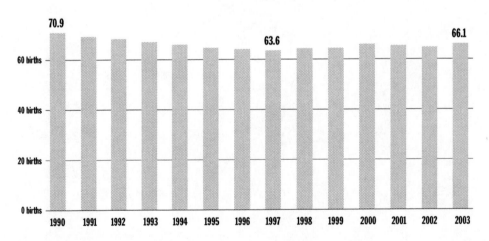

Table 5.14 Average Age of Mother by Race and Hispanic Origin, 2000

(average age of mothers giving birth, and average age at first birth, by race and Hispanic origin, 2000; in years)

	all births	first birth
Total mothers	**27.2**	**24.9**
American Indian	25.1	21.6
Black, non-Hispanic	25.2	22.3
Central and South American	27.5	24.8
Chinese	31.6	30.1
Cuban	28.8	26.5
Filipino	29.5	27.3
Hawaiian	25.7	22.6
Japanese	31.8	30.6
Mexican	25.4	22.2
Puerto Rican	25.0	22.4
White, non-Hispanic	28.0	25.9

Source: National Center for Health Statistics, Mean Age of Mother, 1970–2000, *National Vital Statistics Report, Vol. 51, No. 1, 2002*

Table 5.15 Birth Rates by Age of Mother, 1990 to 2003

(number of live births per 1,000 women in age group and percent change in rate, 1990 to 2003)

	total*	15 to 19	20 to 24	25 to 29	30 to 34	35 to 39	40 to 44	45 to 49
2003	66.1	41.7	102.6	115.7	95.2	43.8	8.7	0.5
2002	64.8	43.0	103.6	113.6	91.5	41.4	8.3	0.5
2001	65.3	45.3	106.2	113.4	91.9	40.6	8.1	0.5
2000	65.9	47.7	109.7	113.5	91.2	39.7	8.0	0.5
1999	64.4	48.8	107.9	111.2	87.1	37.8	7.4	0.4
1998	64.3	50.3	108.4	110.2	85.2	36.9	7.4	0.4
1997	63.6	51.3	107.3	108.3	83.0	35.7	7.1	0.4
1996	64.1	53.5	107.8	108.6	82.1	34.9	6.8	0.3
1995	64.6	56.0	107.5	108.8	81.1	34.0	6.6	0.3
1994	65.9	58.2	109.2	111.0	80.4	33.4	6.4	0.3
1993	67.0	59.0	111.3	113.2	79.9	32.7	6.1	0.3
1992	68.4	60.3	113.7	115.7	79.6	32.3	5.9	0.3
1991	69.3	61.8	115.3	117.2	79.2	31.9	5.5	0.2
1990	70.9	59.9	116.5	120.2	80.8	31.7	5.5	0.2

Percent change

	total*	15 to 19	20 to 24	25 to 29	30 to 34	35 to 39	40 to 44	45 to 49
1990 to 2003	–6.8%	–30.4%	–11.9%	–3.7%	17.8%	38.2%	58.2%	150.0%

* Total is the number of births per 1,000 women aged 15 to 44.
Source: National Center for Health Statistics, Births: Final Data for 2002, *National Vital Statistics Reports, Vol. 52, No. 10, 2003; and* Births: Preliminary Data for 2003, *National Vital Statistics Reports, Vol. 53, No. 9, 2004; Internet site http://www.cdc.gov/nchs/products/pubs/pubd/nvsr/nvsr.htm; calculations by New Strategist*

More than One Million Women Had Their First Baby in 2002

Among women having a first birth, 36 percent were unmarried.

Of the 3.8 million women who gave birth in 2002, nearly 70 percent were aged 20 to 34. Although older mothers frequently garner media attention, only 16 percent of women giving birth in 2002 were aged 35 or older. Those having their first child were even younger, with 72 percent aged 15 to 29.

Although non-Hispanic whites comprise 65 percent of all women aged 15 to 44, they account for a smaller 60 percent share of births. Hispanics, in contrast, account for 15 percent of women in the age group but for 20 percent of births. This suggests that the Hispanic population will continue to grow as a share of the U.S. population.

Most women who give birth are married, but the married share is a relatively small 63 percent. Most unmarried women who have children have never been married. This suggests that a sizable proportion of women have "uncoupled" childbearing from marriage. No doubt some have unmarried partners who will help them raise their child, but many are likely going it alone.

■ Although many women become single mothers as a result of divorce, a sizable number are having children without ever walking down the aisle.

Women giving birth are almost evenly split by education

(percent distribution of women giving birth by educational attainment, 2002)

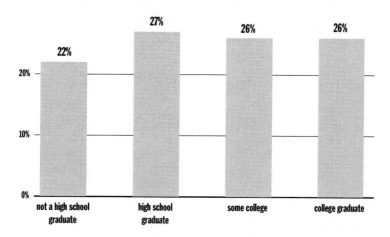

Table 5.16 Characteristics of Women Aged 15 to 44 Giving Birth in the Past Year, 2002

(number, percent, and percent distribution of women who gave birth in the past year and who had a first birth in past year, by selected characteristics, 2002; numbers in thousands)

		giving birth in past year			first birth in past year		
	total	number	percent of population	percent distribution	number	percent of population	percent distribution
Total women	**61,361**	**3,766**	**6.1%**	**100.0%**	**1,415**	**2.3%**	**100.0%**
Age							
Aged 15 to 19	9,809	549	5.6	14.6	272	2.8	19.2
Aged 20 to 24	9,683	872	9.0	23.2	438	4.5	31.0
Aged 25 to 29	9,221	897	9.7	23.8	306	3.3	21.6
Aged 30 to 34	10,284	859	8.4	22.8	272	2.6	19.2
Aged 35 to 39	10,803	452	4.2	12.0	85	0.8	6.0
Aged 40 to 44	11,561	137	1.2	3.6	42	0.4	3.0
Marital status							
Married, husband present	27,828	2,382	8.6	63.3	825	3.0	58.3
Married, husband absent	2,446	124	5.1	3.3	42	1.7	3.0
Widowed or divorced	5,303	143	2.7	3.8	35	0.7	2.5
Never married	25,782	1,118	4.3	29.7	513	2.0	36.3
Race and Hispanic origin							
Asian	3,267	181	5.5	4.8	89	2.7	6.3
Black	8,846	571	6.5	15.2	197	2.2	13.9
Hispanic	9,141	750	8.2	19.9	278	3.0	19.6
Non-Hispanic white	40,017	2,262	5.7	60.1	854	2.1	60.4
Educational attainment							
Not a high school graduate	13,096	812	6.2	21.6	264	2.0	18.7
High school graduate	16,644	1,005	6.0	26.7	380	2.3	26.9
Some college or associate's degree	17,564	971	5.5	25.8	377	2.1	26.6
Bachelor's degree or more	14,057	977	7.0	25.9	394	2.8	27.8
Labor force status							
In labor force	43,360	2,056	4.7	54.6	846	2.0	59.8
Not in labor force	18,001	1,710	9.5	45.4	568	3.2	40.1
Household income							
Under $25,000	13,311	1,042	7.8	27.7	401	3.0	28.3
$25,000 to $34,999	7,076	458	6.5	12.2	139	2.0	9.8
$35,000 to $49,999	8,477	457	5.4	12.1	161	1.9	11.4
$50,000 to $74,999	10,613	554	5.2	14.7	247	2.3	17.5
$75,000 or more	13,771	826	6.0	21.9	294	2.1	20.8
Region							
Northeast	11,616	694	6.0	18.4	247	2.1	17.5
Midwest	14,041	780	5.6	20.7	303	2.2	21.4
South	21,680	1,453	6.7	38.6	561	2.6	39.6
West	14,024	838	6.0	22.3	305	2.2	21.6
Nativity							
Native born	52,428	3,129	6.0	83.1	1,153	2.2	81.5
Foreign born	8,933	637	7.1	16.9	262	2.9	18.5

Note: Numbers by income will not sum to total because not reported is not shown.
Source: Bureau of the Census, Fertility of American Women: June 2002, detailed tables, Internet site http://www.census.gov/population/www/socdemo/fertility/cps2002.html

More than One-Third of Newborns Are Hispanic or Black

Babies born today promise great diversity tomorrow.

Of the 4 million babies born in 2003, 22 percent were born to Hispanic women and 15 percent to black women. Another 5 percent were born to Asian women. Only 57 percent of babies were born to non-Hispanic whites. As today's children grow up, they will create an increasingly multicultural society with no single racial or ethnic group claiming the majority of the U.S. population.

Among all women who gave birth in 2003, 52 percent were in their twenties. The proportion was an even higher 56 to 57 percent among black and Hispanic mothers, respectively. Among non-Hispanic whites, however, slightly less than half of those giving birth in 2003 were in their twenties. Among Asians, the figure was just 43 percent. Behind these differing age patterns is educational attainment. Asian and non-Hispanic white women, who attain higher levels of education, delay childbearing while they earn their degrees.

■ Hispanic women have more children than Asians, blacks, or non-Hispanic whites, driving growth in the Hispanic population.

Most babies are born to women in their twenties
(percent distribution of births, by age of mother, 2003)

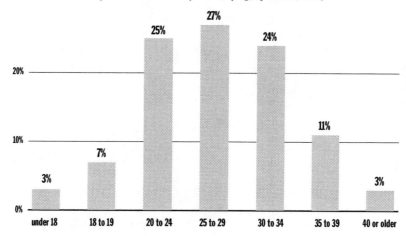

Table 5.17 Births by Age, Race, and Hispanic Origin, 2003

(number and percent distribution of births by age, race, and Hispanic origin of mother, 2003)

	total	American Indian	Asian	black	Hispanic	non-Hispanic white
Total births	**4,091,063**	**42,647**	**221,247**	**599,414**	**912,256**	**2,320,778**
Under age 15	6,665	156	105	2,722	2,349	1,402
Aged 15–17	134,617	2,648	2,307	36,855	46,949	46,899
Aged 18–19	280,344	4,969	5,351	64,009	81,523	125,827
Aged 20–24	1,032,337	14,480	30,639	196,112	273,258	521,712
Aged 25–29	1,086,898	10,421	64,336	139,853	246,388	627,373
Aged 30–34	975,964	6,372	75,546	97,526	169,056	626,245
Aged 35–39	467,520	2,900	35,107	49,810	75,812	303,008
Aged 40–44	100,873	660	7,405	11,880	16,169	64,414
Aged 45–54	5,845	43	451	645	753	3,897

PERCENT DISTRIBUTION BY RACE AND HISPANIC ORIGIN

	total	American Indian	Asian	black	Hispanic	non-Hispanic white
Total births	**100.0%**	**1.0%**	**5.4%**	**14.7%**	**22.3%**	**56.7%**
Under age 15	100.0	2.3	1.6	40.8	35.2	21.0
Aged 15–17	100.0	2.0	1.7	27.4	34.9	34.8
Aged 18–19	100.0	1.8	1.9	22.8	29.1	44.9
Aged 20–24	100.0	1.4	3.0	19.0	26.5	50.5
Aged 25–29	100.0	1.0	5.9	12.9	22.7	57.7
Aged 30–34	100.0	0.7	7.7	10.0	17.3	64.2
Aged 35–39	100.0	0.6	7.5	10.7	16.2	64.8
Aged 40–44	100.0	0.7	7.3	11.8	16.0	63.9
Aged 45–54	100.0	0.7	7.7	11.0	12.9	66.7

PERCENT DISTRIBUTION BY AGE

	total	American Indian	Asian	black	Hispanic	non-Hispanic white
Total births	**100.0%**	**100.0%**	**100.0%**	**100.0%**	**100.0%**	**100.0%**
Under age 15	0.2	0.4	0.1	0.5	0.3	0.1
Aged 15–17	3.3	6.2	1.0	6.1	5.1	2.0
Aged 18–19	6.9	11.7	2.4	10.7	8.9	5.4
Aged 20–24	25.2	34.0	13.8	32.7	30.0	22.5
Aged 25–29	26.6	24.4	29.1	23.3	27.0	27.0
Aged 30–34	23.9	14.9	34.1	16.3	18.5	27.0
Aged 35–39	11.4	6.8	15.9	8.3	8.3	13.1
Aged 40–44	2.5	1.5	3.3	2.0	1.8	2.8
Aged 45–54	0.1	0.1	0.2	0.1	0.1	0.2

Note: Births by race and Hispanic origin will not add to total because Hispanics may be of any race and "not stated" is not shown.
Source: National Center for Health Statistics, Births: Preliminary Data for 2003, National Vital Statistics Reports, Vol. 53, No. 9, 2004; Internet site http://www.cdc.gov/nchs/products/pubs/pubd/nvsr/nvsr.htm; calculations by New Strategist

Table 5.18 Births to Hispanics by Age and Hispanic Origin, 2002

(number and percent distribution of births by age and Hispanic origin of mother, 2002)

	total	Mexican	Puerto Rican	Cuban	Central and South American	other Hispanic
Total Hispanic births	**876,642**	**627,505**	**57,465**	**14,232**	**125,981**	**51,459**
Under age 20	130,321	99,593	10,211	1,159	10,750	8,608
Aged 20 to 24	265,235	196,864	18,724	2,410	31,547	15,690
Aged 25 to 29	236,143	170,146	13,841	4,025	35,429	12,702
Aged 30 to 34	157,887	106,177	9,415	3,881	29,222	9,192
Aged 35 to 39	71,480	45,129	4,385	2,283	15,366	4,317
Aged 40 to 44	14,809	9,137	836	442	3,481	913
Aged 45 or older	767	459	53	32	186	37
PERCENT DISTRIBUTION BY HISPANIC ORIGIN						
Total Hispanic births	**100.0%**	**71.6%**	**6.6%**	**1.6%**	**14.4%**	**5.9%**
Under age 20	100.0	76.4	7.8	0.9	8.2	6.6
Aged 20 to 24	100.0	74.2	7.1	0.9	11.9	5.9
Aged 25 to 29	100.0	72.1	5.9	1.7	15.0	5.4
Aged 30 to 34	100.0	67.2	6.0	2.5	18.5	5.8
Aged 35 to 39	100.0	63.1	6.1	3.2	21.5	6.0
Aged 40 to 44	100.0	61.7	5.6	3.0	23.5	6.2
Aged 45 or older	100.0	59.8	6.9	4.2	24.3	4.8
PERCENT DISTRIBUTION BY AGE						
Total Hispanic births	**100.0%**	**100.0%**	**100.0%**	**100.0%**	**100.0%**	**100.0%**
Under age 20	14.9	15.9	17.8	8.1	8.5	16.7
Aged 20 to 24	30.3	31.4	32.6	16.9	25.0	30.5
Aged 25 to 29	26.9	27.1	24.1	28.3	28.1	24.7
Aged 30 to 34	18.0	16.9	16.4	27.3	23.2	17.9
Aged 35 to 39	8.2	7.2	7.6	16.0	12.2	8.4
Aged 40 to 44	1.7	1.5	1.5	3.1	2.8	1.8
Aged 45 or older	0.1	0.1	0.1	0.2	0.1	0.1

Note: Births will not add to total because "not stated" is not shown.
Source: National Center for Health Statistics, Births: Final Data for 2002, National Vital Statistics Reports, Vol. 52, No. 10, 2003; Internet site http://www.cdc.gov/nchs/products/pubs/pubd/nvsr/nvsr.htm; calculations by New Strategist

Thirty-Four Percent of Births Are to Unmarried Women

More than two-thirds of black women giving birth in 2002 were not married.

Overall, about one-third of women who gave birth in 2002 were not married. But the percentage of unwed mothers varies greatly by race and Hispanic origin. Only 15 percent of Asian women giving birth were unmarried. The share was a somewhat larger 23 percent among non-Hispanic white women. Among Hispanics, however, a substantial 44 percent were not married. The majority of American Indian and black women who had a child in 2002 were not married.

Regardless of race or Hispanic origin, the great majority of teenage mothers are unmarried. Overall, 97 percent of women under age 15 and 80 percent of those aged 15 to 19 who gave birth in 2002 were not married. After the teenage years, however, sizable differences in nonmarital births emerge by race and Hispanic origin. Thirty-six percent of Asian women aged 20 to 24 who gave birth in 2002 were not married versus an enormous 81 percent of black women in the age group.

■ Many single mothers will eventually marry, although already having a child in tow can make marriage more difficult.

Most births to women under age 25 are out-of-wedlock

(percent of births to unmarried women by age, 2002)

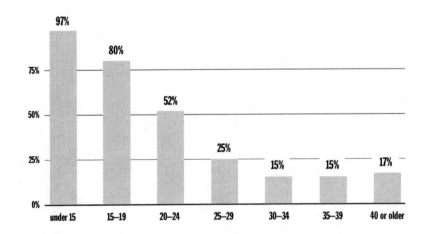

Table 5.19 Births to Unmarried Women by Age, Race, and Hispanic Origin of Mother, 2002

(total number of births and number and percent to unmarried women, by age, race, and Hispanic origin of mother, 2002)

	total	American Indian	Asian	black	Hispanic	non-Hispanic white
Total births	**4,021,726**	**42,368**	**210,907**	**593,691**	**876,642**	**2,298,156**
Under age 15	7,315	133	110	3,188	2,421	1,493
Aged 15 to 19	425,493	7,707	8,003	103,795	127,900	179,511
Aged 20 to 24	1,022,106	14,343	30,059	194,704	265,235	519,153
Aged 25 to 29	1,060,391	10,139	62,519	136,591	236,143	614,909
Aged 30 to 34	951,219	6,338	70,340	95,006	157,887	620,173
Aged 35 to 39	453,927	2,976	32,730	48,388	71,480	297,436
Aged 40 or older	101,275	732	7,146	12,019	15,576	65,481
BIRTHS TO UNMARRIED WOMEN						
Total births to unmarried women	**1,365,966**	**25,297**	**31,344**	**404,864**	**381,466**	**528,535**
Under age 15	7,093	129	107	3,174	2,266	1,446
Aged 15 to 19	340,186	6,678	5,726	99,375	94,483	135,313
Aged 20 to 24	527,657	9,548	10,672	158,276	136,369	214,529
Aged 25 to 29	268,312	4,993	7,318	79,946	83,035	94,304
Aged 30 to 34	139,208	2,475	4,670	40,375	42,254	50,150
Aged 35 to 39	66,036	1,176	2,218	18,958	18,566	25,472
Aged 40 or older	17,474	298	633	4,760	4,493	7,321
PERCENT OF BIRTHS TO UNMARRIED WOMEN						
Total births to unmarried women	**34.0%**	**59.7%**	**14.9%**	**68.2%**	**43.5%**	**23.0%**
Under age 15	97.0	97.0	97.3	99.6	93.6	96.9
Aged 15 to 19	80.0	86.6	71.5	95.7	73.9	75.4
Aged 20 to 24	51.6	66.6	35.5	81.3	51.4	41.3
Aged 25 to 29	25.3	49.2	11.7	58.5	35.2	15.3
Aged 30 to 34	14.6	39.1	6.6	42.5	26.8	8.1
Aged 35 to 39	14.5	39.5	6.8	39.2	26.0	8.6
Aged 40 or older	17.3	40.7	8.9	39.6	28.8	11.2

Note: Births by race and Hispanic origin will not add to total because Hispanics may be of any race and "not stated" is not shown.
Source: National Center for Health Statistics, Births: Final Data for 2002, *National Vital Statistics Reports, Vol. 52, No. 10, 2003; Internet site http://www.cdc.gov/nchs/products/pubs/pubd/nvsr/nvsr.htm; calculations by New Strategist*

Delayed Childbearing Can Lead to Difficulties

Older mothers are more likely to have Caesareans.

First births account for the largest share of births—40 percent in 2003. Thirty-three percent of births are second children, while 27 percent are third or later children. As one would expect, the older the mother the more likely she is to be having her second or later child.

Older women who give birth are more likely than their younger counterparts to have a college degree. Among all women giving birth in 2002, 26 percent were college graduates. Among women aged 30 or older who gave birth, more than 40 percent had a college degree. Many delayed having children until they completed their college education.

Delayed childbearing has its advantages, but it also has risks. Older mothers are much more likely to have a Caesarean delivery. The Caesarean rate increases with age, from 18 percent among teenagers to 40 percent among women aged 40 or older. Older mothers are also more likely to give birth to twins or higher-order multiple deliveries. Many older women use fertility technologies to conceive and bear a child, which can result in multiple births.

■ Although the risks associated with having children later in life are well known, many women wait to begin their families because they are finishing their education or establishing a career.

More than 40 percent of births to women aged 40 or older are by Caesarean

(percent of babies born by Caesarean delivery, by age of mother, 2002)

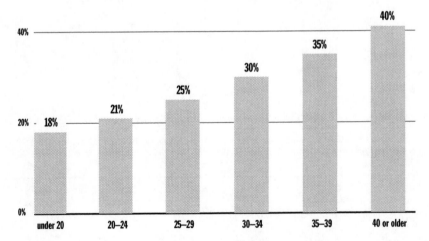

Table 5.20 Births by Age and Birth Order, 2003

(number and percent distribution of births by age and birth order, 2003)

	total	first child	second child	third child	fourth or later child
Total births	**4,091,063**	**1,647,451**	**1,331,672**	**682,289**	**422,715**
Under age 15	6,665	6,533	120	4	2
Aged 15 to 19	414,961	331,983	70,204	10,716	1,306
Aged 20 to 24	1,032,337	485,430	354,366	140,513	50,243
Aged 25 to 29	1,086,898	397,815	370,265	202,155	114,943
Aged 30 to 34	975,964	290,985	351,494	198,783	133,213
Aged 35 to 39	467,520	110,663	154,561	108,184	93,203
Aged 40 to 44	100,873	22,530	29,170	20,976	27,947
Aged 45 to 54	5,845	1,512	1,493	957	1,857

PERCENT DISTRIBUTION BY BIRTH ORDER

Total births	**100.0%**	**40.3%**	**32.6%**	**16.7%**	**10.3%**
Under age 15	100.0	98.0	1.8	0.1	0.0
Aged 15 to 19	100.0	80.0	16.9	2.6	0.3
Aged 20 to 24	100.0	47.0	34.3	13.6	4.9
Aged 25 to 29	100.0	36.6	34.1	18.6	10.6
Aged 30 to 34	100.0	29.8	36.0	20.4	13.7
Aged 35 to 39	100.0	23.7	33.1	23.1	19.9
Aged 40 to 44	100.0	22.3	28.9	20.8	27.7
Aged 45 to 54	100.0	25.9	25.5	16.4	31.8

PERCENT DISTRIBUTION BY AGE

Total births	**100.0%**	**100.0%**	**100.0%**	**100.0%**	**100.0%**
Under age 15	0.2	0.4	0.0	0.0	0.0
Aged 15 to 19	10.1	20.2	5.3	1.6	0.3
Aged 20 to 24	25.2	29.5	26.6	20.6	11.9
Aged 25 to 29	26.6	24.1	27.8	29.6	27.2
Aged 30 to 34	23.9	17.7	26.4	29.1	31.5
Aged 35 to 39	11.4	6.7	11.6	15.9	22.0
Aged 40 to 44	2.5	1.4	2.2	3.1	6.6
Aged 45 to 54	0.1	0.1	0.1	0.1	0.4

Note: Numbers will not add to total because "not stated" is not shown.
Source: National Center for Health Statistics, Births: Preliminary Data for 2003, *National Vital Statistics Reports, Vol. 53, No. 9, 2004; Internet site http://www.cdc.gov/nchs/products/pubs/pubd/nvsr/nvsr.htm; calculations by New Strategist*

Table 5.21 Births by Age and Educational Attainment of Mother, 2002

(number and percent distribution of births by age and educational attainment of mother, 2002)

	total	not a high school graduate	high school graduate only	some college	college graduate
Total births	**4,021,726**	**854,582**	**1,234,726**	**851,732**	**1,026,819**
Under age 20	432,808	257,203	146,680	21,817	–
Aged 20 to 24	1,022,106	278,335	445,622	227,368	57,339
Aged 25 to 29	1,060,391	167,398	315,029	271,475	293,155
Aged 30 to 34	951,219	96,271	206,783	211,563	424,862
Aged 35 to 39	453,927	43,949	98,280	98,235	207,087
Aged 40 or older	101,275	11,426	22,332	21,274	44,376

PERCENT DISTRIBUTION BY EDUCATIONAL ATTAINMENT

Total births	**100.0%**	**21.2%**	**30.7%**	**21.2%**	**25.5%**
Under age 20	100.0	59.4	33.9	5.0	–
Aged 20 to 24	100.0	27.2	43.6	22.2	5.6
Aged 25 to 29	100.0	15.8	29.7	25.6	27.6
Aged 30 to 34	100.0	10.1	21.7	22.2	44.7
Aged 35 to 39	100.0	9.7	21.7	21.6	45.6
Aged 40 or older	100.0	11.3	22.1	21.0	43.8

PERCENT DISTRIBUTION BY AGE

Total births	**100.0%**	**100.0%**	**100.0%**	**100.0%**	**100.0%**
Under age 20	10.8	30.1	11.9	2.6	–
Aged 20 to 24	25.4	32.6	36.1	26.7	5.6
Aged 25 to 29	26.4	19.6	25.5	31.9	28.6
Aged 30 to 34	23.7	11.3	16.7	24.8	41.4
Aged 35 to 39	11.3	5.1	8.0	11.5	20.2
Aged 40 or older	2.5	1.3	1.8	2.5	4.3

Note: Births by education will not add to total because "not stated" is not shown. (–) means sample is too small to make a reliable estimate.
Source: National Center for Health Statistics, Births: Final Data for 2002, *National Vital Statistics Reports, Vol. 52, No. 10, 2003; Internet site http://www.cdc.gov/nchs/products/pubs/pubd/nvsr/nvsr.htm; calculations by New Strategist*

Table 5.22 Births by Age of Mother and Method of Delivery, 2002

(number and percent distribution of births by age and method of delivery, 2002)

| | | vaginal | | Caesarean | | |
	total births	total	after previous Caesarean	total	primary	repeat
Total births	**4,021,726**	**2,958,423**	**59,248**	**1,043,846**	**634,426**	**409,420**
Under age 20	432,808	353,653	1,506	77,563	67,741	9,822
Aged 20 to 24	1,022,106	799,537	10,910	218,239	144,947	73,292
Aged 25 to 29	1,060,391	788,776	16,294	266,452	159,869	106,583
Aged 30 to 34	951,219	663,566	17,976	282,576	156,159	126,417
Aged 35 to 39	453,927	293,251	10,278	158,005	82,497	75,508
Aged 40 or older	101,275	59,640	2,284	41,011	23,213	17,798

PERCENT DISTRIBUTION BY METHOD OF DELIVERY

Total births	**100.0%**	**73.6%**	**1.5%**	**26.0%**	**15.8%**	**10.2%**
Under age 20	100.0	81.7	0.3	17.9	15.7	2.3
Aged 20 to 24	100.0	78.2	1.1	21.4	14.2	7.2
Aged 25 to 29	100.0	74.4	1.5	25.1	15.1	10.1
Aged 30 to 34	100.0	69.8	1.9	29.7	16.4	13.3
Aged 35 to 39	100.0	64.6	2.3	34.8	18.2	16.6
Aged 40 or older	100.0	58.9	2.3	40.5	22.9	17.6

PERCENT DISTRIBUTION BY AGE

Total births	**100.0%**	**100.0%**	**100.0%**	**100.0%**	**100.0%**	**100.0%**
Under age 20	10.8	12.0	2.5	7.4	10.7	2.4
Aged 20 to 24	25.4	27.0	18.4	20.9	22.8	17.9
Aged 25 to 29	26.4	26.7	27.5	25.5	25.2	26.0
Aged 30 to 34	23.7	22.4	30.3	27.1	24.6	30.9
Aged 35 to 39	11.3	9.9	17.3	15.1	13.0	18.4
Aged 40 or older	2.5	2.0	3.9	3.9	3.7	4.3

Note: Numbers will not add to total because not stated is not shown.
Source: National Center for Health Statistics, Births: Final Data for 2002, National Vital Statistics Reports, Vol. 52, No. 10, 2003; Internet site http://www.cdc.gov/nchs/products/pubs/pubd/nvsr/nvsr.htm; calculations by New Strategist

Table 5.23 Births by Age and Plurality, 2002

(number and percent distribution of births by age and plurality, 2002)

	total	single deliveries	twin deliveries	higher order multiple deliveries
Total births	**4,021,726**	**3,889,191**	**125,134**	**7,401**
Under age 20	432,808	425,880	6,835	93
Aged 20 to 24	1,022,106	998,739	22,856	511
Aged 25 to 29	1,060,391	1,028,038	30,725	1,628
Aged 30 to 34	951,219	911,431	36,956	2,832
Aged 35 to 39	453,927	430,447	21,637	1,843
Aged 40 to 44	95,788	90,378	5,033	377
Aged 45 or older	5,487	4,278	1,092	117
PERCENT DISTRIBUTION BY PLURALITY				
Total births	**100.0%**	**96.7%**	**3.1%**	**0.2%**
Under age 20	100.0	98.4	1.6	0.0
Aged 20 to 24	100.0	97.7	2.2	0.0
Aged 25 to 29	100.0	96.9	2.9	0.2
Aged 30 to 34	100.0	95.8	3.9	0.3
Aged 35 to 39	100.0	94.8	4.8	0.4
Aged 40 or older	100.0	94.4	5.3	0.4
PERCENT DISTRIBUTION BY AGE				
Total births	**100.0%**	**100.0%**	**100.0%**	**100.0%**
Under age 20	10.8	11.0	5.5	1.3
Aged 20 to 24	25.4	25.7	18.3	6.9
Aged 25 to 29	26.4	26.4	24.6	22.0
Aged 30 to 34	23.7	23.4	29.5	38.3
Aged 35 to 39	11.3	11.1	17.3	24.9
Aged 40 or older	2.4	2.3	4.0	5.1

Source: National Center for Health Statistics, Births: Final Data for 2002, *National Vital Statistics Reports, Vol. 52, No. 10, 2003; Internet site http://www.cdc.gov/nchs/products/pubs/pubd/nvsr/nvsr.htm; calculations by New Strategist*

Less-Educated Women Take Risks during Pregnancy

One in five American Indian women smoked during her pregnancy.

Eighty-four percent of women giving birth in 2002 sought prenatal care during the first trimester of their pregnancy. Fewer than 1 percent admitted to drinking alcoholic beverages while pregnant, but 11 percent smoked.

American Indian mothers are most likely to engage in risky behavior while pregnant. Only 70 percent received prenatal care during the first trimester. Twenty percent smoked, and nearly 3 percent admitted to drinking alcohol. American Indian women are among the least educated, which may help to explain these high-risk behaviors.

Cubans are the best-educated Hispanics, and they are more likely than other Hispanics to obtain prenatal care early in their pregnancy. Among Asians, Hawaiian women are the least educated. They are more likely than other Asian women to smoke during pregnancy.

Although a mother's behavior during pregnancy can influence the health of her fetus, most congenital anomalies are genetic or of unclear origin. The most common problems are heart malformations and other circulatory/respiratory problems.

■ Despite significant public health efforts to inform women of healthy behavior during pregnancy, many women still engage in practices that could harm their babies.

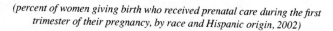

Non-Hispanic white women are most likely to receive prenatal care during the first trimester

(percent of women giving birth who received prenatal care during the first trimester of their pregnancy, by race and Hispanic origin, 2002)

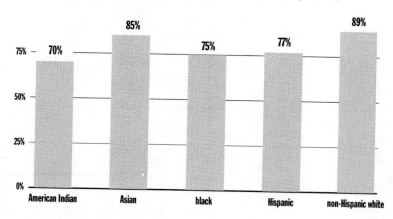

Table 5.24 Births by Selected Characteristics, Race, and Hispanic Origin, 2002

(total number of births, births per 1,000 women aged 15 to 44, average number of births in lifetime, and percent of births by selected characteristics, by race and Hispanic origin, 2002)

	total	American Indian	Asian	black	Hispanic	non-Hispanic white
Total births	4,021,726	42,368	210,907	593,691	876,642	2,298,156
Births per 1,000 women aged 15 to 44	64.8	58.0	64.1	65.8	94.4	57.4
Average number of births in lifetime	2.0	1.7	1.8	2.0	2.7	1.8
Percent of births by selected characteristics						
Births to mothers under age 20	10.8%	18.5%	3.8%	18.0%	14.9%	7.9%
Fourth and higher-order births	10.8	19.1	6.5	15.3	13.6	8.9
Births to unmarried women	34.0	59.7	14.9	68.2	43.5	23.0
Mothers completing high school	78.5	69.2	89.7	75.6	51.9	88.3
Mothers born in 50 states or D.C.	76.7	94.4	16.9	87.0	36.7	94.2
Prenatal care beginning in first trimester	83.7	69.8	84.8	75.2	76.7	88.6
Late or no prenatal care	3.6	8.0	3.1	6.2	5.5	2.2
Smoker	11.4	19.7	2.5	8.7	3.0	15.0
Drinker	0.8	2.5	0.3	0.9	0.5	0.9
Caesarean delivery	26.1	23.1	25.0	27.6	25.2	26.2

Note: Average number of births in lifetime is the total fertility rate divided by 1000.
Source: National Center for Health Statistics, Births: Final Data for 2002, *National Vital Statistics Reports, Vol. 52, No. 10, 2003; Internet site http://www.cdc.gov/nchs/products/pubs/pubd/nvsr/nvsr.htm; calculations by New Strategist*

Table 5.25 Births to Hispanics by Selected Characteristics and Hispanic Origin, 2002

(total number of births to Hispanics, births per 1,000 women aged 15 to 44, average number of births in lifetime, and percent of births by selected characteristics, by Hispanic origin, 2002)

	total	Mexican	Puerto Rican	Cuban	Central and South American	other Hispanic
Total births to Hispanics	876,642	627,505	57,465	14,232	125,981	51,459
Births per 1,000 women aged 15 to 44	94.4	102.8	65.4	59.0	86.1	–
Average number of births in lifetime	2.7	2.9	1.9	1.9	2.6	–
Percent of births by selected characteristics						
Births to mothers under age 20	14.9%	15.9%	17.8%	8.1%	8.5%	16.7%
Fourth and higher-order births	13.6	14.7	12.2	4.9	10.8	11.8
Births to unmarried women	43.5	42.1	59.1	29.8	44.8	44.4
Mothers completing high school	51.9	45.8	68.5	88.2	64.2	68.3
Mothers born in 50 states or D.C.	36.7	36.1	65.8	45.0	11.5	71.7
Prenatal care beginning in first trimester	76.7	75.7	79.9	92.0	78.7	76.7
Late or no prenatal care	5.5	5.8	4.1	1.3	4.9	5.3
Smoker	3.0	2.2	9.0	2.8	1.3	6.5
Drinker	0.5	0.5	0.7	0.3	0.3	0.9
Caesarean delivery	25.2	24.5	26.2	36.9	27.0	24.6

Note: Average number of births in lifetime is the total fertility rate divided by 1000. (–) means data are not available.
Source: National Center for Health Statistics, Births: Final Data for 2002, National Vital Statistics Reports, Vol. 52, No. 10, 2003; Internet site http://www.cdc.gov/nchs/products/pubs/pubd/nvsr/nvsr.htm; calculations by New Strategist

Table 5.26 Births to Asians by Selected Characteristics and Asian Origin, 2002

(number and percent distribution of births to Asians by Asian origin, and percent of births by selected characteristics and Asian origin, 2002)

	total	Chinese	Japanese	Hawaiian	Filipino	other
Total births to Asians	**210,907**	**33,673**	**9,264**	**6,772**	**33,016**	**128,182**
Percent distribution of births by Asian origin	**100.0%**	**16.0%**	**4.4%**	**3.2%**	**15.7%**	**60.8%**
Percent of births by selected characteristics						
Births to mothers under age 20	3.8%	0.9%	1.7%	14.6%	4.5%	4.0%
Fourth and higher-order births	6.5	2.1	3.9	16.3	7.3	7.1
Births to unmarried women	14.9	9.0	10.3	50.4	20.0	13.5
Mothers completing high school	89.7	88.7	97.8	85.7	94.7	88.4
Mothers born in 50 states or D.C.	16.9	10.0	40.4	97.4	21.5	11.6
Prenatal care beginning in first trimester	84.8	87.2	90.5	78.1	85.4	83.9
Late or no prenatal care	3.1	2.1	2.1	4.7	2.8	3.5
Smoker	2.5	0.5	4.0	13.7	2.9	2.1
Drinker	0.3	0.1	0.8	1.1	0.4	0.3
Caesarean delivery	25.0	23.9	20.8	22.4	28.5	24.8

Source: National Center for Health Statistics, Births: Final Data for 2002, *National Vital Statistics Reports, Vol. 52, No. 10, 2003; Internet site http://www.cdc.gov/nchs/products/pubs/pubd/nvsr/nvsr.htm; calculations by New Strategist*

Table 5.27 Births with Selected Congenital Anomalies, 2002

(number of births in 49 reporting states and the District of Columbia with selected congenital anomalies, and rate per 100,000 live births, 2002)

	number	rate per 100,000 live births
Total live births in reporting states	**3,993,973**	–
Anencephalus	391	9.9
Spina bifida/meningocele	793	20.0
Hydrocephalus	892	22.5
Microcephalus	219	5.5
Other central nervous system anomalies	881	22.2
Heart malformations	5,152	129.9
Other circulatory/respiratory anomalies	5,222	131.7
Rectal atresia/senosis	329	8.3
Tracheo-esophageal fistula/esophageal atresia	430	10.8
Omphalocele/gastroschisis	1,203	30.3
Other gastrointestinal anomalies	1,432	36.1
Malformed genitalia	3,433	86.6
Renal agenesis	612	15.4
Other urogenital anomalies	4,036	101.8
Cleft lip/palate	3,114	78.5
Polydactyly/syndactyly/adactyly	3,259	82.2
Clubfoot	2,363	59.6
Diaphragmatic hernia	479	12.1
Other musculoskeletal/ integumental anomalies	9,077	228.9
Down's syndrome	1,850	46.7
Other chromosomal anomalies	1,253	31.6

Note: (–) means not applicable.
Source: National Center for Health Statistics, **Births: Final Data for 2002,** *National Vital Statistics Reports, Vol. 52, No. 10, 2003; Internet site http://www.cdc.gov/nchs/products/pubs/pubd/nvsr/nvsr.htm; calculations by New Strategist*

6

Coverage and Cost

■ **Americans spend more for health care than the citizens of any other country.**

Per capita spending in the United States topped $5,000 in 2001, with Switzerland coming in a distant second at $3,322.

■ **Only 16 percent of health care costs are paid for out-of-pocket.**

Prescription drug expenses are most likely to be paid for out-of-pocket (30 percent), hospital care the least (3 percent).

■ **Sixty percent of Americans have health insurance through an employer.**

Twelve percent are covered by Medicaid (health insurance for the poor), 14 percent by Medicare (health insurance for people aged 65 or older), and 16 percent have no insurance.

■ **Cost is the primary reason for being uninsured.**

Fifty-three percent of the uninsured say they do not have health insurance because it costs too much.

■ **Sixty-nine percent of workers in private industry have access to health insurance through their employer.**

Among service workers, however, only 42 percent have access to health insurance through their employer.

■ **Health care spending rises with age.**

Householders under age 25 spend an average of only $546 a year on health care, while householders aged 75 or older spend $3,856.

Health Care Costs Have Grown Rapidly

As costs rise, individuals are paying a smaller share of the total.

Between 1960 and 2002, the nation's spending on health care soared, climbing from just $27 billion to $1.6 trillion. The U.S. spends more than any other country on health care, fully $5,021 per person in 2001. Switzerland, in second place, spent just $3,322 per capita on health care.

As the number of dollars spent on health care has grown, the allocation of those dollars has remained remarkably stable. In 1960, 35 percent of health care expenditures went to hospital care. The share was only a slightly smaller 31 percent in 2002. Prescription drugs accounted for 10.1 percent of health care spending in 1960 and 10.4 percent in 2002.

As health care costs have increased, more of the financial burden has shifted to public funds. In 1965 private funds paid for fully 75 percent of health care expenditures. In 2002, the share was a much smaller 54 percent. Individuals are also bearing a smaller proportion of the costs, with out-of-pocket expenditures accounting for 16 percent of total health care expenditures in 2002—down from the 55 percent majority in 1960. The biggest change has been in prescription drugs, with the out-of-pocket share falling from 96 to just 30 percent between 1960 and 2002.

■ With costs rising far faster than overall inflation—and incomes—health care would bankrupt many families if they had to pay the same share of health care expenses out-of-pocket as they did in 1960.

Only 30 percent of prescription drug expenses are paid for out-of-pocket

(percent of total health care expenditures paid for out-of-pocket, by type of expenditure, 1960 and 2002)

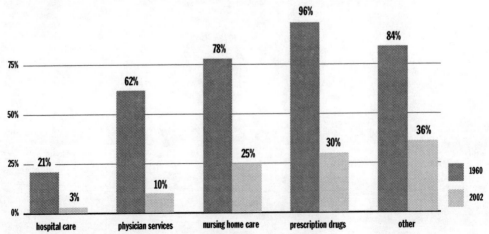

Table 6.1 National Health Care Expenditures, 1960 to 2002

(total national health care expenditures and average annual percent change, 1960 to 2002)

	total (billions)	average annual percent change from previous year shown
2002	$1,553.0	9.3%
2001	1,420.7	8.5
2000	1,309.4	7.1
1999	1,222.6	5.4
1995	990.2	7.3
1990	696.0	11.0
1980	245.8	12.9
1970	73.1	10.6
1960	26.7	–

Source: National Center for Health Statistics, Health, United States, 2004; *Internet site http://www.cdc.gov/nchs/hus.htm; calculations by New Strategist*

Table 6.2 National Health Care Expenditures by Type of Expenditure, 1960 and 2002

(national health care expenditures and percent distribution by type of expenditure, 1960 and 2002)

	2002		1960	
	total (billions)	percent distribution	total (billions)	percent distribution
Total national health care spending	**$1,553.0**	**100.0%**	**$26.7**	**100.0%**
Health services and supplies	**1,496.3**	**96.3**	**25.0**	**93.6**
Personal health care	1,340.2	86.3	23.4	87.6
Hospital care	486.5	31.3	9.2	34.5
Professional services	501.5	32.3	8.3	31.1
Physician services	339.5	21.9	5.4	20.2
Other professional services	45.9	3.0	0.4	1.5
Dental services	70.3	4.5	2.0	7.5
Other personal health care	45.8	2.9	0.6	2.2
Nursing home and home health	139.3	9.0	0.9	3.4
Home health care	36.1	2.3	0.1	0.4
Nursing home care	103.2	6.6	0.8	3.0
Retail outlet sales of medical pdts.	212.9	13.7	5.0	18.7
Prescription drugs	162.4	10.5	2.7	10.1
Other medical products	50.5	3.3	2.3	8.6
Government administration and net cost of private health insurance	105.0	6.8	1.2	4.5
Government public health activities	51.2	3.3	0.4	1.5
Investment	**56.7**	**3.7**	**1.7**	**6.4**
Research	34.3	2.2	0.7	2.6
Construction	22.4	1.4	1.0	3.7

Source: National Center for Health Statistics, Health, United States, 2004; *Internet site http://www.cdc.gov/nchs/hus.htm; calculations by New Strategist*

Table 6.3 Trends in Public vs. Private Funding of National Health Care, 1965 to 2002

(total GDP, total national health care expenditures, per capita expenditures, and percent of GDP, by public and private funding, 1965 to 2002)

	GDP (billions)	total (billions)	per capita	percent of GDP	private funds total (billions)	per capita	percent of total	public funds total (billions)	per capita	percent of total
2002	$10,446	$1,553.0	$5,440	14.9%	$839.6	$2,941	54.1%	$713.4	$2,499	45.9%
2001	10,082	1,424.5	5,035	14.1	777.9	2,749	54.6	646.7	2,286	45.4
2000	9,825	1,310.0	4,672	13.3	718.7	2,563	54.9	591.3	2,109	45.1
1999	9,274	1,219.7	4,392	13.2	669.7	2,411	54.9	550.0	1,980	45.1
1998	8,781	1,150.0	4,178	13.1	628.4	2,283	54.6	521.6	1,895	45.4
1997	8,318	1,092.7	4,007	13.1	589.2	2,160	53.9	503.6	1,846	46.1
1996	7,813	1,039.4	3,847	13.3	557.5	2,063	53.6	481.9	1,784	46.4
1995	7,400	990.1	3,697	13.4	532.5	1,988	53.8	457.7	1,709	46.2
1994	7,054	937.2	3,534	13.3	509.8	1,922	54.4	427.3	1,611	45.6
1993	6,642	888.1	3,381	13.4	497.7	1,895	56.0	390.4	1,486	44.0
1992	6,319	827.0	3,184	13.1	468.5	1,803	56.6	358.5	1,380	43.4
1991	5,986	761.8	2,966	12.7	441.3	1,718	57.9	320.6	1,248	42.1
1990	5,803	696.0	2,738	12.0	413.5	1,627	59.4	282.5	1,111	40.6
1989	5,489	622.7	2,477	11.3	370.9	1,476	59.6	251.8	1,002	40.4
1988	5,108	558.1	2,243	10.9	331.7	1,333	59.4	226.4	910	40.6
1987	4,742	498.0	2,020	10.5	289.3	1,174	58.1	208.8	847	41.9
1986	4,453	457.2	1,872	10.3	266.9	1,093	58.4	190.4	780	41.6
1985	4,213	426.8	1,765	10.1	252.2	1,043	59.1	174.6	722	40.9
1984	3,933	390.1	1,628	9.9	229.3	957	58.8	160.8	671	41.2
1983	3,535	353.5	1,489	10.0	206.1	868	58.3	147.5	621	41.7
1982	3,259	321.0	1,366	9.8	186.7	794	58.2	134.3	571	41.8
1981	3,131	285.1	1,225	9.1	163.9	704	57.5	121.2	521	42.5
1980	2,796	245.8	1,067	8.8	140.9	612	57.3	104.8	455	42.7
1975	1,635	129.8	590	7.9	74.8	340	57.6	55.0	250	42.4
1970	1,040	73.1	348	7.0	45.4	216	62.2	27.6	131	37.8
1967	834	50.7	249	6.1	31.8	156	62.8	18.9	93	37.2
1966	789	45.1	224	5.7	31.6	156	69.9	13.6	67	30.1
1965	720	41.0	205	5.7	30.8	154	75.1	10.2	51	24.9

Source: Centers for Medicare and Medicaid Services, 2003 Data Compendium, Internet site http://www.cms.hhs.gov/researchers/pubs/datacompendium/current/; and Health, United States, 2004; Internet site http://www.cdc.gov/nchs/hus.htm; calculations by New Strategist

Table 6.4   Personal Health Care Expenditures, 1960 to 2002

(total and per capita personal health care expenditures and percent distribution by source of funds, 1960 to 2002)

	total personal health care expenditures (billions)	per capita personal health care expenditures	percent distribution by source of payment				
						government	
			total	out-of-pocket	private health insurance	federal	state and local
2002	$1,340.2	$4,695	100.0%	15.9%	35.8%	33.6%	10.6%
2001	1,231.4	4,352	100.0	16.3	35.5	33.5	10.4
2000	1,135.3	4,049	100.0	17.0	35.1	32.8	10.4
1999	1,065.0	3,835	100.0	17.3	34.4	32.6	10.3
1995	865.7	3,233	100.0	16.9	33.4	34.1	10.5
1990	609.4	2,398	100.0	22.5	33.4	28.6	10.5
1980	214.6	931	100.0	27.1	28.3	29.3	11.1
1970	63.2	301	100.0	39.7	22.3	22.9	12.3
1960	23.4	126	100.0	55.2	21.4	8.7	12.6

Note: Numbers will not add to total because other private funds are not shown.
Source: National Center for Health Statistics, Health, United States, 2004; Internet site http://www.cdc.gov/nchs/hus.htm

Table 6.5 Out-of-Pocket Payments for Personal Health Care Expenditures, 1960 to 2002

(total personal health care expenditures and percent paid out-of-pocket by type of expenditure, 1960 to 2002)

	total		hospital care		physician services		nursing home care		prescription drugs		other expenditures	
	amount (billions)	percent paid out-of-pocket	amount (billions)	percent paid out-of-pocket	amount (billions)	percent paid out-of-pocket	amount (billions)	percent paid out-of-pocket	amount (billions)	percent paid out-of-pocket	amount (billions)	percent paid out-of-pocket
2002	$1,340.2	15.9%	$486.5	3.0%	$339.5	10.1%	$103.2	25.1%	$162.4	29.9%	$248.6	35.8%
2001	1,231.4	16.3	444.3	2.9	315.1	10.5	99.1	26.9	140.8	30.2	232.0	36.7
2000	1,135.3	17.0	413.2	3.1	290.3	11.1	93.8	27.9	121.5	31.5	216.5	38.4
1999	1,065.0	17.3	393.5	3.2	270.9	11.7	89.6	28.1	104.4	32.9	206.6	39.1
1995	865.7	16.9	343.6	3.1	220.5	11.9	74.6	26.9	60.8	42.7	166.2	38.3
1990	609.4	22.5	253.9	4.4	157.5	19.3	52.7	37.5	40.3	59.1	104.9	49.6
1980	214.6	27.1	101.5	5.2	47.1	30.2	17.7	40.0	12.0	69.4	36.3	64.3
1970	63.2	39.7	27.6	9.1	14.0	46.1	4.2	53.6	5.5	82.4	11.9	78.6
1960	23.4	55.2	9.2	20.8	5.4	61.6	0.8	77.9	2.7	96.0	5.3	84.2

Note: Other expenditures include dental services, other professional services, home health care, nonprescription drugs and other medical nondurables, vision products and other medical durables.
Source: National Center for Health Statistics. Health, United States, 2004; Internet site http://www.cdc.gov/nchs/hus.htm

Table 6.6 Consumer Price Index for Health Care by Type of Product or Service, 2003

(consumer price index for all items, for major categories, and for components of medical care, 2003; 1982–84 = 100 unless otherwise noted)

	2003
All items	**184.0**
Food	180.0
Apparel	120.9
Housing	184.8
Energy	136.5
Medical care	297.1
Components of medical care	
Medical care services	306.0
Professional services	261.2
Physician services	267.7
Dental services	292.5
Eyeglasses and eyecare*	155.9
Services by other medical professionals*	177.1
Hospital and related services	394.8
Hospital services**	144.7
Inpatient hospital services**	140.1
Outpatient hospital services*	337.9
Nursing homes and adult day care	135.2
Medical care products	262.8
Prescription drugs and medical supplies	326.3
Nonprescription drugs and medical supplies*	152.0
Internal and respiratory over-the-counter drugs	181.2
Nonprescription medical equipment and supplies	178.1

* 1986 = 100
** 1996 = 100
Source: National Center for Health Statistics, **Health, United States, 2004***; Internet site http://www.cdc.gov/nchs/hus.htm*

Table 6.7 Health Care Spending by Country, 2001

(health care expenditures as a percent of gross domestic product, and per capita and indexed per capita health care expenditures, for the United States and selected countries, 2001)

	health care expenditures as a percent of GDP	per capita health care expenditures	indexed per capita health care expenditures
United States	**14.1%**	**$5,021**	**100**
Australia	9.2	2,513	50
Austria	7.7	2,191	44
Belgium	9.0	2,490	50
Canada	9.7	2,792	56
Czech Republic	7.3	1,106	22
Denmark	8.6	2,503	50
Finland	7.0	1,841	37
France	9.5	2,561	51
Germany	10.7	2,808	56
Greece	9.4	1,511	30
Hungary	6.8	911	18
Iceland	9.2	2,643	53
Ireland	6.5	1,935	39
Italy	8.4	2,212	44
Japan	8.0	2,131	42
Mexico	6.0	536	11
Netherlands	8.9	2,626	52
New Zealand	8.1	1,710	34
Norway	8.0	2,920	58
Poland	6.3	629	13
Portugal	9.2	1,613	32
Slovak Republic	5.7	682	14
Spain	7.5	1,600	32
Sweden	8.7	2,270	45
Switzerland	11.1	3,322	66
United Kingdom	7.6	1,992	40

Note: Per capita health expenditures for each country have been adjusted to U.S. dollars using gross domestic product purchasing power parities.
Source: National Center for Health Statistics, Health, United States, 2004; Internet site http://www.cdc.gov/nchs/hus.htm; calculations by New Strategist

Americans Are Less Likely to Have Employment-Based Health Insurance Coverage

The percentage of people under age 65 with employment-based coverage fell from 69 to 65 percent between 1984 and 2003.

In 2003, 60 percent of the U.S. population had health insurance through their or a family member's employer. Just 9 percent purchased health insurance on their own, down from 12 percent in 1994. One reason for the decline in private purchasing may be rising premiums, making private insurance increasingly unaffordable. The percentage of the population covered by the poverty-based Medicaid program grew from 8 to 12 percent between 1987 and 2003. Fourteen percent of the population is covered by Medicare, the government's health insurance program for people aged 65 or older. Sixteen percent of the population is without any type of health insurance, up from 13 percent in 1987.

The share of people under age 65 with employment-based health insurance coverage fell in nearly every age group between 1984 and 2002. The largest declines were among people aged 25 to 44, down more than 6 percentage points during those years.

People aged 18 to 24 are most likely to be without any type of health insurance, in part because many forego obtaining insurance since they do not yet feel vulnerable to health problems. A growing number of middle-aged and older adults are also without coverage. Between 1987 and 2003, the number of uninsured 45-to-54-year-olds more than doubled.

■ Rising health insurance premiums are forcing many businesses to ask their employees to contribute more toward the cost. Employees who cannot afford to pay more are dropping their coverage.

The ranks of the uninsured are growing

(percent of U.S. population without health insurance, by age, 1987 and 2003)

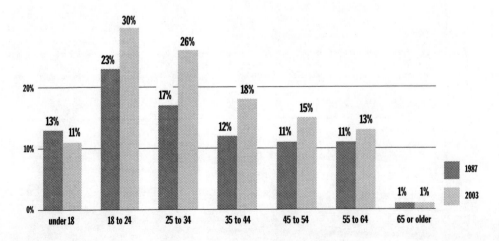

Table 6.8 Health Insurance Coverage by Type, 1987 to 2003

(number and percent distribution of people by health insurance coverage status, 1987 to 2003; numbers in thousands)

			covered by private or government health insurance							
			private health insurance			government health insurance				
	total people	total	total	employment based	direct purchase	total	Medicaid	Medicare	military	not covered
2003	288,280	243,320	197,869	174,020	26,486	76,755	35,647	39,456	9,979	44,961
2002	285,933	242,360	198,973	175,296	26,639	73,624	33,246	38,448	10,063	43,574
2001	282,082	240,875	199,860	176,551	26,057	71,295	31,601	38,043	9,552	41,207
2000	279,517	239,714	201,060	177,848	26,524	69,037	29,533	37,740	9,099	39,804
1999	276,804	236,576	198,841	175,101	27,415	67,683	28,506	36,923	8,648	40,228
1998	271,743	227,462	190,861	168,576	25,948	66,087	27,854	35,887	8,747	44,281
1997	269,094	225,646	188,532	165,091	27,158	66,685	28,956	35,590	8,527	43,448
1996	266,792	225,077	187,395	163,221	28,335	69,000	31,451	35,227	8,712	41,716
1995	264,314	223,733	185,881	161,453	30,188	69,776	31,877	34,655	9,375	40,582
1994	262,105	222,387	184,318	159,634	31,349	70,163	31,645	33,901	11,165	39,718
1993	259,753	220,040	182,351	148,318	–	68,554	31,749	33,097	9,560	39,713
1992	256,830	218,189	181,466	148,796	–	66,244	29,416	33,230	9,510	38,641
1991	251,447	216,003	181,375	150,077	–	63,882	26,880	32,907	9,820	35,445
1990	248,886	214,167	182,135	150,215	–	60,965	24,261	32,260	9,922	34,719
1989	246,191	212,807	183,610	151,644	–	57,382	21,185	31,495	9,870	33,385
1988	243,685	211,005	182,019	150,940	–	56,850	20,728	30,925	10,105	32,680
1987	241,187	210,161	182,160	149,739	–	56,282	20,211	30,458	10,542	31,026

Percent distribution

2003	100.0%	84.4%	68.6%	60.4%	9.2%	26.6%	12.4%	13.7%	3.5%	15.6%
2002	100.0	84.8	69.6	61.3	9.3	25.7	11.6	13.4	3.5	15.2
2001	100.0	85.4	70.9	62.6	9.2	25.3	11.2	13.5	3.4	14.6
2000	100.0	85.8	71.9	63.6	9.5	24.7	10.6	13.5	3.3	14.2
1999	100.0	85.5	71.8	63.3	9.9	24.5	10.3	13.3	3.1	14.5
1998	100.0	83.7	70.2	62.0	9.5	24.3	10.3	13.2	3.2	16.3
1997	100.0	83.9	70.1	61.4	10.1	24.8	10.8	13.2	3.2	16.1
1996	100.0	84.4	70.2	61.2	10.6	25.9	11.8	13.2	3.3	15.6
1995	100.0	84.6	70.3	61.1	11.4	26.4	12.1	13.1	3.5	15.4
1994	100.0	84.8	70.3	60.9	12.0	26.8	12.1	12.9	4.3	15.2
1993	100.0	84.7	70.2	57.1	–	26.4	12.2	12.7	3.7	15.3
1992	100.0	85.0	70.7	57.9	–	25.8	11.5	12.9	3.7	15.0
1991	100.0	85.9	72.1	59.7	–	25.4	10.7	13.1	3.9	14.1
1990	100.0	86.1	73.2	60.4	–	24.5	9.7	13.0	4.0	13.9
1989	100.0	86.4	74.6	61.6	–	23.3	8.6	12.8	4.0	13.6
1988	100.0	86.6	74.7	61.9	–	23.3	8.5	12.7	4.1	13.4
1987	100.0	87.1	75.5	62.1	–	23.3	8.4	12.6	4.4	12.9

Note: (–) means data not available.

Source: Bureau of the Census, Current Population Survey, Internet site http://www.census.gov/hhes/hlthins/historic/index.html

Table 6.9 People with Employment-Based Private Health Insurance by Age, 1984 and 2002

(percent of people under age 65 with employment-based private health insurance coverage, by age, 1984 and 2002; percentage point change, 1984–2002)

	2002	1984	percentage point change 1984–2002
Total with insurance	**65.2%**	**69.1%**	**–3.9**
Under age 18	60.5	66.5	–6.0
Aged 18 to 24	54.8	58.7	–3.9
Aged 25 to 34	64.6	71.2	–6.6
Aged 35 to 44	71.0	77.4	–6.4
Aged 45 to 54	72.9	74.6	–1.7
Aged 55 to 64	69.1	69.0	0.1

Note: Private insurance includes that obtained through a present or former employer, union, self-employment, or a professional association.
Source: National Center for Health Statistics, Health, United States, 2004; Internet site http://www.cdc.gov/nchs/hus.htm

Table 6.10 People without Health Insurance by Age, 1987 and 2003

(number and percent of people without health insurance coverage by age, 1987 and 2003; percent change in number and percentage point change in share, 1987–2003; numbers in thousands)

	2003	1987	percent change 1987–2003
Number without coverage	**44,961**	**31,026**	**44.9%**
Under age 18	8,373	8,193	2.2
Aged 18 to 24	8,414	6,108	37.8
Aged 25 to 34	10,345	7,308	41.6
Aged 35 to 44	7,885	4,135	90.7
Aged 45 to 54	5,961	2,695	121.2
Aged 55 to 64	3,696	2,281	62.0
Aged 65 or older	286	306	–6.5
			percentage point change 1987–2003
Percent without coverage	**15.6%**	**12.9%**	**2.7**
Under age 18	11.4	12.9	–1.5
Aged 18 to 24	30.2	23.4	6.8
Aged 25 to 34	26.4	17.0	9.4
Aged 35 to 44	18.1	11.9	6.2
Aged 45 to 54	14.5	11.3	3.2
Aged 55 to 64	13.0	10.5	2.5
Aged 65 or older	0.8	1.1	–0.2

Source: Bureau of the Census, Internet site http://www.census.gov/hhes/hlthins/historic/index.html; calculations by New Strategist

Hispanics Are Most Likely to Be Uninsured

Many do not have access to employment-based health care coverage.

Most working-age Americans have health insurance through an employer. Among people aged 18 to 24, however, only 48 percent have employment-based coverage. Fully 30 percent of 18-to-24-year-olds have no health insurance coverage. People aged 25 to 34 account for the largest share of the uninsured—23 percent in 2003.

Females are slightly more likely than males to be covered under a government health insurance program. Women tend to have lower incomes, which is one reason for their greater participation in the Medicaid program. But women also make up the majority of older adults, and are therefore more likely to be covered by Medicare.

The biggest differences in health insurance coverage are by race and Hispanic origin. Blacks and Hispanics are much less likely than Asians and non-Hispanic whites to have employer-provided health insurance. One reason for the disparity is that many blacks and Hispanics work in service industries, where health insurance is less likely to be offered. Hispanics are particularly unlikely to have any type of health insurance, one-third being uninsured.

■ As Hispanic immigrants become acculturated and move into the middle class, the percentage of those covered by health insurance is likely to increase.

Fewer than half of Hispanics have employment-based coverage

(percent of population with employment-based health insurance, by race and Hispanic origin, 2003)

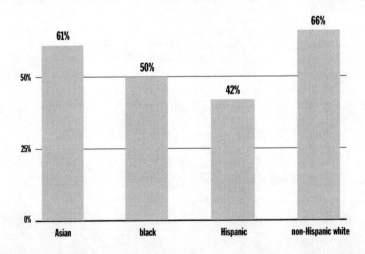

Table 6.11 Health Insurance Coverage by Age, 2003

(number and percent distribution of people by age and health insurance coverage status, 2003; numbers in thousands)

		covered by private or government health insurance								
		private health insurance				**government health insurance**				
	total	total	total	employment based	direct purchase	total	Medicaid	Medicare	military	not covered
Total people	288,280	243,320	197,869	174,020	26,486	76,755	35,647	39,456	9,979	44,961
Under age 18	73,580	65,207	48,475	45,004	3,893	21,389	19,392	483	2,021	8,373
Aged 18–24	27,824	19,410	16,526	13,434	1,596	3,929	3,016	176	902	8,414
Aged 25–34	39,201	28,856	25,606	23,946	2,058	4,210	3,073	538	898	10,345
Aged 35–44	43,573	35,688	32,533	30,386	2,793	4,420	2,860	940	1,111	7,885
Aged 45–54	41,068	35,108	32,000	29,722	3,198	4,569	2,359	1,569	1,369	5,961
Aged 55–64	28,375	24,679	21,569	19,324	2,987	4,893	1,757	2,494	1,471	3,696
Aged 65+	34,659	34,373	21,159	12,204	9,962	33,345	3,190	33,257	2,206	286

Percent distribution by coverage status

Total people	100.0%	84.4%	68.6%	60.4%	9.2%	26.6%	12.4%	13.7%	3.5%	15.6%
Under age 18	100.0	88.6	65.9	61.2	5.3	29.1	26.4	0.7	2.7	11.4
Aged 18–24	100.0	69.8	59.4	48.3	5.7	14.1	10.8	0.6	3.2	30.2
Aged 25–34	100.0	73.6	65.3	61.1	5.2	10.7	7.8	1.4	2.3	26.4
Aged 35–44	100.0	81.9	74.7	69.7	6.4	10.1	6.6	2.2	2.5	18.1
Aged 45–54	100.0	85.5	77.9	72.4	7.8	11.1	5.7	3.8	3.3	14.5
Aged 55–64	100.0	87.0	76.0	68.1	10.5	17.2	6.2	8.8	5.2	13.0
Aged 65+	100.0	99.2	61.0	35.2	28.7	96.2	9.2	96.0	6.4	0.8

Percent distribution by age

Total people	100.0%	100.0%	100.0%	100.0%	100.0%	100.0%	100.0%	100.0%	100.0%	100.0%
Under age 18	25.5	26.8	24.5	25.9	14.7	27.9	54.4	1.2	20.3	18.6
Aged 18–24	9.7	8.0	8.4	7.7	6.0	5.1	8.5	0.4	9.0	18.7
Aged 25–34	13.6	11.9	12.9	13.8	7.8	5.5	8.6	1.4	9.0	23.0
Aged 35–44	15.1	14.7	16.4	17.5	10.5	5.8	8.0	2.4	11.1	17.5
Aged 45–54	14.2	14.4	16.2	17.1	12.1	6.0	6.6	4.0	13.7	13.3
Aged 55–64	9.8	10.1	10.9	11.1	11.3	6.4	4.9	6.3	14.7	8.2
Aged 65+	12.0	14.1	10.7	7.0	37.6	43.4	8.9	84.3	22.1	0.6

Note: Numbers may not add to total because some people have more than one type of health insurance coverage.
Source: Bureau of the Census, 2004 Current Population Survey, Internet site http://www.census.gov/hhes/hlthins/historic/index. html; calculations by New Strategist

Table 6.12 Health Insurance Coverage by Sex, 2003

(number and percent distribution of people by sex and health insurance coverage status, 2003; numbers in thousands)

			covered by private or government health insurance							
			private health insurance			government health insurance				not covered
	total	total	total	employment based	direct purchase	total	Medicaid	Medicare	military	
Total people	**288,280**	**243,320**	**197,869**	**174,020**	**26,486**	**76,755**	**35,647**	**39,456**	**9,979**	**44,961**
Females	147,053	125,880	100,892	87,541	14,327	42,059	19,706	22,125	4,624	21,173
Males	141,227	117,440	96,977	86,479	12,159	34,695	15,941	17,330	5,356	23,788

Percent distribution by coverage status

Total people	**100.0%**	**84.4%**	**68.6%**	**60.4%**	**9.2%**	**26.6%**	**12.4%**	**13.7%**	**3.5%**	**15.6%**
Females	100.0	85.6	68.6	59.5	9.7	28.6	13.4	15.0	3.1	14.4
Males	100.0	83.2	68.7	61.2	8.6	24.6	11.3	12.3	3.8	16.8

Percent distribution by sex

Total people	**100.0%**	**100.0%**	**100.0%**	**100.0%**	**100.0%**	**100.0%**	**100.0%**	**100.0%**	**100.0%**	**100.0%**
Females	51.0	51.7	51.0	50.3	54.1	54.8	55.3	56.1	46.3	47.1
Males	49.0	48.3	49.0	49.7	45.9	45.2	44.7	43.9	53.7	52.9

Note: Numbers may not add to total because some people have more than one type of health insurance coverage.
Source: Bureau of the Census, 2004 Current Population Survey, Internet site http://www.census.gov/hhes/hlthins/historic/index.html; calculations by New Strategist

Table 6.13 Health Insurance Coverage by Race and Hispanic Origin, 2003

(number and percent distribution of people by race, Hispanic origin, and health insurance coverage status, 2003; numbers in thousands)

		covered by private or government health insurance								
		private health insurance			government health insurance					
	total	total	total	employment based	direct purchase	total	Medicaid	Medicare	military	not covered
Total people	288,280	243,320	197,869	174,020	26,486	76,755	35,647	39,456	9,979	44,961
Asian	12,905	10,504	8,826	7,829	1,159	2,478	1,385	1,096	355	2,401
Black	37,651	30,344	20,136	18,669	1,732	13,195	9,292	4,080	1,283	7,307
Hispanic	40,425	27,188	18,183	16,788	1,551	10,716	8,505	2,462	639	13,237
Non-Hispanic white	194,877	173,295	149,084	129,261	21,865	49,743	16,247	31,458	7,563	21,582

Percent distribution by coverage status

Total people	100.0%	84.4%	68.6%	60.4%	9.2%	26.6%	12.4%	13.7%	3.5%	15.6%
Asian	100.0	81.4	68.4	60.7	9.0	19.2	10.7	8.5	2.8	18.6
Black	100.0	80.6	53.5	49.6	4.6	35.0	24.7	10.8	3.4	19.4
Hispanic	100.0	67.3	45.0	41.5	3.8	26.5	21.0	6.1	1.6	32.7
Non-Hispanic white	100.0	88.9	76.5	66.3	11.2	25.5	8.3	16.1	3.9	11.1

Percent distribution by race and Hispanic origin

Total people	100.0%	100.0%	100.0%	100.0%	100.0%	100.0%	100.0%	100.0%	100.0%	100.0%
Asian	4.5	4.3	4.5	4.5	4.4	3.2	3.9	2.8	3.6	5.3
Black	13.1	12.5	10.2	10.7	6.5	17.2	26.1	10.3	12.9	16.3
Hispanic	14.0	11.2	9.2	9.6	5.9	14.0	23.9	6.2	6.4	29.4
Non-Hispanic white	67.6	71.2	75.3	74.3	82.6	64.8	45.6	79.7	75.8	48.0

Note: Numbers by race and Hispanic origin may not sum to total because not all races are shown, Hispanics may be of any race, and some people have more than one type of health insurance coverage.
Source: Bureau of the Census, 2004 Current Population Survey, Internet site http://www.census.gov/hhes/hlthins/historic/index. html; calculations by New Strategist

Cost Is the Primary Reason for Being Uninsured

Employment-related reasons rank second as a cause.

The number-one reason given by the uninsured for their lack of coverage is cost, cited by 53 percent. Some of the uninsured do not have access to insurance through an employer and are ineligible for other programs, such as Medicaid or Medicare. They must purchase an individual health insurance policy or go without. Since individual policies do not benefit from the lower premiums available to groups of insured people, the cost can be prohibitive. For other uninsured, employer-provided health insurance is available, but the contribution required of the employee is out of their reach.

Forty-five percent of people without insurance cite employment-related reasons for their lack of coverage. Thirty percent say they have no health insurance because of a job loss or change in employment. Fifteen percent say their company does not offer insurance or refuses to cover them.

■ As health insurance costs rise, a growing share of Americans will be without insurance.

Job loss is an important reason why people aged 18 to 64 are without health insurance

*(percent of uninsured who do not have health insurance because of
a job loss or change in employment, by age, 2002)*

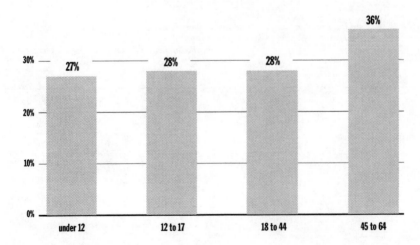

Table 6.14   Reason for Lack of Health Insurance Coverage, 2002

(number of people under age 65 without health insurance and percent distribution by reason for lack of coverage, by selected characteristics, 2002; numbers in thousands)

	total		cost	lost job or change in employment	employer didn't offer or company refused	Medicaid stopped	ineligible due to age or left school	change in marital status or death of parent	other
	number	percent							
Total < 65 withou health insurance	**40,127**	**100.0%**	**52.7%**	**29.7%**	**15.1%**	**8.7%**	**7.6%**	**3.1%**	**6.9%**
Sex									
Female	18,475	100.0	52.9	29.5	12.2	12.1	5.2	4.1	7.2
Male	21,652	100.0	53.8	30.3	15.7	7.1	6.2	2.2	7.4
Age									
Under age 12	4,842	100.0	51.6	27.0	7.5	16.6	0.7	2.0	10.2
Aged 12 to 17	2,940	100.0	55.4	27.6	7.1	11.8	2.2	2.5	8.5
Aged 18 to 44	23,962	100.0	50.6	28.3	16.6	8.5	11.7	2.7	6.4
Aged 45 to 64	8,383	100.0	58.9	35.9	17.5	3.9	0.6	4.8	6.4
Race and Hispanic origin									
Asian	1,706	100.0	50.7	20.5	13.7	7.1	6.3	0.8	14.8
Black	5,796	100.0	47.6	32.1	12.1	14.5	6.3	2.7	5.5
Hispanic	10,872	100.0	58.3	19.9	16.8	10.1	2.2	1.5	9.3
Non-Hispanic white	20,699	100.0	52.1	36.2	13.3	6.9	7.6	4.4	5.9
Education									
Less than high school	6,676	100.0	59.5	24.8	19.1	8.4	1.0	2.9	7.2
High school graduate	7,954	100.0	55.9	36.4	16.8	6.1	1.8	4.5	5.7
Some college	5,700	100.0	53.0	41.7	18.3	5.9	3.3	5.0	5.7
College graduate	2,792	100.0	51.6	39.2	16.4	2.1	5.4	3.4	9.3
Household income									
Less than $20,000	10,835	100.0	52.9	24.0	14.7	15.4	5.7	3.0	7.8
$20,000 to $34,999	8,026	100.0	55.1	32.7	14.3	8.6	4.1	3.0	5.5
$35,000 to $54,999	5,943	100.0	52.8	37.4	12.3	5.7	5.9	3.2	7.0
$55,000 to $74,999	2,538	100.0	47.4	43.4	15.0	4.5	6.3	2.8	7.6
$75,000 or more	2,255	100.0	43.4	42.0	11.9	3.7	10.7	2.2	8.2

Note: Numbers may not sum to total because people can report more than one reason. Other includes moved, self-employed, never had coverage, did not want or need coverage, and other unspecified reasons.
Source: National Center for Health Statistics, Summary Health Statistics for the U.S. Population: National Health Interview Survey, 2002, *Vital and Health Statistics, Series 10, No. 220, 2004; Internet site http://www.cdc.gov/nchs/nhis.htm*

Most Children Get Health Insurance through a Family Member's Employment

More than one-quarter, however, are insured through Medicaid.

Like their parents, children are most likely to be covered by employment-based health insurance policies. But more than one in four children is covered through Medicaid, the health insurance program for the poor. Medicaid coverage is much greater for blacks and Hispanics than it is for non-Hispanic whites. Among black children, 44 percent have health insurance through Medicaid, as do 40 percent of Hispanic children. Fewer than half of black or Hispanic children are covered by employment-based insurance.

Eleven percent of children under age 18 had no health insurance coverage in 2003. Among Hispanics, the figure is a much higher 21 percent. Sixteen percent of American Indian children are without health insurance, as are 14 percent of black children. Many black and Hispanic parents work for employers who do not provide health insurance coverage.

■ Without Medicaid, a large proportion of the nation's children would be unable to obtain necessary medical care.

Only 7 percent of non-Hispanic white children are without health insurance

(percent of children without health insurance, by race and Hispanic origin, 2003)

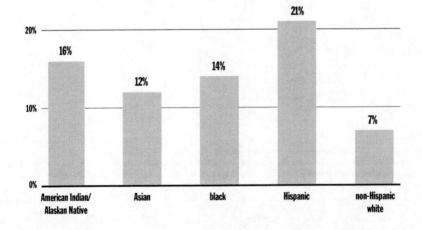

Table 6.15 Health Insurance Coverage of Children, 2003

(number and percent distribution of children under age 18 by selected characteristics and health insurance coverage status, 2003; numbers in thousands)

	total	covered by private or government health insurance	private health insurance			government health insurance				not covered
		total	total	employment based	direct purchase	total	Medicaid	Medicare	military	
Total children	73,580	65,207	48,475	45,004	3,893	21,389	19,392	483	2,021	8,373
Age										
Under age 3	11,451	10,253	6,879	6,508	533	4,117	3,762	113	348	1,197
Aged 3 to 5	12,383	11,131	7,900	7,456	609	4,071	3,728	103	333	1,252
Aged 6 to 11	23,921	21,288	15,848	14,903	1,263	6,892	6,281	147	610	2,633
Aged 12 to 17	25,826	22,535	17,848	16,137	1,487	6,309	5,620	120	730	3,290
Race and Hispanic origin										
American Indian and Alaskan Native	1,653	1,387	811	756	70	719	661	25	53	266
Asian	3,632	3,208	2,586	2,360	268	836	723	34	105	424
Black	12,363	10,636	5,879	5,550	359	5,775	5,417	167	362	1,727
Hispanic	13,854	10,944	5,824	5,483	389	5,817	5,585	120	190	2,911
Non-Hispanic white	43,432	40,222	33,989	31,422	2,861	8,917	7,637	165	1,351	3,210
Family income										
Less than $25,000	16,828	13,753	4,166	3,525	515	10,785	10,452	255	326	3,075
$25,000 to $49,999	18,520	15,878	11,371	10,434	974	6,069	5,494	143	584	2,642
$50,000 to $74,999	14,182	13,008	11,669	10,949	890	2,182	1,759	41	427	1,174
$75,000 or more	22,601	21,487	20,692	19,585	1,487	1,767	1,133	29	657	1,114
Family status										
In families	72,131	64,126	47,899	44,493	3,866	20,804	18,838	469	1,994	8,005
Married-couple families	51,189	46,388	38,754	36,451	3,114	10,661	9,035	221	1,677	4,801
Female householder, no spouse present	17,069	14,639	7,165	6,317	520	8,779	8,509	211	249	2,431
Male householder, no spouse present	3,872	3,099	1,979	1,725	231	1,364	1,293	36	68	773
Family reference person work status										
Worked during year	58,081	52,334	41,831	39,032	3,241	14,245	12,704	319	1,561	5,747
Full-time	49,288	44,480	36,517	34,311	2,634	11,150	9,812	279	1,335	4,807
Part-time	8,794	7,854	5,314	4,721	607	3,095	2,892	41	226	940
Did not work	14,049	11,792	6,067	5,461	625	6,559	6,133	149	433	2,257
Nativity										
Native	70,483	63,249	47,233	43,861	3,781	20,525	18,563	464	1,991	7,234
Foreign born	3,098	1,958	1,242	1,143	112	864	830	19	30	1,139
Naturalized citizen	452	386	310	283	29	107	92	2	15	66
Not a citizen	2,645	1,572	932	861	83	757	738	17	15	1,073

(continued)

| | | covered by private or government health insurance | | | | | | | | |
| | | | private health insurance | | | government health insurance | | | | |
	total	total	total	employment based	direct purchase	total	Medicaid	Medicare	military	not covered
PERCENT DISTRIBUTION										
Total children	**100.0%**	**88.6%**	**65.9%**	**61.2%**	**5.3%**	**29.1%**	**26.4%**	**0.7%**	**2.7%**	**11.4%**
Age										
Under age 3	100.0	89.5	60.1	56.8	4.7	36.0	32.9	1.0	3.0	10.5
Aged 3 to 5	100.0	89.9	63.8	60.2	4.9	32.9	30.1	0.8	2.7	10.1
Aged 6 to 11	100.0	89.0	66.3	62.3	5.3	28.8	26.3	0.6	2.6	11.0
Aged 12 to 17	100.0	87.3	69.1	62.5	5.8	24.4	21.8	0.5	2.8	12.7
Race and Hispanic origin										
American Indian and Alaskan Native	100.0	83.9	49.1	45.7	4.2	43.5	40.0	1.5	3.2	16.1
Asian	100.0	88.3	71.2	65.0	7.4	23.0	19.9	0.9	2.9	11.7
Black	100.0	86.0	47.6	44.9	2.9	46.7	43.8	1.4	2.9	14.0
Hispanic	100.0	79.0	42.0	39.6	2.8	42.0	40.3	0.9	1.4	21.0
Non-Hispanic white	100.0	92.6	78.3	72.3	6.6	20.5	17.6	0.4	3.1	7.4
Family income										
Less than $25,000	100.0	81.7	24.8	20.9	3.1	64.1	62.1	1.5	1.9	18.3
$25,000 to $49,999	100.0	85.7	61.4	56.3	5.3	32.8	29.7	0.8	3.2	14.3
$50,000 to $74,999	100.0	91.7	82.3	77.2	6.3	15.4	12.4	0.3	3.0	8.3
$75,000 or more	100.0	95.1	91.6	86.7	6.6	7.8	5.0	0.1	2.9	4.9
Family status										
In families	100.0	88.9	66.4	61.7	5.4	28.8	26.1	0.7	2.8	11.1
Married-couple families	100.0	90.6	75.7	71.2	6.1	20.8	17.7	0.4	3.3	9.4
Female householder, no spouse present	100.0	85.8	42.0	37.0	3.0	51.4	49.9	1.2	1.5	14.2
Male householder, no spouse present	100.0	80.0	51.1	44.6	6.0	35.2	33.4	0.9	1.8	20.0
Family reference person work status										
Worked during year	100.0	90.1	72.0	67.2	5.6	24.5	21.9	0.5	2.7	9.9
Full-time	100.0	90.2	74.1	69.6	5.3	22.6	19.9	0.6	2.7	9.8
Part-time	100.0	89.3	60.4	53.7	6.9	35.2	32.9	0.5	2.6	10.7
Did not work	100.0	83.9	43.2	38.9	4.4	46.7	43.7	1.1	3.1	16.1
Nativity										
Native	100.0	89.7	67.0	62.2	5.4	29.1	26.3	0.7	2.8	10.3
Foreign born	100.0	63.2	40.1	36.9	3.6	27.9	26.8	0.6	1.0	36.8
Naturalized citizen	100.0	85.4	68.6	62.6	6.4	23.7	20.4	0.4	3.3	14.6
Not a citizen	100.0	59.4	35.2	32.6	3.1	28.6	27.9	0.6	0.6	40.6

Source: Bureau of the Census, Current Population Survey, 2004 Annual Social and Economic Supplement; Internet site http://ferret. bls.census.gov/macro/032004/health/h08_000.htm

Table 6.16 Children without Health Insurance, 2003

(number and percent distribution of children under age 18 without health insurance by selected characteristics, 2003; numbers in thousands)

	number	percent of total children	percent distribution
Children without health insurance	**8,373**	**11.4%**	**100.0%**
Age			
Under age 3	1,197	10.5	14.3
Aged 3 to 5	1,252	10.1	15.0
Aged 6 to 11	2,633	11.0	31.4
Aged 12 to 17	3,290	12.7	39.3
Race and Hispanic origin			
American Indian, Alaskan Native	266	16.1	3.2
Asian	424	11.7	5.1
Black	1,727	14.0	20.6
Hispanic	2,911	21.0	34.8
Non-Hispanic white	3,210	7.4	38.3
Family income			
Less than $25,000	3,075	18.3	36.7
$25,000 to $49,999	2,642	14.3	31.6
$50,000 to $74,999	1,174	8.3	14.0
$75,000 or more	1,114	4.9	13.3
Family status			
In families	8,005	11.1	95.6
Married couple families	4,801	9.4	57.3
Female householder, no spouse present	2,431	14.2	29.0
Male householder, no spouse present	773	20.0	9.2
Family reference person work status			
Worked during year	5,747	9.9	68.6
Full-time	4,807	9.8	57.4
Part-time	940	10.7	11.2
Did not work	2,257	16.1	27.0
Nativity			
Native	7,234	10.3	86.4
Foreign born	1,139	36.8	13.6
Naturalized citizen	66	14.6	0.8
Not a citizen	1,073	40.6	12.8

Source: Bureau of the Census, Current Population Survey, 2004 Annual Social and Economic Supplement; Internet site http://ferret. bls.census.gov/macro/032004/health/h08_000.htm; calculations by New Strategist

Service Workers Are Least Likely to Have Health Insurance

Union members are more likely than nonunion workers to have health insurance.

A sizable 69 percent of workers in private industry have access to medical insurance through their employer. Although more than three-quarters take advantage of this offering, one in four does not. This figure translates into employer-provided health insurance for only 53 percent of all workers in private industry.

The type of work people do influences the likelihood of being offered employment-based health insurance. Those in white- or blue-collar jobs are much more likely than service workers to have access to employer-provided health insurance. Union members are more likely than those who are not in unions to have access to health care benefits. Those in higher-wage jobs ($15 or more per hour) are more likely than lower-paid workers to be offered health insurance.

Three-quarters of workers with employer-provider health insurance must pay some of the cost for individual coverage, while 89 percent must contribute to the cost of family coverage. For individual coverage, workers are required to pay only 18 percent of the premium cost. For family coverage, they are required to pay a much higher 31 percent.

■ Although most workers can obtain health insurance through their employer, few retirees receive these benefits.

Fewer than half of workers in service occupations have access to employer-provided health insurance

(percent of private-industry workers with access to an employer-provided medical plan, by type of occupation, 2004)

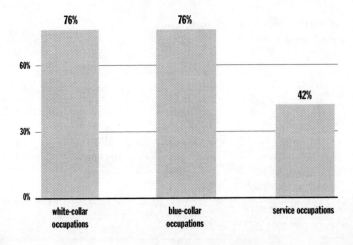

Table 6.17 Health Care Benefits in Private Industry, 2004

(percent of workers with access to and participating in health care benefits by selected characteristics and type of benefit, 2004)

	medical			dental			vision		
	access to	participate in	percent with access who participate	access to	participate in	percent with access who participate	access to	participate in	percent with access who participate
Total workers	**69%**	**53%**	**76.8%**	**46%**	**37%**	**80.4%**	**29%**	**22%**	**75.9%**
Worker characteristics									
White-collar occupations	76	59	77.6	53	43	81.1	33	25	75.8
Blue-collar occupations	76	60	78.9	47	40	85.1	29	25	86.2
Service occupations	42	24	57.1	25	16	64.0	18	11	61.1
Full time	84	66	78.6	56	46	82.1	35	27	77.1
Part time	20	11	55.0	13	8	61.5	8	6	75.0
Union	89	81	91.0	73	68	93.2	56	50	89.3
Nonunion	67	50	74.6	43	33	76.7	26	19	73.1
Average wage less than $15/hour	57	40	70.2	34	26	76.5	20	15	75.0
Average wage $15/hour or more	86	71	82.6	63	53	84.1	41	33	80.5
Establishment characteristics									
Goods producing	83	69	83.1	56	49	87.5	36	30	83.3
Service producing	65	48	73.8	43	33	76.7	27	20	74.1
Fewer than 100 workers	58	43	74.1	31	24	77.4	18	14	77.8
100 or more workers	82	64	78.0	64	52	81.3	42	32	76.2

Source: Bureau of Labor Statistics, National Compensation Survey, Employee Benefits in Private Industry, 2004; *Internet site http://www.bls.gov/ncs/ebs/home.htm; calculations by New Strategist*

Table 6.18 Employee Contributions for Health Care Coverage in Private Industry, 2004

(percent of workers participating in health care benefits who are required to pay for coverage, employee share of premiums, and average monthly contribution, by selected characteristics and single or family coverage, 2004)

	single coverage			family coverage		
	employee contribution required	employee share of premium	average flat monthly contribution	employee contribution required	employee share of premium	average flat monthly contribution
Total workers	**76%**	**18%**	**$67.57**	**89%**	**31%**	**$264.59**
Worker characteristics						
White-collar occupations	78	19	69.07	91	32	271.60
Blue-collar occupations	70	16	63.15	84	28	242.81
Service occupations	81	21	72.40	91	35	294.58
Full time	76	18	67.05	89	31	263.65
Part time	71	21	78.61	83	33	284.66
Union	57	11	56.53	67	17	195.12
Nonunion	79	20	68.98	93	33	273.51
Average wage less than $15/hour	79	20	70.27	92	34	275.81
Average wage $15/hour or more	73	17	65.22	86	28	255.05
Establishment characteristics						
Goods producing	74	16	59.89	85	26	221.25
Service producing	77	19	70.63	90	33	281.44
Fewer than 100 workers	67	18	74.02	87	36	307.78
100 or more workers	83	18	63.33	90	27	231.23

Source: Bureau of Labor Statistics, National Compensation Survey, Employee Benefits in Private Industry, 2004; *Internet site http://www.bls.gov/ncs/ebs/home.htm*

Table 6.19 Retiree Health Care Benefits in Private Industry, 2004

(percent of establishments offering health care benefits for all workers and for retirees, by selected characteristics, 2004)

	benefits for current workers	benefits for retirees	
		under 65	65 or older
Total establishments	**61**%	**5**%	**4**%
Goods producing	64	3	3
Service producing	61	5	4
Fewer than 100 workers	60	4	3
100 or more workers	96	13	12

Note: Health care benefits may include a medical plan or a separate dental, vision, or prescription drug plan.
Source: Bureau of Labor Statistics, National Compensation Survey, Employee Benefits in Private Industry, 2004; *Internet site http://www.bls.gov/ncs/ebs/home.htm*

Health Care Spending Rises with Age

The oldest householders spend 60 percent more than the average household on out-of-pocket health care costs.

American households spent $2,416 in 2003 on out-of-pocket health care costs. But costs rise with age, with the youngest householders spending an average of $546, while the oldest spend $3,856. On some health care categories, the disparity is even greater. Younger householders spend only 16 percent as much as the average household on prescription drugs, for example, while the oldest spend more than twice the average on this item.

In the aggregate, households spent $279 billion out-of-pocket on health care in 2003. They spent $144 billion on health insurance premiums, $68 billion on medical services, $54 billion on drugs, and $12 billion on medical supplies. Householders aged 65 or older accounted for 31 percent of total out-of-pocket health care spending. They accounted for an even larger 42 percent of out-of-pocket spending on prescription drugs. Householders aged 45 to 54 accounted for 29 percent of out-of-pocket spending on lab tests and X-rays, a much greater share than the 12 percent accounted for by householders aged 65 or older.

■ Although virtually everyone aged 65 or older is covered by Medicare, older Americans still must pay a considerable amount out-of-pocket for health care. Many purchase supplemental insurance policies that add to their expenses.

Out-of-pocket health care spending surpasses $3,000 a year in the 55-or-older age groups

(average annual out-of-pocket spending by consumer units on health care, by age, 2003)

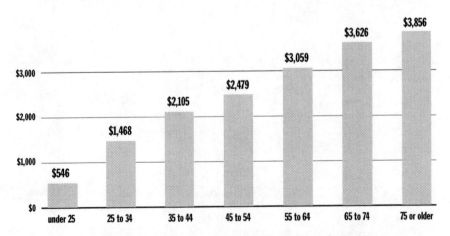

Table 6.20 Out-of-Pocket Spending on Health Care, 2003: Average Household Spending by Age of Householder

(average annual out-of-pocket spending of consumer units (CU) on health care, by age of consumer unit reference person, 2003)

	total consumer units	under 25	25 to 34	35 to 44	45 to 54	55 to 64	aged 65 or older total	65 to 74	75+
Number of consumer units (in thousands, add 000)	115,356	8,584	19,737	24,413	23,131	16,580	22,912	11,495	11,417
Average number of persons per CU	2.5	1.8	2.9	3.2	2.6	2.1	1.7	1.9	1.5
Average before-tax income of CU	$51,128.00	$20,680.00	$50,389.00	$61,091.00	$68,028.00	$58,672.00	$30,437.00	$35,314.00	$25,492.00
Average spending of CU, total	40,817.33	22,395.53	40,525.22	47,175.06	50,100.86	44,190.65	29,376.29	33,629.17	25,016.38
Health care, average spending	2,416.39	546.26	1,467.74	2,104.68	2,479.46	3,059.00	3,741.12	3,625.67	3,856.38
HEALTH INSURANCE	1,251.62	280.62	809.56	1,109.48	1,165.96	1,571.83	2,002.42	1,973.71	2,031.33
Commercial health insurance	249.19	77.76	195.08	307.16	294.30	382.86	156.01	179.51	132.35
Traditional fee-for-service health plan (not BCBS)	81.75	25.36	39.14	83.20	79.71	156.56	85.97	76.71	95.31
Preferred-provider health plan (not BCBS)	167.44	52.40	155.93	223.96	214.59	226.30	70.04	102.80	37.05
Blue Cross, Blue Shield	350.88	81.14	254.96	342.95	380.66	527.14	385.42	350.24	420.85
Traditional fee-for-service health plan	63.91	10.53	30.54	68.02	68.88	121.14	61.83	50.94	72.80
Preferred-provider health plan	124.05	32.11	114.32	129.94	151.13	218.59	64.88	68.88	60.84
Health maintenance organization	109.20	32.92	96.55	129.64	139.97	143.48	71.03	68.10	73.97
Commercial Medicare supplement	46.84	5.46	10.84	9.58	15.12	29.53	177.60	154.47	200.89
Other BCBS health insurance	6.88	0.11	2.71	5.77	5.56	14.40	10.09	7.85	12.35
Health maintenance plans (HMOs)	278.97	80.46	287.53	335.75	349.81	367.08	150.23	175.41	124.87
Medicare payments	215.02	9.89	20.14	35.91	53.80	137.09	869.74	859.04	880.52
Commercial Medicare supplements/ other health insurance	157.55	31.38	51.86	87.72	87.40	157.66	441.02	409.52	472.75
Commercial Medicare supplement (not BCBS)	102.12	14.30	25.90	36.07	34.64	68.25	363.70	325.70	401.96
Other health insurance (not BCBS)	55.43	17.07	25.96	51.65	52.76	89.41	77.32	83.81	70.79

(continued)

	total consumer units	under 25	25 to 34	35 to 44	45 to 54	55 to 64	aged 65 or older		
							total	65 to 74	75+
MEDICAL SERVICES	**$590.82**	**$128.54**	**$394.32**	**$597.84**	**$717.80**	**$742.05**	**$688.33**	**$681.34**	**$695.11**
Physician's services	143.63	41.43	126.67	148.97	182.64	193.74	115.20	132.01	98.28
Dental services	227.24	34.16	121.41	247.22	286.90	274.88	274.77	306.51	242.82
Eye care services	34.60	11.26	30.30	31.44	47.25	41.29	32.82	38.52	27.07
Service by professionals other than physicians	38.54	9.55	20.01	42.93	52.34	49.97	38.50	34.59	42.45
Lab tests, X-rays	28.93	4.18	21.40	35.56	42.04	38.70	17.34	21.13	13.52
Hospital room	26.06	5.45	20.74	24.16	26.00	43.92	27.54	36.05	18.97
Hospital services other than room	43.34	17.66	35.71	46.43	43.18	69.71	37.33	43.88	30.74
Care in convalescent or nursing home	32.80	1.63	2.69	8.32	21.43	13.24	122.13	40.81	204.00
Other medical services	14.40	3.20	15.40	12.82	16.03	16.59	16.19	17.11	15.27
DRUGS	**466.85**	**99.77**	**202.04**	**300.64**	**459.01**	**626.66**	**904.56**	**837.93**	**970.51**
Nonprescription drugs	70.30	33.82	55.03	65.73	67.11	78.46	100.95	108.47	92.91
Nonprescription vitamins	48.02	11.57	26.83	36.58	64.22	62.61	66.30	76.92	54.94
Prescription drugs	348.53	54.38	120.18	198.33	327.69	485.59	737.31	652.54	822.66
MEDICAL SUPPLIES	**107.10**	**37.33**	**61.82**	**96.72**	**136.69**	**118.46**	**145.80**	**132.68**	**159.42**
Eyeglasses and contact lenses	50.97	20.77	32.23	46.75	73.24	62.70	51.95	59.94	43.90
Hearing aids	14.40	2.70	3.21	8.99	15.57	11.86	34.86	16.06	53.79
Topicals and dressings	30.10	12.40	22.00	33.82	31.63	29.41	39.30	32.59	46.47
Medical equipment for general use	3.10	0.62	0.72	1.90	2.98	5.28	5.90	7.36	4.43
Supportive, convalescent medical equipment	5.25	0.55	2.27	3.00	7.23	5.31	9.92	13.64	6.18
Rental of medical equipment	2.13	0.15	0.80	1.11	4.67	2.58	2.21	2.44	1.98
Rental of supportive, convalescent medical equipment	1.15	0.14	0.59	1.15	1.37	1.32	1.66	0.64	2.68

Source: Bureau of Labor Statistics, unpublished data from the 2003 Consumer Expenditure Survey

Table 6.21 Out-of-Pocket Spending on Health Care, 2003: Indexed Household Spending by Age of Householder

(indexed average annual out-of-pocket spending of consumer units (CU) on health care, by age of consumer unit reference person, 2003; index definition: an index of 100 is the average for all consumer units; an index of 132 means that spending by consumer units in that group is 32 percent above the average for all consumer units; an index of 68 indicates spending that is 32 percent below the average for all consumer units)

	total consumer units	under 25	25 to 34	35 to 44	45 to 54	55 to 64	aged 65 or older total	65 to 74	75+
Average spending of CU, total	**$40,817**	**$22,396**	**$40,525**	**$47,175**	**$50,101**	**$44,191**	**$29,376**	**$33,629**	**$25,016**
Average spending of CU, index	**100**	**55**	**99**	**116**	**123**	**108**	**72**	**82**	**61**
Health care, indexed spending	**100**	**23**	**61**	**87**	**103**	**127**	**155**	**150**	**160**
HEALTH INSURANCE	**100**	**22**	**65**	**89**	**93**	**126**	**160**	**158**	**162**
Commercial health insurance	**100**	**31**	**78**	**123**	**118**	**154**	**63**	**72**	**53**
Traditional fee-for-service health plan (not BCBS)	100	31	48	102	98	192	105	94	117
Preferred-provider health plan (not BCBS)	100	31	93	134	128	135	42	61	22
Blue Cross, Blue Shield	**100**	**23**	**73**	**98**	**108**	**150**	**110**	**100**	**120**
Traditional fee-for-service health plan	100	16	48	106	108	190	97	80	114
Preferred-provider health plan	100	26	92	105	122	176	52	56	49
Health maintenance organization	100	30	88	119	128	131	65	62	68
Commercial Medicare supplement	100	12	23	20	32	63	379	330	429
Other BCBS health insurance	100	2	39	84	81	209	147	114	180
Health maintenance plans (HMOs)	**100**	**29**	**103**	**120**	**125**	**132**	**54**	**63**	**45**
Medicare payments	**100**	**5**	**9**	**17**	**25**	**64**	**404**	**400**	**410**
Commercial Medicare supplements/other health insurance	**100**	**20**	**33**	**56**	**55**	**100**	**280**	**260**	**300**
Commercial Medicare supplement (not BCBS)	100	14	25	35	34	67	356	319	394
Other health insurance (not BCBS)	100	31	47	93	95	161	139	151	128

(continued)

	total consumer units	under 25	25 to 34	35 to 44	45 to 54	55 to 64	total	65 to 74	75+
MEDICAL SERVICES	**100**	**22**	**67**	**101**	**121**	**126**	**117**	**115**	**118**
Physician's services	100	29	88	104	127	135	80	92	68
Dental services	100	15	53	109	126	121	121	135	107
Eye care services	100	33	88	91	137	119	95	111	78
Service by professionals other than physicians	100	25	52	111	136	130	100	90	110
Lab tests, X-rays	100	14	74	123	145	134	60	73	47
Hospital room	100	21	80	93	100	169	106	138	73
Hospital services other than room	100	41	82	107	100	161	86	101	71
Care in convalescent or nursing home	100	5	8	25	65	40	372	124	622
Other medical services	100	22	107	89	111	115	112	119	106
DRUGS	**100**	**21**	**43**	**64**	**98**	**134**	**194**	**179**	**208**
Nonprescription drugs	100	48	78	93	95	112	144	154	132
Nonprescription vitamins	100	24	56	76	134	130	138	160	114
Prescription drugs	100	16	34	57	94	139	212	187	236
MEDICAL SUPPLIES	**100**	**35**	**58**	**90**	**128**	**111**	**136**	**124**	**149**
Eyeglasses and contact lenses	100	41	63	92	144	123	102	118	86
Hearing aids	100	19	22	62	108	82	242	112	374
Topicals and dressings	100	41	73	112	105	98	131	108	154
Medical equipment for general use	100	20	23	61	96	170	190	237	143
Supportive, convalescent medical equipment	100	10	43	57	138	101	189	260	118
Rental of medical equipment	100	7	38	52	121	121	104	115	93
Rental of supportive, convalescent medical equipment	100	12	51	100	119	115	144	56	233

Source: Calculations by New Strategist based on the Bureau of Labor Statistics 2003 Consumer Expenditure Survey

Table 6.22 Out-of-Pocket Spending on Health Care, 2003: Total Spending by Age of Householder

(total annual out-of-pocket spending on health care, by consumer unit (CU) age groups, 2003; consumer units and dollars in thousands)

	total consumer units	under 25	25 to 34	35 to 44	45 to 54	55 to 64	aged 65 or older total	aged 65 or older 65 to 74	aged 65 or older 75+
Number of consumer units	115,356	8,584	19,737	24,413	23,131	16,580	22,912	11,495	11,417
Total spending of all CUs ($)	4,708,523,919	192,243,230	799,846,267	1,151,684,740	1,158,882,993	732,680,977	673,069,556	386,567,309	285,612,010
Health care, total spending	278,745,085	4,689,096	28,968,784	51,381,553	57,352,389	50,718,220	85,716,541	41,677,077	44,028,290
HEALTH INSURANCE	144,381,877	2,408,842	15,978,286	27,085,735	26,969,821	26,060,941	45,879,447	22,687,796	23,191,695
Commercial health insurance	28,745,562	667,492	3,850,294	7,498,697	6,807,453	6,347,819	3,574,501	2,063,467	1,511,040
Traditional fee-for-service health plan (not BCBS)	9,430,353	217,690	772,506	2,031,162	1,843,772	2,595,765	1,969,745	881,781	1,088,154
Preferred-provider health plan (not BCBS)	19,315,209	449,802	3,077,590	5,467,535	4,963,681	3,752,054	1,604,756	1,181,686	423,000
Blue Cross, Blue Shield	40,476,113	696,506	5,032,146	8,372,438	8,805,046	8,739,981	8,830,743	4,026,009	4,804,844
Traditional fee-for-service health plan	7,372,402	90,390	602,768	1,660,572	1,593,263	2,008,501	1,416,649	585,555	831,158
Preferred-provider health plan	14,309,912	275,632	2,256,334	3,172,225	3,495,788	3,624,222	1,486,531	791,776	694,610
Health maintenance organization	12,596,875	282,585	1,905,607	3,164,901	3,237,646	2,378,898	1,627,439	782,810	844,515
Commercial Medicare supplement	5,403,275	46,869	213,949	233,877	349,741	489,607	4,069,171	1,775,633	2,293,561
Other BCBS health insurance	793,649	944	53,487	140,863	128,608	238,752	231,182	90,236	141,000
Health maintenance plans (HMOs)	32,180,863	690,669	5,674,980	8,196,665	8,091,455	6,086,186	3,442,070	2,016,338	1,425,641
Medicare payments	24,803,847	84,896	397,503	876,671	1,244,448	2,272,952	19,927,483	9,874,665	10,052,897
Commercial Medicare supplements/ other health insurance	18,174,338	269,366	1,023,561	2,141,508	2,021,649	2,614,003	10,104,650	4,707,432	5,397,387
Commercial Medicare supplement (not BCBS)	11,780,155	122,751	511,188	880,577	801,258	1,131,585	8,333,094	3,743,922	4,589,177
Other health insurance (not BCBS)	6,394,183	146,529	512,373	1,260,931	1,220,392	1,482,418	1,771,556	963,396	808,209

(continued)

	total consumer units	under 25	25 to 34	35 to 44	45 to 54	55 to 64	aged 65 or older		
							total	65 to 74	75+
MEDICAL SERVICES	$68,154,632	$1,103,387	$7,782,694	$14,595,068	$16,603,432	$12,303,189	$15,771,017	$7,832,003	$7,936,071
Physician's services	16,568,582	355,635	2,500,086	3,636,805	4,224,646	3,212,209	2,639,462	1,517,455	1,122,063
Dental services	26,213,497	293,229	2,396,269	6,035,382	6,636,284	4,557,510	6,295,530	3,523,332	2,772,276
Eye care services	3,991,318	96,656	598,031	767,545	1,092,940	684,588	751,972	442,787	309,058
Service by professionals other than physicians	4,445,820	81,977	394,937	1,048,050	1,210,677	828,503	882,112	397,612	484,652
Lab tests, X-rays	3,337,249	35,881	422,372	868,126	972,427	641,646	397,294	242,889	154,358
Hospital room	3,006,177	46,783	409,345	589,818	601,406	728,194	630,996	414,395	216,580
Hospital services other than room	4,999,529	151,593	704,808	1,133,496	998,797	1,155,792	855,305	504,401	350,959
Care in convalescent or nursing home	3,783,677	13,992	53,093	203,116	495,697	219,519	2,798,243	469,111	2,329,068
Other medical services	1,661,126	27,469	303,950	312,975	370,790	275,062	370,945	196,679	174,338
DRUGS	53,853,949	856,426	3,987,663	7,339,524	10,617,360	10,390,023	20,725,279	9,632,005	11,080,313
Nonprescription drugs	8,109,527	290,311	1,086,127	1,604,666	1,552,321	1,300,867	2,312,966	1,246,863	1,060,753
Nonprescription vitamins	5,539,395	99,317	529,544	893,028	1,485,473	1,038,074	1,519,066	884,195	627,250
Prescription drugs	40,205,027	466,798	2,371,993	4,841,830	7,579,797	8,051,082	16,893,247	7,500,947	9,392,309
MEDICAL SUPPLIES	12,354,628	320,441	1,220,141	2,361,225	3,161,776	1,964,067	3,340,570	1,525,157	1,820,098
Eyeglasses and contact lenses	5,879,695	178,290	636,124	1,141,308	1,694,114	1,039,566	1,190,278	689,010	501,206
Hearing aids	1,661,126	23,177	63,356	219,473	360,150	196,639	798,712	184,610	614,120
Topicals and dressings	3,472,216	106,442	434,214	825,648	731,634	487,618	900,442	374,622	530,548
Medical equipment for general use	357,604	5,322	14,211	46,385	68,930	87,542	135,181	84,603	50,577
Supportive, convalescent medical equipment	605,619	4,721	44,803	73,239	167,237	88,040	227,287	156,792	70,557
Rental of medical equipment	245,708	1,288	15,790	27,098	108,022	42,776	50,636	28,048	22,606
Rental of supportive, convalescent medical equipment	132,659	1,202	11,645	28,075	31,689	21,886	38,034	7,357	30,598

Note: Numbers may not add to total because of rounding.
Source: Calculations by New Strategist based on the Bureau of Labor Statistics 2003 Consumer Expenditure Survey

Table 6.23 Out-of-Pocket Spending on Health Care, 2003: Market Shares by Age of Householder

(percentage of total annual out-of-pocket spending on health care accounted for by consumer unit age groups, 2003)

	total consumer units	under 25	25 to 34	35 to 44	45 to 54	55 to 64	aged 65 or older total	65 to 74	75+
Share of total consumer units	100.0%	7.4%	17.1%	21.2%	20.1%	14.4%	19.9%	10.0%	9.9%
Share of total spending	100.0	4.1	17.0	24.5	24.6	15.6	14.3	8.2	6.1
Health care, market shares	100.0	1.7	10.4	18.4	20.6	18.2	30.8	15.0	15.8
HEALTH INSURANCE	100.0	1.7	11.1	18.8	18.7	18.1	31.8	15.7	16.1
Commercial health insurance	100.0	2.3	13.4	26.1	23.7	22.1	12.4	7.2	5.3
Traditional fee-for-service health plan (not BCBS)	100.0	2.3	8.2	21.5	19.6	27.5	20.9	9.4	11.5
Preferred-provider health plan (not BCBS)	100.0	2.3	15.9	28.3	25.7	19.4	8.3	6.1	2.2
Blue Cross, Blue Shield	100.0	1.7	12.4	20.7	21.8	21.6	21.8	9.9	11.9
Traditional fee-for-service health plan	100.0	1.2	8.2	22.5	21.6	27.2	19.2	7.9	11.3
Preferred-provider health plan	100.0	1.9	15.8	22.2	24.4	25.3	10.4	5.5	4.9
Health maintenance organization	100.0	2.2	15.1	25.1	25.7	18.9	12.9	6.2	6.7
Commercial Medicare supplement	100.0	0.9	4.0	4.3	6.5	9.1	75.3	32.9	42.4
Other BCBS health insurance	100.0	0.1	6.7	17.7	16.2	30.1	29.1	11.4	17.8
Health maintenance plans (HMOs)	100.0	2.1	17.6	25.5	25.1	18.9	10.7	6.3	4.4
Medicare payments	100.0	0.3	1.6	3.5	5.0	9.2	80.3	39.8	40.5
Commercial Medicare supplements/other health insurance	100.0	1.5	5.6	11.8	11.1	14.4	55.6	25.9	29.7
Commercial Medicare supplement (not BCBS)	100.0	1.0	4.3	7.5	6.8	9.6	70.7	31.8	39.0
Other health insurance (not BCBS)	100.0	2.3	8.0	19.7	19.1	23.2	27.7	15.1	12.6

(continued)

	total consumer units	under 25	25 to 34	35 to 44	45 to 54	55 to 64	aged 65 or older		
							total	65 to 74	75+
MEDICAL SERVICES	100.0%	1.6%	11.4%	21.4%	24.4%	18.1%	23.1%	11.5%	11.6%
Physician's services	100.0	2.1	15.1	22.0	25.5	19.4	15.9	9.2	6.8
Dental services	100.0	1.1	9.1	23.0	25.3	17.4	24.0	13.4	10.6
Eye care services	100.0	2.4	15.0	19.2	27.4	17.2	18.8	11.1	7.7
Service by professionals other than physicians	100.0	1.8	8.9	23.6	27.2	18.6	19.8	8.9	10.9
Lab tests, X-rays	100.0	1.1	12.7	26.0	29.1	19.2	11.9	7.3	4.6
Hospital room	100.0	1.6	13.6	19.6	20.0	24.2	21.0	13.8	7.2
Hospital services other than room	100.0	3.0	14.1	22.7	20.0	23.1	17.1	10.1	7.0
Care in convalescent or nursing home	100.0	0.4	1.4	5.4	13.1	5.8	74.0	12.4	61.6
Other medical services	100.0	1.7	18.3	18.8	22.3	16.6	22.3	11.8	10.5
DRUGS	100.0	1.6	7.4	13.6	19.7	19.3	38.5	17.9	20.6
Nonprescription drugs	100.0	3.6	13.4	19.8	19.1	16.0	28.5	15.4	13.1
Nonprescription vitamins	100.0	1.8	9.6	16.1	26.8	18.7	27.4	16.0	11.3
Prescription drugs	100.0	1.2	5.9	12.0	18.9	20.0	42.0	18.7	23.4
MEDICAL SUPPLIES	100.0	2.6	9.9	19.1	25.6	15.9	27.0	12.3	14.7
Eyeglasses and contact lenses	100.0	3.0	10.8	19.4	28.8	17.7	20.2	11.7	8.5
Hearing aids	100.0	1.4	3.8	13.2	21.7	11.8	48.1	11.1	37.0
Topicals and dressings	100.0	3.1	12.5	23.8	21.1	14.0	25.9	10.8	15.3
Medical equipment for general use	100.0	1.5	4.0	13.0	19.3	24.5	37.8	23.7	14.1
Supportive, convalescent medical equipment	100.0	0.8	7.4	12.1	27.6	14.5	37.5	25.9	11.7
Rental of medical equipment	100.0	0.5	6.4	11.0	44.0	17.4	20.6	11.4	9.2
Rental of supportive, convalescent medical equipment	100.0	0.9	8.8	21.2	23.9	16.5	28.7	5.5	23.1

Note: Numbers may not add to total because of rounding.
Source: Calculations by New Strategist based on the Bureau of Labor Statistics 2003 Consumer Expenditure Survey

Nineteen Percent of Health Care Costs Are Paid for Out-of-Pocket

The out-of-pocket share is lowest for preschoolers and the elderly.

Eighty-five percent of Americans had health care expenses in 2002, totaling a median of $960, according to the federal government's Medical Expenditure Panel Survey. Average per person spending on health care was far higher than the median, at $3,302. The large difference between the median and the average indicates great variability in individual health care costs. Not surprisingly, as people get older, the cost of their health care rises sharply. For the 89 percent of children under age 6 with expenses, the median expenditure was just $384 in 2002. For the 96 percent of people aged 65 or older with expenses, the median was a much higher $3,540.

Overall, 19 percent of health care spending is paid for out-of-pocket. Private insurance covers 40 percent of costs, Medicare (the federal government's health insurance program for people aged 65 or older) covers 22 percent, and Medicaid (the federal government's health insurance program for the poor) covers 11 percent. For children under age 6, only 9 percent of health care costs are paid for out-of-pocket. Many states have health care programs that cover expenses for small children, such as vaccinations. People aged 65 or older pay for just 17 percent of their health care expenses out-of-pocket.

■ Among the uninsured, only 49 percent of health care costs are paid for out-of-pocket. The rest of the expense is shouldered by society as a whole.

Government insurance programs pay for one-third of health care expenses

(percent distribution of total health care expenses by source of payment, 2002)

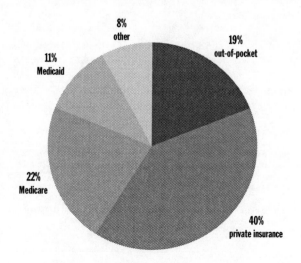

8%
other

19%
out-of-pocket

11%
Medicaid

22%
Medicare

40%
private insurance

Table 6.24 Total Spending on All Health Services by Selected Characteristics, 2002

(total number of people, percent with health care expense, median and average expense per person with expense, total health care expenses, and percent distribution of total expenses by source of payment, by selected characteristics, 2002)

All health services	total (thousands)	percent w/ expense	spending per person with expense		total expenses (millions)	percent distribution of total expenses by source of payment					
			median	average		total	out-of-pocket	private insurance	Medicare	Medicaid	other
Total people	**288,182**	**85.2%**	**$960**	**$3,302**	**$810,724**	**100.0%**	**19.1%**	**39.7%**	**22.0%**	**10.8%**	**8.3%**
Age											
Under age 65	251,926	83.6	766	2,557	538,458	100.0	20.3	52.2	5.0	13.7	8.9
Under age 6	23,292	88.8	384	1,364	28,204	100.0	9.1	47.5	0.3	36.1	6.9
Aged 6 to 17	49,455	83.6	401	1,228	50,786	100.0	25.6	44.2	0.3	23.3	6.6
Aged 18 to 44	111,219	78.5	738	2,233	195,017	100.0	20.7	52.1	4.0	14.6	8.6
Aged 45 to 64	67,960	90.0	1,710	4,321	264,451	100.0	20.2	54.3	7.1	8.7	9.7
Aged 65 or older	36,256	96.3	3,540	7,797	272,266	100.0	16.9	15.2	55.7	5.1	7.1
Sex											
Male	140,802	80.1	774	3,116	351,351	100.0	17.0	39.2	23.6	9.7	10.5
Female	147,380	90.1	1,138	3,461	459,373	100.0	20.8	40.2	20.8	11.7	6.6
Race and Hispanic origin											
Hispanic	39,665	70.7	460	2,223	62,330	100.0	16.3	28.1	14.2	28.5	12.9
Black, non-Hispanic	34,875	77.7	643	3,124	84,635	100.0	13.1	33.5	21.3	21.9	10.3
Asian, non-Hispanic	11,478	77.0	606	1,906	16,836	100.0	21.3	43.6	19.7	10.3	5.1
White/other, non-Hispanic	202,164	89.8	1,145	3,564	646,923	100.0	20.2	41.6	22.9	7.7	7.6
Health insurance: under age 65											
Any private	183,560	88.2	841	2,484	402,292	100.0	21.4	69.8	2.2	1.5	5.1
Public only	34,687	84.5	577	3,663	107,351	100.0	8.5	–	16.9	62.9	11.8
Uninsured	33,679	57.4	396	1,491	28,815	100.0	49.3	–	–	–	50.7
Health insurance: aged 65 or older											
Medicare only	10,540	95.1	3,303	7,090	71,059	100.0	21.4	–	63.9	–	14.8
Medicare/private	21,606	97.5	3,548	7,736	162,987	100.0	16.9	25.3	53.4	0.4	3.9
Medicare/other public	3,920	95.1	4,742	10,222	38,100	100.0	8.4	–	50.6	34.7	6.2
Income status											
Poor	35,618	78.3	823	3,811	106,314	100.0	13.3	12.4	26.3	37.0	11.0
Near poor	12,469	80.7	754	3,778	38,000	100.0	16.0	17.4	37.8	18.9	9.9
Low income	40,170	79.5	845	3,863	123,397	100.0	16.7	27.0	30.5	13.6	12.2
Middle income	91,063	84.5	838	3,089	237,792	100.0	19.3	44.3	20.4	8.5	7.5
High income	108,862	90.6	1,137	3,095	305,221	100.0	22.5	53.6	16.4	1.3	6.2

Note: Uninsured refers to people uninsured for the entire year. Tricare (armed-forces related coverage) is considered private insurance in these data. Other insurance includes Department of Veterans Affairs (except Tricare), American Indian Health Service, state and local clinics, worker's compensation, homeowner's and automobile insurance, etc. Poor refers to incomes below poverty level. Near poor encompasses incomes from poverty level through 125 percent of poverty level. Low income is more than 125 percent of poverty level through 200 percent of poverty level. Middle income is more than 200 percent of poverty level through 400 percent of poverty level. High income is more than 400 percent of poverty level. (–) means not applicable or sample too small to make a reliable estimate.

Source: Center for Financing, Access and Cost Trends, Agency for Healthcare Research and Quality: Medical Expenditure Panel Survey, 2002; Internet site http://www.meps.ahrq.gov/CompendiumTables/TC_TOC.htm

Insurance Covers Most of the Cost of Physician Visits

Older Americans pay the least out-of-pocket to see a doctor.

More than two-thirds of Americans went to the doctor in 2002, spending a median of $245 per person on physician visits. Sixteen percent of the cost of physician visits is paid for by individuals out-of-pocket. Private insurance covers 41 percent of the cost, while Medicare's share is 23 percent and Medicaid's 9 percent.

The oldest Americans are most likely to visit the doctor. Eighty-nine percent of people aged 65 or older visited a physician in 2002, spending a median of $575 per person on doctor visits during the year. Older Americans paid only 8 percent of the cost of their doctor visits out-of-pocket, compared with a 20 percent share paid for out-of-pocket by people under age 65.

Private health insurance covers 50 percent of the cost of physician visits for people under age 65, while Medicaid accounts for a 12 percent share. Among people aged 65 or older, Medicare covers 63 percent of the cost of their physician visits, while private health insurance accounts for a 19 percent share.

■ Health insurance coverage is not evolving as rapidly as the health care industry. Americans spend more on prescription drugs than on physician visits, but health insurance covers a much greater share of the cost of physician visits than prescription drugs.

People aged 18 to 44 are least likely to see a doctor

(percent of people with expenses for visiting a physician, by age, 2002)

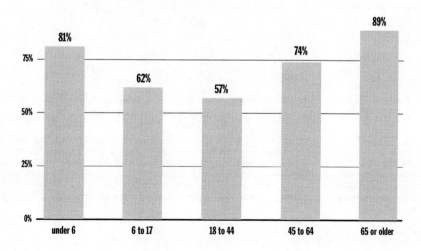

Table 6.25 Spending on Physician Visits by Selected Characteristics, 2002

(total number of people, percent with physician visit expense, median and average expense per person with expense, total physician visit expenses, and percent distribution of total expenses by source of payment, by selected characteristics, 2002)

Physician visits	total (thousands)	percent w/ expense	spending per person with expense median	spending per person with expense average	total expenses (millions)	total	percent distribution of total expenses by source of payment out-of-pocket	private insurance	Medicare	Medicaid	other
Total people	**288,182**	**67.8%**	**$245**	**$667**	**$130,330**	**100.0%**	**16.0%**	**40.7%**	**22.7%**	**9.4%**	**11.2%**
Age											
Under age 65	251,926	64.8	211	558	91,076	100.0	19.6	50.1	5.4	12.4	12.5
Under age 6	23,292	81.0	214	353	6,649	100.0	14.2	50.2	0.8	26.3	8.5
Aged 6 to 17	49,455	61.6	138	313	9,540	100.0	17.7	48.8	0.7	24.9	7.8
Aged 18 to 44	111,219	57.1	197	549	34,912	100.0	21.0	49.2	4.8	12.2	12.9
Aged 45 to 64	67,960	74.1	323	794	39,974	100.0	19.7	51.1	7.8	7.3	14.0
Aged 65 or older	36,256	88.9	575	1,218	39,254	100.0	7.7	18.8	62.8	2.4	8.2
Sex											
Male	140,802	60.9	216	622	53,321	100.0	14.8	40.3	22.2	8.4	14.4
Female	147,380	74.4	273	702	77,009	100.0	16.8	40.9	23.0	10.1	9.1
Race and Hispanic origin											
Hispanic	39,665	54.1	180	515	11,058	100.0	12.9	27.8	14.5	28.9	16.0
Black, non-Hispanic	34,875	59.3	188	601	12,426	100.0	9.7	31.5	20.8	23.0	15.0
Asian, non-Hispanic	11,478	59.0	188	587	3,976	100.0	13.6	44.6	24.0	10.7	7.1
White/other, non-Hispanic	202,164	72.5	270	702	102,870	100.0	17.2	43.0	23.8	5.6	10.4
Health insurance: under age 65											
Any private	183,560	69.6	217	543	69,420	100.0	21.5	65.7	2.0	1.0	9.8
Public only	34,687	68.0	222	722	17,025	100.0	5.0	–	20.5	62.5	12.0
Uninsured	33,679	35.1	140	392	4,630	100.0	44.7	–	–	–	55.4
Health insurance: aged 65 or older											
Medicare only	10,540	87.5	545	1,071	9,884	100.0	8.9	–	75.8	–	15.3
Medicare/private	21,606	90.6	596	1,294	25,327	100.0	7.8	29.2	57.4	0.1	5.5
Medicare/other public	3,920	86.5	559	1,190	4,033	100.0	3.4	–	65.6	23.1	7.8
Income status											
Poor	35,618	60.9	250	725	15,730	100.0	8.3	11.7	27.0	39.4	13.6
Near poor	12,469	64.7	220	736	5,937	100.0	12.5	17.0	39.1	21.0	10.4
Low income	40,170	62.7	251	721	18,145	100.0	11.0	27.5	33.3	15.2	13.1
Middle income	91,063	66.7	228	601	36,506	100.0	17.2	44.4	21.1	4.6	12.7
High income	108,862	73.3	259	677	54,012	100.0	19.5	53.5	17.2	0.8	9.0

Note: Uninsured refers to people uninsured for the entire year. Tricare (armed-forces related coverage) is considered private insurance in these data. Other insurance includes Department of Veterans Affairs (except Tricare), American Indian Health Service, state and local clinics, worker's compensation, homeowner's and automobile insurance, etc. Poor refers to incomes below poverty level. Near poor encompasses incomes from poverty level through 125 percent of poverty level. Low income is more than 125 percent of poverty level through 200 percent of poverty level. Middle income is more than 200 percent of poverty level through 400 percent of poverty level. High income is more than 400 percent of poverty level. (–) means not applicable or sample too small to make a reliable estimate.
Source: Center for Financing, Access and Cost Trends, Agency for Healthcare Research and Quality: Medical Expenditure Panel Survey, 2002; Internet site http://www.meps.ahrq.gov/CompendiumTables/TC_TOC.htm

Insurance Payments Cover Nearly All Hospital Inpatient Expenses

Few Americans could afford a hospital stay if they had to foot the bill.

Overall, 7.5 percent of the population had expenses for hospital inpatient stays in 2002, spending a median of $5,734 on this service. One of the primary purposes of health insurance is to cover potentially catastrophic costs that can arise from serious accidents or illnesses, typically the types of events associated with an inpatient hospital stay. Health insurance generally does its job well in these cases. Individuals pay only 2.5 percent of the costs of inpatient hospital stays out-of-pocket, with some form of insurance covering the remainder. Even those without health insurance do not pay the full costs of inpatient hospitalization. Their out-of-pocket share is just 15 percent.

Seventeen percent of the population used hospital outpatient services in 2002, spending a median of $582 on them. Individuals paid 6 percent of the costs of their hospital outpatient services out-of-pocket. The uninsured paid a 30 percent share out-of-pocket.

Thirteen percent of the population used emergency room services during 2002, spending a median of $377 on them. Eleven percent of emergency room costs were paid for out-of-pocket, with the uninsured paying a 52 percent share of their emergency room costs out-of-pocket.

■ Affordable "hospitalization only" health insurance policies could protect the uninsured from devastating medical bills and hospitals from losses when the uninsured are unable to pay.

The uninsured pay only a fraction of their bills

(percent of hospital inpatient, outpatient, and emergency room services paid for out-of-pocket by the uninsured, 2002)

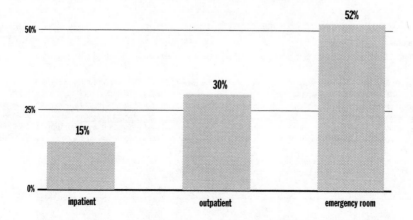

Tabel 6.26 Spending on Hospital Inpatient Services by Selected Characteristics, 2002

(total number of people, percent with hospital inpatient expense, median and average expense per person with expense, total hospital inpatient expenses, and percent distribution of total expenses by source of payment, by selected characteristics, 2002)

Hosptal inpatient services	total (thousands)	percent w/ expense	spending per person with expense — median	spending per person with expense — average	total expenses (millions)	percent distribution of total expenses by source of payment — total	out-of-pocket	private insurance	Medicare	Medicaid	other
Total people	288,182	7.5%	$5,734	$11,855	$256,059	100.0%	2.5%	38.9%	39.8%	10.4%	8.5%
Age											
Under age 65	251,926	5.7	5,154	10,219	146,554	100.0	3.4	60.2	9.2	17.1	10.1
Under age 6	23,292	4.4	2,718	12,721	12,981	100.0	1.3	46.5	0.1	45.2	6.9
Aged 6 to 17	49,455	2.0	4,634	7,480	7,441	100.0	4.5	54.0	0.3	30.0	11.3
Aged 18 to 44	111,219	6.2	4,807	7,608	52,052	100.0	4.6	58.9	6.4	21.7	8.5
Aged 45 to 64	67,960	8.1	6,497	13,508	74,080	100.0	2.9	64.1	13.7	7.6	11.8
Aged 65 or older	36,256	20.0	8,063	15,087	109,505	100.0	1.3	10.5	80.7	1.4	6.2
Sex											
Male	140,802	5.9	6,749	14,221	118,436	100.0	2.0	37.1	41.9	8.6	10.4
Female	147,380	9.0	5,440	10,371	137,622	100.0	2.9	40.5	38.0	11.9	6.7
Race and Hispanic origin											
Hispanic	39,665	5.2	4,431	9,850	20,314	100.0	4.0	29.0	23.7	27.4	16.0
Black, non-Hispanic	34,875	8.1	5,522	10,604	29,995	100.0	2.7	35.2	34.6	18.5	9.0
Asian, non-Hispanic	11,478	3.5	–	–	–	100.0	–	–	–	–	–
White/other, non-Hispanic	202,164	8.1	6,049	12,425	202,586	100.0	2.3	40.4	42.1	7.4	7.7
Health insurance: under age 65											
Any private	183,560	5.2	5,400	10,436	100,500	100.0	3.4	87.7	4.3	2.0	2.7
Public only	34,687	10.5	4,478	10,379	37,680	100.0	1.0	–	24.5	61.0	13.4
Uninsured	33,679	3.2	3,388	7,746	8,374	100.0	14.6	–	–	–	85.4
Health insurance: aged 65 or older											
Medicare only	10,540	21.8	7,383	13,913	31,973	100.0	1.7	–	83.5	–	14.8
Medicare/private	21,606	18.7	8,262	15,860	64,007	100.0	1.1	18.0	78.4	0.1	2.4
Medicare/other public	3,920	23.4	8,825	14,692	13,487	100.0	0.8	–	84.9	10.6	3.7
Income status											
Poor	35,618	10.5	5,290	10,847	40,656	100.0	2.9	16.8	41.1	29.3	9.8
Near poor	12,469	9.3	5,300	11,995	13,939	100.0	1.0	19.4	61.7	10.4	7.6
Low income	40,170	9.3	5,908	13,317	49,495	100.0	1.8	30.6	44.5	8.5	14.5
Middle income	91,063	7.0	5,705	11,935	76,544	100.0	2.5	44.8	37.0	10.2	5.5
High income	108,862	6.0	6,030	11,500	75,426	100.0	3.0	53.9	34.8	1.5	6.9

Note: Uninsured refers to people uninsured for the entire year. Tricare (armed-forces related coverage) is considered private insurance in these data. Other insurance includes Department of Veterans Affairs (except Tricare), American Indian Health Service, state and local clinics, worker's compensation, homeowner's and automobile insurance, etc. Poor refers to incomes below poverty level. Near poor encompasses incomes from poverty level through 125 percent of poverty level. Low income is more than 125 percent of poverty level through 200 percent of poverty level. Middle income is more than 200 percent of poverty level through 400 percent of poverty level. High income is more than 400 percent of poverty level. (–) means not applicable or sample too small to make a reliable estimate.

Source: Center for Financing, Access and Cost Trends, Agency for Healthcare Research and Quality: Medical Expenditure Panel Survey, 2002; Internet site http://www.meps.ahrq.gov/CompendiumTables/TC_TOC.htm

Table 6.27 Spending on Hospital Outpatient Services by Selected Characteristics, 2002

(total number of people, percent with hospital outpatient service expense, median and average expense per person with expense, total hospital outpatient service expenses, and percent distribution of total expenses by source of payment, by selected characteristics, 2002)

Hospital outpatient services	total (thousands)	percent w/ expense	spending per person with expense		total expenses (millions)	percent distribution of total expenses by source of payment					
			median	average		total	out-of-pocket	private insurance	Medicare	Medicaid	other
Total people	**288,182**	**16.7%**	**$582**	**$1,642**	**$78,915**	**100.0%**	**6.3%**	**58.2%**	**19.3%**	**6.4%**	**9.8%**
Age											
Under age 65	251,926	13.9	615	1,708	59,641	100.0	7.1	68.7	6.2	7.9	10.0
Under age 6	23,292	8.1	536	1,162	2,203	100.0	6.9	68.2	1.0	20.1	3.8
Aged 6 to 17	49,455	5.9	390	1,103	3,223	100.0	8.9	56.6	0.5	25.5	8.5
Aged 18 to 44	111,219	12.0	593	1,662	22,196	100.0	6.7	69.1	6.7	8.1	9.4
Aged 45 to 64	67,960	24.6	726	1,912	32,019	100.0	7.3	69.7	6.7	5.2	11.1
Aged 65 or older	36,256	36.2	509	1,467	19,275	100.0	3.7	25.6	60.0	1.6	9.0
Sex											
Male	140,802	13.0	722	1,833	33,528	100.0	5.3	57.1	20.8	5.0	11.7
Female	147,380	20.2	502	1,525	45,387	100.0	7.0	59.0	18.3	7.3	8.4
Race and Hispanic origin											
Hispanic	39,665	8.2	623	1,685	5,475	100.0	8.7	40.9	11.4	21.8	17.1
Black, non-Hispanic	34,875	11.9	556	2,060	8,567	100.0	3.4	50.1	20.2	15.5	10.7
Asian, non-Hispanic	11,478	9.3	321	1,312	1,402	100.0	7.6	79.6	6.7	1.5	4.5
White/other, non-Hispanic	202,164	19.6	586	1,604	63,472	100.0	6.5	60.3	20.2	3.9	9.2
Health insurance: under age 65											
Any private	183,560	15.5	650	1,743	49,478	100.0	6.4	82.9	3.0	1.0	6.7
Public only	34,687	13.2	502	1,744	7,974	100.0	5.4	–	27.9	52.6	14.1
Uninsured	33,679	5.8	325	1,199	2,189	100.0	29.7	–	–	–	70.3
Health insurance: aged 65 or older											
Medicare only	10,540	32.1	336	1,112	3,762	100.0	4.4	–	64.7	–	30.9
Medicare/private	21,606	39.2	572	1,619	13,723	100.0	3.7	36.0	57.3	0.1	2.9
Medicare/other public	3,920	32.6	417	1,393	1,780	100.0	2.7	–	71.6	15.9	9.7
Income status											
Poor	35,618	14.1	479	1,733	8,731	100.0	6.4	11.1	33.4	31.8	17.2
Near poor	12,469	15.3	438	1,419	2,703	100.0	3.6	35.6	26.6	12.1	22.2
Low income	40,170	16.1	452	1,345	8,684	100.0	6.8	37.6	33.7	8.8	13.1
Middle income	91,063	15.9	639	1,687	24,496	100.0	6.4	64.6	15.5	3.0	10.6
High income	108,862	18.5	640	1,704	34,302	100.0	6.3	72.7	14.3	1.2	5.5

Note: Uninsured refers to people uninsured for the entire year. Tricare (armed-forces related coverage) is considered private insurance in these data. Other insurance includes Department of Veterans Affairs (except Tricare), American Indian Health Service, state and local clinics, worker's compensation, homeowner's and automobile insurance, etc. Poor refers to incomes below poverty level. Near poor encompasses incomes from poverty level through 125 percent of poverty level. Low income is more than 125 percent of poverty level through 200 percent of poverty level. Middle income is more than 200 percent of poverty level through 400 percent of poverty level. High income is more than 400 percent of poverty level. (–) means not applicable or sample too small to make a reliable estimate.
Source: Center for Financing, Access and Cost Trends, Agency for Healthcare Research and Quality: Medical Expenditure Panel Survey, 2002; Internet site http://www.meps.ahrq.gov/CompendiumTables/TC_TOC.htm

Table 6.28 Spending on Emergency Room Services by Selected Characteristics, 2002

(total number of people, percent with emergency room services expense, median and average expense per person with expense, total emergency room service expenses, and percent distribution of total expenses by source of payment, by selected characteristics, 2002)

Emergency room services	total (thousands)	percent w/ expense	spending per person with expense — median	spending per person with expense — average	total expenses (millions)	percent distribution — total	out-of-pocket	private insurance	Medicare	Medicaid	other
Total people	**288,182**	**13.4%**	**$377**	**$723**	**$27,879**	**100.0%**	**11.4%**	**50.6%**	**15.9%**	**9.3%**	**12.8%**
Age											
Under age 65	251,926	12.5	381	719	22,647	100.0	13.1	58.7	3.0	11.1	14.2
Under age 6	23,292	16.9	279	410	1,614	100.0	14.4	57.9	0.7	20.6	6.4
Aged 6 to 17	49,455	11.4	329	490	2,753	100.0	12.4	63.8	0.8	15.2	7.9
Aged 18 to 44	111,219	12.5	412	770	10,691	100.0	15.4	57.9	1.2	9.8	15.6
Aged 45 to 64	67,960	11.8	488	945	7,588	100.0	9.7	58.0	6.7	9.4	16.1
Aged 65 or older	36,256	19.5	355	739	5,232	100.0	4.3	15.4	71.8	1.6	6.9
Sex											
Male	140,802	12.5	386	727	12,740	100.0	11.7	54.0	15.5	5.6	13.2
Female	147,380	14.3	371	720	15,139	100.0	11.2	47.7	16.2	12.4	12.5
Race and Hispanic origin											
Hispanic	39,665	10.9	312	718	3,115	100.0	13.3	43.0	12.4	17.8	13.5
Black, non-Hispanic	34,875	15.3	334	599	3,196	100.0	11.5	41.9	16.3	17.3	13.1
Asian, non-Hispanic	11,478	6.1	–	–	–	100.0	–	–	–	–	–
White/other, non-Hispanic	202,164	13.9	391	745	21,005	100.0	11.2	52.8	16.5	7.0	12.5
Health insurance: under age 65											
Any private	183,560	11.7	438	786	16,873	100.0	9.8	78.7	0.6	1.1	9.7
Public only	34,687	20.5	236	534	3,796	100.0	7.1	–	15.0	61.2	16.7
Uninsured	33,679	8.6	350	682	1,978	100.0	52.1	–	–	–	47.9
Health insurance: aged 65 or older											
Medicare only	10,540	20.5	355	809	1,744	100.0	6.1	–	79.6	–	14.3
Medicare/private	21,606	18.4	357	714	2,835	100.0	3.8	28.5	64.7	0.1	2.9
Medicare/other public	3,920	24.3	324	681	650	100.0	2.1	–	81.8	12.2	3.9
Income status											
Poor	35,618	18.7	269	574	3,828	100.0	14.7	10.5	19.3	38.7	16.9
Near poor	12,469	17.7	302	605	1,337	100.0	11.4	22.6	24.9	17.5	23.6
Low income	40,170	15.8	342	686	4,347	100.0	11.1	35.4	24.7	12.3	16.5
Middle income	91,063	12.9	401	759	8,919	100.0	11.8	62.5	12.3	2.6	10.7
High income	108,862	10.6	439	815	9,448	100.0	9.9	66.4	12.6	1.2	9.9

Note: Uninsured refers to people uninsured for the entire year. Tricare (armed-forces related coverage) is considered private insurance in these data. Other insurance includes Department of Veterans Affairs (except Tricare), American Indian Health Service, state and local clinics, worker's compensation, homeowner's and automobile insurance, etc. Poor refers to incomes below poverty level. Near poor encompasses incomes from poverty level through 125 percent of poverty level. Low income is more than 125 percent of poverty level through 200 percent of poverty level. Middle income is more than 200 percent of poverty level through 400 percent of poverty level. High income is more than 400 percent of poverty level. (–) means not applicable or sample too small to make a reliable estimate.
Source: Center for Financing, Access and Cost Trends, Agency for Healthcare Research and Quality: Medical Expenditure Panel Survey, 2002; Internet site http://www.meps.ahrq.gov/CompendiumTables/TC_TOC.htm

Older Adults Pay the Most for Prescription Drugs

They have the greatest need for medication, and they also incur the highest costs.

Sixty-four percent of Americans had prescription drug expenses in 2002, with a median cost of $271 per person with the expense. Individuals paid fully 42 percent of that amount out-of-pocket, while private insurance covered just 37 percent.

Regardless of age, most people had prescription drug expenses in 2002. The proportion ranged from a low of 50 percent among school-aged children to a high of 91 percent among people aged 65 or older. People under age 65 pay for 37 percent of their prescription drug costs out-of-pocket. People aged 65 or older must pay for a larger 54 percent of the cost of their prescription drugs out-of-pocket. This proportion is likely to shrink once the new Medicare prescription drug benefit goes into effect in 2006. Among people aged 65 or older with prescription drug costs, the median expense was a lofty $1,036.

The uninsured paid 87 percent of their prescription drug costs out-of-pocket. Median prescription drug expenses for the uninsured were $130 in 2002 versus $205 for those under age 65 with private insurance. This suggests that many uninsured people are foregoing medication because they cannot afford it.

■ Prescription medications are increasingly central to the treatment of many health conditions, yet prescription drug coverage can be spotty.

People under age 65 are more likely to have insurance coverage for prescription drugs

(percent of prescription drug expenses paid out-of-pocket, by age, 2002)

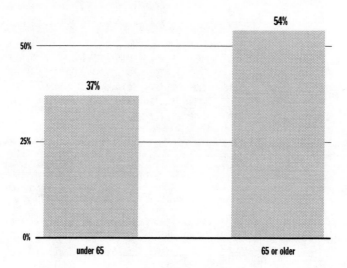

Table 6.29 Spending on Prescription Drugs by Selected Characteristics, 2002

(total number of people, percent with prescription drug expense, median and average expense per person with expense, total prescription drug expenses, and percent distribution of total expenses by source of payment, by selected characteristics, 2002)

Prescription drugs	total (thousands)	percent w/ expense	spending per person with expense — median	spending per person with expense — average	total expenses (millions)	percent distribution of total expenses by source of payment — total	out-of-pocket	private insurance	Medicare	Medicaid	other
Total people	288,182	64.4%	$271	$812	$15,616	100.0%	42.3%	37.2%	4.3%	12.5%	3.7%
Age											
Under age 65	251,926	60.6	191	660	100,725	100.0	36.7	45.5	1.1	14.0	2.6
Under age 6	23,292	58.4	47	130	1,767	100.0	33.4	36.5	–	29.9	0.2
Aged 6 to 17	49,455	50.0	76	284	7,015	100.0	30.2	39.1	–	30.2	0.5
Aged 18 to 44	111,219	56.8	165	501	31,628	100.0	38.1	43.9	1.1	15.3	1.6
Aged 45 to 64	67,960	75.3	565	1,178	60,315	100.0	36.8	47.4	1.3	11.0	3.5
Aged 65 or older	36,256	90.5	1,036	1,521	49,892	100.0	53.7	20.5	10.6	9.4	5.8
Sex											
Male	140,802	57.2	217	766	61,681	100.0	38.0	38.3	5.2	10.8	7.6
Female	147,380	71.2	311	847	88,936	100.0	45.3	36.5	3.6	13.6	1.0
Race and Hispanic origin											
Hispanic	39,665	47.6	118	544	10,260	100.0	41.5	23.9	4.0	28.8	1.9
Black, non-Hispanic	34,875	54.4	204	764	14,507	100.0	39.2	28.5	2.5	26.5	3.3
Asian, non-Hispanic	11,478	48.5	150	484	2,695	100.0	39.4	28.6	9.7	20.9	1.4
White/other, non-Hispanic	202,164	70.3	321	867	123,155	100.0	42.8	39.6	4.4	9.3	3.9
Health insurance: under age 65											
Any private	183,560	64.9	205	623	74,195	100.0	34.8	61.8	0.7	1.3	1.3
Public only	34,687	59.6	155	978	20,200	100.0	28.0	–	2.9	65.0	4.1
Uninsured	33,679	38.1	130	493	6,330	100.0	86.5	–	–	–	13.5
Health insurance: age 65 or older											
Medicare only	10,540	89.4	942	1,397	13,162	100.0	74.6	–	14.9	–	10.4
Medicare/private	21,606	91.8	1,034	1,464	29,039	100.0	50.4	35.2	8.8	1.1	4.5
Medicare/other public	3,920	88.8	1,409	2,203	7,664	100.0	30.0	–	10.0	56.8	3.1
Income status											
Poor	35,618	57.8	249	971	19,994	100.0	37.8	9.3	3.4	45.2	4.4
Near poor	12,469	62.3	301	1,002	7,790	100.0	46.8	12.5	9.1	25.9	5.8
Low income	40,170	60.2	281	928	22,452	100.0	50.2	21.4	6.0	17.3	5.1
Middle income	91,063	63.2	226	752	43,233	100.0	43.5	41.0	5.4	6.8	3.4
High income	108,862	69.3	310	758	57,147	100.0	39.3	53.8	2.4	1.6	2.9

Note: Uninsured refers to people uninsured for the entire year. Tricare (armed-forces related coverage) is considered private insurance in these data. Other insurance includes Department of Veterans Affairs (except Tricare), American Indian Health Service, state and local clinics, worker's compensation, homeowner's and automobile insurance, etc. Poor refers to incomes below poverty level. Near poor encompasses incomes from poverty level through 125 percent of poverty level. Low income is more than 125 percent of poverty level through 200 percent of poverty level. Middle income is more than 200 percent of poverty level through 400 percent of poverty level. High income is more than 400 percent of poverty level. (–) means not applicable or sample too small to make a reliable estimate.
Source: Center for Financing, Access and Cost Trends, Agency for Healthcare Research and Quality: Medical Expenditure Panel Survey, 2002; Internet site http://www.meps.ahrq.gov/CompendiumTables/TC_TOC.htm

Eyeglasses and Contact Lenses Usually Are Not Covered by Insurance

Most of these expenses are paid for out-of-pocket.

Just as dental care is considered separate from general medical care—and is much less likely to be covered by insurance—vision care is largely omitted from most insurance plans. In 2002, nearly half (47 percent) of the total expense for optometrist office visits was paid for out-of-pocket. The out-of-pocket proportion was 51 percent for people under age 65 and a smaller 31 percent for those aged 65 or older. Overall, 5 percent of Americans visited an optometrist in 2002, spending a median of $75 doing so.

Fifteen percent of the population spent on vision aids in 2002, a category dominated by eyeglasses and contact lenses. The median expense for those buying vision aids was $189. Seventy-three percent of that cost was paid for out-of-pocket.

■ Vision aids are not part of most health insurance plans because the out-of-pocket costs for these items are relatively modest.

Seventy-three percent of the cost of vision aids is paid for out-of-pocket

(percent of total expenses for optometrist office visits and vision aids paid for out-of-pocket, 2002)

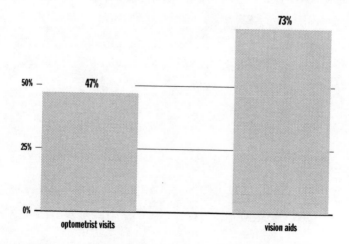

Table 6.30 Spending on Optometrist Office Visits by Selected Characteristics, 2002

(total number of people, percent with optometrist visit expense, median and average expense per person with expense, total optometrist visit expenses, and percent distribution of total expenses by source of payment, by selected characteristics, 2002)

Optometrist office visits	total (thousands)	percent w/ expense	spending per person with expense median	spending per person with expense average	total expenses (millions)	percent distribution of total expenses by source of payment total	out-of-pocket	private insurance	Medicare	Medicaid	other
Total people	**288,182**	**5.4%**	**$75**	**$157**	**$2,436**	**100.0%**	**46.8%**	**38.4%**	**6.5%**	**3.6%**	**4.6%**
Age											
Under age 65	251,926	5.2	72	146	1,897	100.0	51.4	42.2	0.2	4.0	2.2
Under age 6	23,292	1.1	–	–	–	100.0	–	–	–	–	–
Aged 6 to 17	49,455	4.6	65	101	230	100.0	50.7	31.0	–	13.7	4.6
Aged 18 to 44	111,219	4.9	79	125	683	100.0	53.5	41.2	–	3.5	1.8
Aged 45 to 64	67,960	7.3	69	193	964	100.0	50.7	45.3	0.5	1.6	2.0
Aged 65 or older	36,256	7.1	88	209	539	100.0	30.7	25.3	28.7	2.1	13.2
Sex											
Male	140,802	4.5	74	170	1,089	100.0	42.1	37.2	10.6	2.0	8.1
Female	147,380	6.2	76	147	1,347	100.0	50.6	39.4	3.3	4.8	1.9
Race and Hispanic origin											
Hispanic	39,665	2.5	72	110	108	100.0	48.0	25.2	3.0	19.1	4.8
Black, non-Hispanic	34,875	2.9	75	145	145	100.0	37.5	42.3	4.5	14.2	1.4
Asian, non-Hispanic	11,478	3.5	–	–	–	100.0	–	–	–	–	–
White/other, non-Hispanic	202,164	6.5	75	162	2,129	100.0	47.0	39.0	7.0	2.1	5.0
Health insurance: under age 65											
Any private	183,560	6.0	75	154	1,714	100.0	51.1	46.7	0.2	0.6	1.4
Public only	34,687	3.2	60	88	99	100.0	23.9	–	1.6	65.7	8.7
Uninsured	33,679	2.2	–	–	–	100.0	–	–	–	–	–
Health insurance: aged 65 or older											
Medicare only	10,540	5.9	–	–	–	100.0	–	–	–	–	–
Medicare/private	21,606	8.3	87	240	429	100.0	27.0	31.7	28.9	–	12.3
Medicare/other public	3,920	4.2	–	–	–	100.0	–	–	–	–	–
Income status											
Poor	35,618	3.1	63	94	105	100.0	38.8	14.2	6.9	37.2	2.8
Near poor	12,469	3.9	–	–	–	100.0	–	–	–	–	–
Low income	40,170	3.7	75	118	174	100.0	44.9	29.7	8.4	10.6	6.4
Middle income	91,063	5.8	79	153	812	100.0	40.8	39.2	12.9	2.3	4.7
High income	108,862	6.6	74	178	1,277	100.0	51.2	42.1	2.0	0.1	4.5

Note: Uninsured refers to people uninsured for the entire year. Tricare (armed-forces related coverage) is considered private insurance in these data. Other insurance includes Department of Veterans Affairs (except Tricare), American Indian Health Service, state and local clinics, worker's compensation, homeowner's and automobile insurance, etc. Poor refers to incomes below poverty level. Near poor encompasses incomes from poverty level through 125 percent of poverty level. Low income is more than 125 percent of poverty level through 200 percent of poverty level. Middle income is more than 200 percent of poverty level through 400 percent of poverty level. High income is more than 400 percent of poverty level. (–) means not applicable or sample too small to make a reliable estimate.
Source: Center for Financing, Access and Cost Trends, Agency for Healthcare Research and Quality: Medical Expenditure Panel Survey, 2002; Internet site http://www.meps.ahrq.gov/CompendiumTables/TC_TOC.htm

Table 6.31 Spending on Vision Aids by Selected Characteristics, 2002

(total number of people, percent with vision aid expense, median and average expense per person with expense, total vision aid expenses, and percent distribution of total expenses by source of payment, by selected characteristics, 2002)

Vision aids	total (thousands)	percent w/ expense	spending per person with expense — median	spending per person with expense — average	total expenses (millions)	percent distribution of total expenses by source of payment — total	out-of-pocket	private insurance	Medicare	Medicaid	other
Total people	**288,182**	**15.2%**	**$189**	**$222**	**$9,712**	**100.0%**	**72.5%**	**18.7%**	**1.4%**	**4.5%**	**2.8%**
Age											
Under age 65	251,926	14.6	182	218	8,020	100.0	72.1	20.6	0.1	4.7	2.5
Under age 6	23,292	0.9	–	–	–	100.0	–	–	–	–	–
Aged 6 to 17	49,455	11.5	160	184	1,049	100.0	63.4	18.9	0.1	14.8	2.8
Aged 18 to 44	111,219	15.1	160	199	3,324	100.0	74.6	20.9	–	3.0	1.6
Aged 45 to 64	67,960	20.8	225	255	3,606	100.0	72.3	20.9	0.3	3.3	3.2
Aged 65 or older	36,256	19.3	200	242	1,692	100.0	74.8	9.9	7.6	3.3	4.4
Sex											
Male	140,802	12.3	197	228	3,964	100.0	71.1	19.6	1.8	3.5	3.9
Female	147,380	17.9	182	218	5,748	100.0	73.5	18.1	1.2	5.2	2.1
Race and Hispanic origin											
Hispanic	39,665	10.3	150	191	778	100.0	66.5	15.3	2.8	11.9	3.6
Black, non-Hispanic	34,875	12.1	180	212	893	100.0	58.4	22.1	1.9	13.4	4.2
Asian, non-Hispanic	11,478	13.7	180	206	323	100.0	64.6	27.4	–	4.9	3.1
White/other, non-Hispanic	202,164	16.8	197	228	7,717	100.0	75.1	18.3	1.3	2.7	2.6
Health insurance: under age 65											
Any private	183,560	16.4	195	226	6,833	100.0	73.9	24.2	0.1	0.5	1.4
Public only	34,687	10.3	150	181	646	100.0	38.8	–	1.1	52.9	7.3
Uninsured	33,679	9.0	150	179	540	100.0	89.1	–	–	–	10.9
Health insurance: aged 65 or older											
Medicare only	10,540	16.7	189	225	395	100.0	79.9	–	12.7	–	7.4
Medicare/private	21,606	21.3	215	249	1,145	100.0	77.1	14.7	5.6	0.2	2.4
Medicare/other public	3,920	15.9	185	243	152	100.0	43.7	–	9.3	35.0	12.0
Income status											
Poor	35,618	10.6	150	186	700	100.0	52.8	7.6	2.2	32.5	4.9
Near poor	12,469	10.4	155	188	243	100.0	66.5	11.7	2.9	15.2	3.7
Low income	40,170	11.3	167	209	949	100.0	72.1	10.7	2.6	7.8	6.8
Middle income	91,063	14.4	177	216	2,826	100.0	72.2	20.1	1.8	3.0	3.0
High income	108,862	19.3	200	237	4,994	100.0	75.9	21.4	0.8	0.2	1.7

Note: Uninsured refers to people uninsured for the entire year. Tricare (armed-forces related coverage) is considered private insurance in these data. Other insurance includes Department of Veterans Affairs (except Tricare), American Indian Health Service, state and local clinics, worker's compensation, homeowner's and automobile insurance, etc. Poor refers to incomes below poverty level. Near poor encompasses incomes from poverty level through 125 percent of poverty level. Low income is more than 125 percent of poverty level through 200 percent of poverty level. Middle income is more than 200 percent of poverty level through 400 percent of poverty level. High income is more than 400 percent of poverty level. (–) means not applicable or sample too small to make a reliable estimate.

Source: Center for Financing, Access and Cost Trends, Agency for Healthcare Research and Quality: Medical Expenditure Panel Survey, 2002; Internet site http://www.meps.ahrq.gov/CompendiumTables/TC_TOC.htm

Nearly Half the Cost of Dental Visits Is Paid for Out-of-Pocket

People aged 65 or older are especially likely to pay out-of-pocket for dental care.

Most Americans have health insurance, but a much smaller share have dental insurance. This is readily apparent in the fact that 47 percent of expenditures for dental office visits in 2002 were paid for out-of-pocket. Among people under age 65, 41 percent of dental expenses were paid out of pocket. Among people aged 65 or older, the proportion was a much larger 74 percent. Overall, 40 percent of Americans had dental visit expenses in 2002, averaging $174 per person.

Only 2 percent of Americans visited an orthodontist in 2002, and most of them were aged 6 to 17. Within the 6-to-17 age group, 8 percent saw an orthodontist, spending a median of $800. Sixty-two percent of orthodontia care is paid for out-of-pocket (not shown in table).

■ With escalating health care costs cutting into company profits, it's unlikely employers will be adding more generous dental benefits to their health care plans anytime soon.

Children pay the least out-of-pocket for dental care

(percent of total spending on general dentist office visits paid for out-of-pocket, by age, 2002)

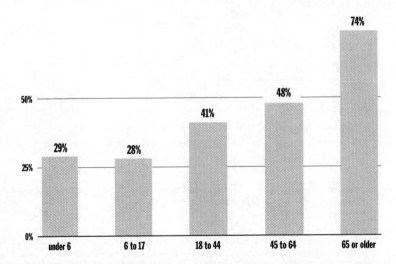

Table 6.32 Spending on Visits to General Dentists by Selected Characteristics, 2002

(total number of people, percent with general dentist office visit expenses, median and average expense per person with expense, total general dentist office visit expenses, and percent distribution of total expenses by source of payment, by selected characteristics, 2002)

General dentists	total (thousands)	percent w/ expense	spending per person with expense		total expenses (millions)	percent distribution of total expenses by source of payment					
			median	average		total	out-of-pocket	private insurance	Medicare	Medicaid	other
Total people	**288,182**	**39.5%**	**$174**	**$411**	**$46,736**	**100.0%**	**46.8%**	**43.0%**	**0.6%**	**4.5%**	**5.0%**
Age											
Under age 65	251,926	39.7	170	394	39,351	100.0	41.8	47.9	0.1	5.0	5.2
Under age 6	23,292	19.4	103	192	867	100.0	28.9	48.2	–	18.7	4.3
Aged 6 to 17	49,455	48.5	141	256	6,144	100.0	28.4	49.4	–	15.1	7.0
Aged 18 to 44	111,219	36.1	164	364	14,614	100.0	40.5	51.3	–	3.3	4.8
Aged 45 to 64	67,960	46.0	216	567	17,727	100.0	48.1	44.6	0.1	2.3	4.9
Aged 65 or older	36,256	38.3	200	532	7,384	100.0	73.8	16.9	3.4	1.7	4.2
Sex											
Male	140,802	36.4	174	410	21,008	100.0	45.8	43.6	0.3	4.1	6.1
Female	147,380	42.5	174	411	25,728	100.0	47.7	42.5	0.8	4.8	4.2
Race and Hispanic origin											
Hispanic	39,665	23.3	125	284	2,622	100.0	42.8	39.7	0.5	6.9	10.1
Black, non-Hispanic	34,875	25.4	130	312	2,764	100.0	32.3	42.7	0.2	13.5	11.3
Asian, non-Hispanic	11,478	32.8	193	470	1,768	100.0	42.8	43.8	1.2	7.6	4.7
White/other, non-Hispanic	202,164	45.5	181	430	39,582	100.0	48.3	43.2	0.6	3.6	4.3
Health insurance: under age 65											
Any private	183,560	46.5	180	406	34,721	100.0	41.3	54.3	–	0.6	3.8
Public only	34,687	26.5	95	273	2,506	100.0	17.4	–	0.7	70.7	11.2
Uninsured	33,679	15.8	165	399	2,124	100.0	79.0	–	–	–	21.0
Health insurance: aged 65 or older											
Medicare only	10,540	30.3	195	599	1,909	100.0	86.2	–	8.0	–	5.8
Medicare/private	21,606	46.2	203	518	5,170	100.0	70.6	24.2	1.7	0.1	3.3
Medicare/other public	3,920	17.6	200	435	300	100.0	50.3	–	2.9	38.5	8.2
Income status											
Poor	35,618	23.2	118	342	2,819	100.0	44.1	14.9	1.6	31.4	8.0
Near poor	12,469	24.4	138	308	938	100.0	49.3	22.4	0.7	22.6	4.9
Low income	40,170	27.5	147	343	3,787	100.0	53.7	27.3	1.7	12.8	4.5
Middle income	91,063	37.0	169	388	13,068	100.0	46.0	45.5	0.5	2.6	5.4
High income	108,862	53.1	191	452	26,123	100.0	46.5	47.8	0.3	0.7	4.6

Note: Uninsured refers to people uninsured for the entire year. Tricare (armed-forces related coverage) is considered private insurance in these data. Other insurance includes Department of Veterans Affairs (except Tricare), American Indian Health Service, state and local clinics, worker's compensation, homeowner's and automobile insurance, etc. Poor refers to incomes below poverty level. Near poor encompasses incomes from poverty level through 125 percent of poverty level. Low income is more than 125 percent of poverty level through 200 percent of poverty level. Middle income is more than 200 percent of poverty level through 400 percent of poverty level. High income is more than 400 percent of poverty level. (–) means not applicable or sample too small to make a reliable estimate.

Source: Center for Financing, Access and Cost Trends, Agency for Healthcare Research and Quality: Medical Expenditure Panel Survey, 2002; Internet site http://www.meps.ahrq.gov/CompendiumTables/TC_TOC.htm

Table 6.33 Spending on Orthodontic Office Visits by Selected Characteristics, 2002

(total number of people, percent with orthodontic office visit expense, median and average expense per person with expense, and total orthodontic visit expenses, by selected characteristics, 2002)

Orthodontic office visits	total people (thousands)	percent with expense	spending per person with expense		total spending (millions)
			median	average	
Total people	**288,182**	**2.0%**	**$600**	**$1,608**	**$9,499**
Age					
Under age 65	251,926	2.3	600	1,620	9,412
Under age 6	23,292	0.3	–	–	–
Aged 6 to 17	49,455	8.2	800	1,771	7,215
Aged 18 to 44	111,219	1.2	393	1,259	1,641
Aged 45 to 64	67,960	0.5	–	–	–
Aged 65 or older	36,256	0.3	–	–	–
Sex					
Male	140,802	1.7	585	1,625	3,847
Female	147,380	2.4	600	1,596	5,652
Race and Hispanic origin					
Hispanic	39,665	1.5	392	1,083	646
Black, non-Hispanic	34,875	1.3	–	–	–
Asian, non-Hispanic	11,478	2.7	–	–	–
White and other, non-Hispanic	202,164	2.2	603	1,719	7,801
Health insurance: under age 65					
Any private	183,560	2.8	700	1,750	8,855
Public only	34,687	1.1	–	–	–
Uninsured	33,679	1.1	–	–	–
Health insurance: aged 65 or older					
Medicare only	10,540	–	–	–	–
Medicare and private	21,606	–	–	–	–
Medicare and other public	3,920	–	–	–	–
Income status					
Poor	35,618	0.9	–	–	–
Near poor	12,469	1.0	–	–	–
Low income	40,170	1.0	–	–	–
Middle income	91,063	2.1	696	1,786	3,398
High income	108,862	2.9	700	1,689	5,355

Note: Uninsured refers to people uninsured for the entire year. Tricare (armed-forces related coverage) is considered private insurance in these data. Poor refers to incomes below poverty level. Near poor encompasses incomes from poverty level through 125 percent of poverty level. Low income is more than 125 percent of poverty level through 200 percent of poverty level. Middle income is more than 200 percent of poverty level through 400 percent of poverty level. High income is more than 400 percent of poverty level. (–) means not applicable or sample too small to make a reliable estimate.
Source: Center for Financing, Access and Cost Trends, Agency for Healthcare Research and Quality: Medical Expenditure Panel Survey, 2002; Internet site http://www.meps.ahrq.gov/CompendiumTables/TC_TOC.htm

Few Patients See Physician's Assistants

Only 4 percent of Americans visited a chiropractor in 2002.

In 2002, only 2 percent of the population visited a physician's assistant for medical care. About the same proportion saw a physical therapist or used home health care services. A larger 4 percent visited a chiropractor, and 9 percent visited a nurse or nurse practitioner. People aged 65 or older are more likely to use each of these types of services than are those under age 65. Ten percent of people aged 65 or older used home health care in 2002, for example, compared with fewer than 1 percent of those under age 65. Five percent of people aged 65 or older used a chiropractor, and 4 percent saw a physical therapist.

Among those using home health care services in 2002, median costs were a substantial $2,220. Because most of those using home health care are aged 65 or older, Medicare pays for a large portion of the cost. For people who saw a physical therapist in 2002, the median expense was $595. For those who saw chiropractors, the median was $207. Expenses for visits to nurses or physician's assistants were much lower—a median of just $70 per person for visits to nurses and $80 per person for visits to physician's assistants.

■ Many health insurance providers now cover the cost of visits to nonphysician health care providers in an effort to lower overall costs.

Nonphysician health care providers are not yet commonly used

(percent of people visiting health care provider, by type, 2002)

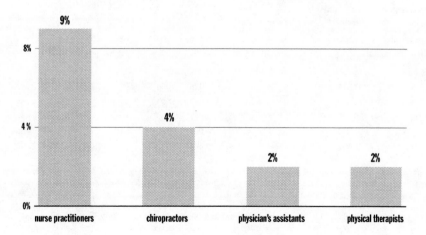

Table 6.34 Spending on Home Health Care Services by Selected Characteristics, 2002

(total number of people, percent with home health care expense, median and average expense per person with expense, total home health care expenses, and percent distribution of total expenses by source of payment, by selected characteristics, 2002)

Home health care services	total (thousands)	percent w/ expense	spending per person with expense		total expenses (millions)	percent distribution of total expenses by source of payment					
			median	average		total	out-of-pocket	private insurance	Medicare	Medicaid	other
Total people	**288,182**	**2.1%**	**$2,220**	**$5,811**	**$34,817**	**100.0%**	**7.6%**	**6.5%**	**30.6%**	**44.8%**	**10.4%**
Age											
Under age 65	251,926	0.9	1,230	5,999	13,371	100.0	1.8	6.5	6.5	73.4	11.8
Under age 6	23,292	1.0	–	–	–	100.0	–	–	–	–	–
Aged 6 to 17	49,455	0.3	–	–	–	100.0	–	–	–	–	–
Aged 18 to 44	111,219	0.6	–	–	–	100.0	–	–	–	–	–
Aged 45 to 64	67,960	1.7	1,251	5,260	6,119	100.0	3.4	7.0	11.4	65.7	12.4
Aged 65 or older	36,256	10.4	2,735	5,700	21,446	100.0	11.2	6.4	45.7	27.1	9.6
Sex											
Male	140,802	1.7	2,109	6,617	16,109	100.0	5.8	7.5	29.6	48.1	9.0
Female	147,380	2.4	2,455	5,259	18,708	100.0	9.2	5.6	31.5	42.0	11.6
Race and Hispanic origin											
Hispanic	39,665	1.2	3,198	9,577	4,543	100.0	1.0	1.4	11.8	77.1	8.6
Black, non-Hispanic	34,875	2.3	4,043	7,172	5,686	100.0	4.7	5.1	20.3	53.9	15.9
Asian, non-Hispanic	11,478	0.5	–	–	–	100.0	–	–	–	–	–
White/other, non-Hispanic	202,164	2.3	2,004	5,183	24,215	100.0	9.6	7.8	36.3	36.9	9.5
Health insurance: under age 65											
Any private	183,560	0.6	600	2,412	2,530	100.0	2.9	34.5	10.0	45.9	6.8
Public only	34,687	3.3	2,608	9,346	10,789	100.0	1.5	–	5.7	80.2	12.6
Uninsured	33,679	0.1	–	–	–	100.0	–	–	–	–	–
Health insurance: age 65 or older											
Medicare only	10,540	9.3	1,538	3,484	3,407	100.0	12.1	–	72.4	–	15.5
Medicare/private	21,606	8.2	2,584	5,185	9,136	100.0	19.8	15.1	56.6	2.3	6.2
Medicare/other public	3,920	26.1	5,282	8,703	8,903	100.0	2.2	–	24.2	62.8	10.8
Income status											
Poor	35,618	3.4	2,584	6,233	7,448	100.0	3.7	2.1	21.6	61.5	11.1
Near poor	12,469	4.6	–	–	–	100.0	–	–	–	–	–
Low income	40,170	3.3	2,945	6,002	7,963	100.0	5.6	1.8	33.4	44.2	14.9
Middle income	91,063	1.7	1,601	6,460	10,004	100.0	12.0	4.0	21.2	55.6	7.1
High income	108,862	1.2	2,004	5,064	6,808	100.0	9.3	22.1	50.9	9.7	8.0

Note: Uninsured refers to people uninsured for the entire year. Tricare (armed-forces related coverage) is considered private insurance in these data. Other insurance includes Department of Veterans Affairs (except Tricare), American Indian Health Service, state and local clinics, worker's compensation, homeowner's and automobile insurance, etc. Poor refers to incomes below poverty level. Near poor encompasses incomes from poverty level through 125 percent of poverty level. Low income is more than 125 percent of poverty level through 200 percent of poverty level. Middle income is more than 200 percent of poverty level through 400 percent of poverty level. High income is more than 400 percent of poverty level. (–) means not applicable or sample too small to make a reliable estimate.

Source: Center for Financing, Access and Cost Trends, Agency for Healthcare Research and Quality: Medical Expenditure Panel Survey, 2002; Internet site http://www.meps.ahrq.gov/CompendiumTables/TC_TOC.htm

Table 6.35 Spending on Visits to Nurses or Nurse Practitioners by Selected Characteristics, 2002

(total number of people, percent with nurse/nurse practitioner visit expense, median and average expense per person with expense, total nurse/nurse practitioner visit expenses, and percent distribution of total expenses by source of payment, by selected characteristics, 2002)

Nurse visits	total (thousands)	percent w/ expense	spending per person with expense median	spending per person with expense average	total expenses (millions)	percent distribution of total expenses by source of payment total	out-of-pocket	private insurance	Medicare	Medicaid	other
Total people	**288,182**	**8.9%**	**$70**	**$327**	**$8,391**	**100.0%**	**15.7%**	**39.7%**	**28.4%**	**6.7%**	**9.5%**
Age											
Under age 65	251,926	8.0	66	277	5,565	100.0	21.3	50.7	8.6	9.3	10.0
Under age 6	23,292	8.3	53	120	233	100.0	14.5	36.8	0.4	36.8	11.4
Aged 6 to 17	49,455	5.9	50	187	550	100.0	14.4	54.8	0.6	10.3	19.9
Aged 18 to 44	111,219	7.8	75	305	2,636	100.0	28.5	48.7	5.5	11.0	6.4
Aged 45 to 64	67,960	9.7	72	327	2,146	100.0	15.1	53.7	15.5	4.1	11.7
Aged 65 or older	36,256	15.4	89	508	2,827	100.0	4.7	18.2	67.3	1.5	8.4
Sex											
Male	140,802	6.1	54	362	3,095	100.0	9.4	31.5	40.0	7.1	12.0
Female	147,380	11.6	76	309	5,296	100.0	19.4	44.6	21.6	6.5	8.0
Race and Hispanic origin											
Hispanic	39,665	4.2	66	356	600	100.0	8.7	24.0	32.3	18.3	16.7
Black, non-Hispanic	34,875	6.0	69	747	1,553	100.0	4.4	42.2	30.9	9.6	12.9
Asian, non-Hispanic	11,478	5.2	–	–	–	100.0	–	–	–	–	–
White/other, non-Hispanic	202,164	10.5	71	284	6,058	100.0	19.4	40.5	27.6	4.8	7.7
Health insurance: under age 65											
Any private	183,560	8.6	65	275	4,369	100.0	24.7	64.6	3.2	0.9	6.7
Public only	34,687	8.3	73	351	1,017	100.0	3.3	–	33.7	47.3	15.8
Uninsured	33,679	3.9	63	135	179	100.0	42.9	–	–	–	57.2
Health insurance: aged 65 or older											
Medicare only	10,540	14.6	65	358	549	100.0	3.4	–	76.6	–	20.0
Medicare/private	21,606	16.9	96	595	2,166	100.0	5.1	23.7	65.5	0.3	5.4
Medicare/other public	3,920	10.0	–	–	–	100.0	–	–	–	–	–
Income status											
Poor	35,618	7.9	75	234	663	100.0	9.0	5.0	20.8	45.1	20.2
Near poor	12,469	8.1	75	471	473	100.0	3.7	5.8	63.1	10.9	16.5
Low income	40,170	9.0	75	286	1,031	100.0	9.5	43.3	27.5	6.6	13.1
Middle income	91,063	8.3	68	338	2,539	100.0	15.4	40.2	30.9	5.5	8.1
High income	108,862	9.8	67	344	3,685	100.0	20.5	49.1	23.8	0.1	6.5

Note: Uninsured refers to people uninsured for the entire year. Tricare (armed-forces related coverage) is considered private insurance in these data. Other insurance includes Department of Veterans Affairs (except Tricare), American Indian Health Service, state and local clinics, worker's compensation, homeowner's and automobile insurance, etc. Poor refers to incomes below poverty level. Near poor encompasses incomes from poverty level through 125 percent of poverty level. Low income is more than 125 percent of poverty level through 200 percent of poverty level. Middle income is more than 200 percent of poverty level through 400 percent of poverty level. High income is more than 400 percent of poverty level. (–) means not applicable or sample too small to make a reliable estimate.
Source: Center for Financing, Access and Cost Trends, Agency for Healthcare Research and Quality: Medical Expenditure Panel Survey, 2002; Internet site http://www.meps.ahrq.gov/CompendiumTables/TC_TOC.htm

Table 6.36 Spending on Physician's Assistant Visits by Selected Characteristics, 2002

(total number of people, percent with physician's assistant visit expense, median and average expense per person with expense, and total physician's assistant visit expenses, by selected characteristics, 2002)

Physician's assistant visits	total people (thousands)	percent with expense	spending per person with expense		total spending (millions)
			median	average	
Total people	**288,182**	**2.3%**	**$80**	**$178**	**$1,205**
Age					
Under age 65	251,926	2.3	78	166	973
Under age 6	23,292	1.7	–	–	–
Aged 6 to 17	49,455	1.6	50	104	83
Aged 18 to 44	111,219	2.3	75	187	471
Aged 45 to 64	67,960	3.1	88	172	365
Aged 65 or older	36,256	2.6	144	251	232
Sex					
Male	140,802	1.6	80	174	380
Female	147,380	3.1	80	180	824
Race and Hispanic origin					
Hispanic	39,665	0.7	–	–	–
Black, non-Hispanic	34,875	1.0	–	–	–
Asian, non-Hispanic	11,478	0.8	–	–	–
White and other, non-Hispanic	202,164	3.0	80	178	1,078
Health insurance: under age 65					
Any private	183,560	2.7	75	160	784
Public only	34,687	1.7	–	–	–
Uninsured	33,679	1.0	–	–	–
Health insurance: aged 65 or older					
Medicare only	10,540	2.0	–	–	–
Medicare and private	21,606	3.1	–	–	–
Medicare and other public	3,920	1.1			
Income status					
Poor	35,618	1.4	–	–	–
Near poor	12,469	1.8	–	–	–
Low income	40,170	2.1	100	229	191
Middle income	91,063	2.6	81	166	400
High income	108,862	2.6	80	166	468

Note: Uninsured refers to people uninsured for the entire year. Tricare (armed-forces related coverage) is considered private insurance in these data. Poor refers to incomes below poverty level. Near poor encompasses incomes from poverty level through 125 percent of poverty level. Low income is more than 125 percent of poverty level through 200 percent of poverty level. Middle income is more than 200 percent of poverty level through 400 percent of poverty level. High income is more than 400 percent of poverty level. (–) means not applicable or sample too small to make a reliable estimate.
Source: Center for Financing, Access and Cost Trends, Agency for Healthcare Research and Quality: Medical Expenditure Panel Survey, 2002; Internet site http://www.meps.ahrq.gov/CompendiumTables/TC_TOC.htm

Table 6.37 Spending on Chiropractic Office Visits by Selected Characteristics, 2002

(total number of people, percent with chiropractic office visit expense, median and average expense per person with expense, and total chiropractic office visit expenses, by selected characteristics, 2002)

Chiropractic office visits	total people (thousands)	percent with expense	spending per person with expense		total spending millions)
			median	average	
Total people	**288,182**	**4.0%**	**$207**	**$442**	**$5,124**
Age					
Under age 65	251,926	3.8	200	426	4,113
Under age 6	23,292	0.2	–	–	–
Aged 6 to 17	49,455	1.2	–	–	–
Aged 18 to 44	111,219	4.5	180	383	1,898
Aged 45 to 64	67,960	6.0	253	506	2,053
Aged 65 or older	36,256	5.3	264	522	1,011
Sex					
Male	140,802	3.5	153	380	1,861
Female	147,380	4.5	245	488	3,264
Race and Hispanic origin					
Hispanic	39,665	1.3	–	–	–
Black, non-Hispanic	34,875	0.8	–	–	–
Asian, non-Hispanic	11,478	1.9	–	–	–
White and other, non-Hispanic	202,164	5.2	204	435	4,594
Health insurance: under age 65					
Any private	183,560	4.6	211	443	3,705
Public only	34,687	1.3	–	–	–
Uninsured	33,679	2.5	–	–	–
Health insurance: aged 65 or older					
Medicare only	10,540	4.3	249	518	719
Medicare and private	21,606	6.4	–	–	–
Medicare and other public	3,920	2.2	–	–	–
Income status					
Poor	35,618	1.9	–	–	–
Near poor	12,469	3.4	–	–	–
Low income	40,170	2.8	146	461	516
Middle income	91,063	4.1	207	433	1,623
High income	108,862	5.2	240	452	2,538

Note: Uninsured refers to people uninsured for the entire year. Tricare (armed-forces related coverage) is considered private insurance in these data. Poor refers to incomes below poverty level. Near poor encompasses incomes from poverty level through 125 percent of poverty level. Low income is more than 125 percent of poverty level through 200 percent of poverty level. Middle income is more than 200 percent of poverty level through 400 percent of poverty level. High income is more than 400 percent of poverty level. (–) means not applicable or sample too small to make a reliable estimate.
Source: Center for Financing, Access and Cost Trends, Agency for Healthcare Research and Quality: Medical Expenditure Panel Survey, 2002; Internet site http://www.meps.ahrq.gov/CompendiumTables/TC_TOC.htm

Table 6.38 Spending on Physical Therapist Visits by Selected Characteristics, 2002

(total number of people, percent with physical therapist visit expense, median and average expense per person with expense, and total physical therapist visit expenses, by selected characteristics, 2002)

Physical therapist visits	total people (thousands)	percent with expense	spending per person with expense		total spending millions)
			median	average	
Total people	**288,182**	**2.3%**	**$595**	**$1,212**	**$8,205**
Age					
Under age 65	251,926	2.1	569	1,112	6,015
Under age 6	23,292	0.4	–	–	–
Aged 6 to 17	49,455	0.8	–	–	–
Aged 18 to 44	111,219	2.1	570	1,148	2,684
Aged 45 to 64	67,960	3.8	632	1,130	2,888
Aged 65 or older	36,256	3.8	760	1,607	2,189
Sex					
Male	140,802	1.9	566	1,271	3,423
Female	147,380	2.8	603	1,173	4,782
Race and Hispanic origin					
Hispanic	39,665	1.1	–	–	–
Black, non-Hispanic	34,875	1.1	–	–	–
Asian, non-Hispanic	11,478	1.2	–	–	–
White and other, non-Hispanic	202,164	2.9	636	1,270	7,364
Health insurance: under age 65					
Any private	183,560	2.6	575	1,125	5,343
Public only	34,687	1.4	–	–	–
Uninsured	33,679	0.5	–	–	–
Health insurance: aged 65 or older					
Medicare only	10,540	3.4	888	1,795	1,702
Medicare and private	21,606	4.4	–	–	–
Medicare and other public	3,920	1.4	–	–	–
Income status					
Poor	35,618	1.2	–	–	–
Near poor	12,469	1.4	–	–	–
Low income	40,170	1.6	–	–	–
Middle income	91,063	2.1	632	1,386	2,703
High income	108,862	3.3	570	1,080	3,836

Note: Uninsured refers to people uninsured for the entire year. Tricare (armed-forces related coverage) is considered private insurance in these data. Poor refers to incomes below poverty level. Near poor encompasses incomes from poverty level through 125 percent of poverty level. Low income is more than 125 percent of poverty level through 200 percent of poverty level. Middle income is more than 200 percent of poverty level through 400 percent of poverty level. High income is more than 400 percent of poverty level. (–) means not applicable or sample too small to make a reliable estimate.
Source: Center for Financing, Access and Cost Trends, Agency for Healthcare Research and Quality: Medical Expenditure Panel Survey, 2002; Internet site http://www.meps.ahrq.gov/CompendiumTables/TC_TOC.htm

Medicaid Rolls Are Growing

The program now covers about one in four children.

Medicare and Medicaid are government programs that provide health insurance to the elderly and disabled (Medicare) and the poor (Medicaid). Medicare is the larger of the two, with expenditures of $234.5 billion in 2001 compared with $208.5 billion spent on Medicaid. Just as the largest health expense that most individuals will encounter is hospital care, the largest share of these programs' expenditures goes to hospitals. More than half of Medicare spending is for hospital care, largely because this program's constituents are older adults who are more likely to need hospitalization and to have longer hospital stays.

The percentage of people under age 65 who are covered by Medicaid grew by 5 percentage points between 1984 and 2002, from 7 percent to 12 percent. The increase was greatest among the young, rising from 12 to 25 percent of children under age 18. One reason for the increase is the shrinking percentage of families covered by employer-provided health insurance. Blacks and Hispanics are considerably more likely than whites to be covered by Medicaid because a larger proportion are poor. By far the largest Medicaid dollar payments to health care vendors per recipient went to facilities that care for the mentally retarded.

■ Little Medicare spending went toward prescription drugs in 2001. This will change after the new Medicare prescription drug benefit goes into effect in 2006.

Medicaid covers a growing share of people in every age group

(percent of people covered by Medicaid, by age, 1984 and 2002)

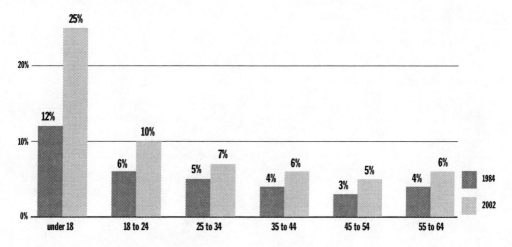

Table 6.39　Medicare and Medicaid Expenses by Type of Service, 2001

(total Medicare and Medicaid expenses and distribution by type of services, 2001)

	Medicare		Medicaid	
	total (billions)	percent	total (billions)	percent
Total expenses	**$234.5**	**100.0%**	**$208.5**	**100.0%**
Hospital care	135.0	57.5	77.1	37.0
Physician and clinical services	63.9	27.3	21.4	10.3
Dentists' services	0.1	–	3.0	1.5
Other professional services	5.4	2.3	1.7	0.8
Home health care	9.9	4.2	7.1	3.4
Prescription drugs	2.4	1.0	24.1	11.6
Other nondurable medical products	1.4	0.6	–	–
Durable medical equipment	4.9	2.1	–	–
Nursing home care	11.6	4.9	47.0	22.5

Note: Other professional services include private duty nurses, chiropractors, optometrists, and other licensed health professionals. (–) means data not available.
Source: Centers for Medicare and Medicaid Services, 2003 Data Compendium, Internet site http://www.cms.hhs.gov/researchers/pubs/datacompendium/current/; calculations by New Strategist

Table 6.40 Medicaid Coverage among People under Age 65, 1984 and 2002

(percent of people under age 65 covered by Medicaid by selected demographic characteristics, 1984 and 2002; percentage point change in share, 1984–2002)

	2002	1984	percentage point change
Percent covered by Medicaid	**11.8%**	**6.8%**	**5.0**
Age			
Under age 18	24.5	11.9	12.6
Aged 18 to 24	9.8	6.4	3.4
Aged 25 to 34	6.6	5.3	1.3
Aged 35 to 44	5.8	3.5	2.3
Aged 45 to 54	5.1	3.2	1.9
Aged 55 to 64	5.8	3.6	2.2
Sex			
Female	13.1	8.0	5.1
Male	10.4	5.2	5.2
Race			
Asian	10.2	9.1	1.1
Black	21.5	18.9	2.6
White	9.5	4.6	4.9
Hispanic origin			
Hispanic	18.9	12.2	6.7
Non-Hispanic white	8.0	3.7	4.3

Source: National Center for Health Statistics, Health, United States, 2004; *Internet site http://www.cdc.gov/nchs/hus.htm*

Table 6.41 Medicaid Recipients by Type of Service, 2001

(number and percent of Medicaid recipients by type of service received and average vendor payment per recipient, 2001)

	number (millions)	percent receiving services	average payment to vendor per recipient
Total Medicaid recipients	**46.0**	**100.0%**	**$4,053**
Inpatient hospital	4.9	10.6	5,313
Mental health facility	0.1	0.2	21,894
Mentally retarded, intermediate care facility	0.1	0.3	83,227
Nursing facility	1.7	3.7	21,894
Physician	20.0	43.5	371
Dental	7.0	15.3	270
Other practitioner	5.1	11.1	149
Outpatient hospital	13.7	29.8	546
Clinic	8.5	18.4	662
Laboratory and radiological	12.3	26.8	131
Home health	1.0	2.2	3,478
Prescribed drugs	21.9	47.6	1,083
Capitated payment services	23.2	50.5	1,257
Primary care case management	6.4	13.9	29
Personal support	5.0	10.8	2,639
Other care	9.9	21.5	1,734

Source: National Center for Health Statistics, Health, United States, 2004; *Internet site http://www.cdc.gov/nchs/hus.htm; calculations by New Strategist*

7

Deaths

■ **A growing share of Americans support the right to die.**

Fifty-eight percent of the public thinks the incurably ill should be permitted to end their life, up from 38 percent in 1977.

■ **Heart disease and cancer are the leading killers.**

The two causes accounted for 51 percent of deaths in 2002. The third leading cause of death, cerebrovascular disease, accounted for just 7 percent of the total.

■ **Most deaths occur to people aged 75 or older.**

Eighty-five percent of deaths occur in the 55-or-older age group, and 57 percent are among people aged 75 or older.

■ **Accidents are the primary cause of death among the young.**

Homicide is the second-leading cause of death among 15-to-24-year-olds, while suicide ranks third.

■ **Accidental death becomes less common with age.**

Among people aged 35 to 44, cancer causes almost as many deaths as accidents. Among people aged 45 to 54, cancer and heart disease rank first and second.

■ **Life expectancy continues to increase.**

Life expectancy reached a record 77.3 years in 2002, up from 68.2 years in 1950. Most of the gain was due to reduced infant mortality.

Skilled Nursing Care Is a Key Component of Hospice Services

But most hospice patients also receive help with housework and personal care.

Hospice services are provided primarily to people who are terminally ill. The primary goal of hospice care is to make the individual as comfortable as possible and to provide support to the patient and family in a variety of ways. This includes help with activities of daily living, such as bathing or dressing in the majority of cases.

Among people who received hospice services in 2000, 80 percent were aged 65 or older. Most of those receiving hospice services were in a private or semiprivate residence, usually their own home or that of a family member.

Most people receiving hospice care have been diagnosed with cancer. The nature of the disease tends to make hospice care appropriate. Unlike a heart attack or stroke, which often results in rapid death, the progression of cancer is relatively slow.

Fully 92 percent of hospice patients received skilled nursing care and the majority (59 percent) received medications. Most also received household or personal care and pastoral or spiritual care.

■ Hospice care allows individuals to avoid hospital or nursing home care in their final days, an advantage both to the individual and to society since hospice care is considerably less expensive than hospitals or nursing homes.

Most hospice patients are elderly

(percent distribution of patients discharged from hospice care, by age, 2000)

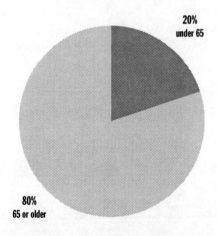

20%
under 65

80%
65 or older

Table 7.1 Hospice Discharges by Selected Characteristics, 2000

(number, percent distribution, average and median length of service for patients discharged from hospice care, by selected characteristics, 2000)

	number	percent distribution	average length of service (days)	median length of service (days)
Total hospice discharges	**621,100**	**100.0%**	**46.9**	**15.6**
Sex				
Females	311,800	50.2	50.9	18.1
Males	309,300	49.8	42.8	14.5
Age				
Under age 65	126,900	20.4	43.9	15.0
Aged 65 or older	494,300	79.6	47.7	16.3
Aged 65 to 74	153,100	24.6	41.2	16.4
Aged 75 to 84	176,400	28.4	50.6	16.5
Aged 85 or older	164,800	26.5	50.5	–
Race				
Black or other	64,300	10.3	–	15.8
White	522,500	84.1	46.7	14.8
Marital status				
Married	293,400	47.2	40.0	11.7
Not married	289,500	46.6	54.1	18.5
Widowed	206,400	33.2	53.5	–
Divorced or separated	35,200	5.7	–	–
Single or never married	47,900	7.7	41.5	–
Unknown	38,300	6.2	45.3	–
Primary source of payment				
Medicare	488,000	78.6	48.1	16.7
All other sources	133,200	21.4	42.4	–
Medicaid	31,400	5.1	24.3	–
Private	80,600	13.0	–	–
Other	21,100	3.4	42.5	–
Residence during care				
Private or semiprivate residence	379,900	61.2	49.7	19.9
Assisted living or residential care facility	21,600	3.5	71.6	–
Health facility (including mental health facility)	217,000	34.9	39.7	6.4
Reason for discharge				
Died	531,000	85.5	42.4	13.6
Did not die	90,200	14.5	73.1	–
Services from agency no longer needed	49,000	7.9	86.2	64.7
Transferred to inpatient care	14,500	2.3	81.7	71.0
Other and unknown	26,700	4.3	44.4	–

Note: (–) means sample is too small to make a reliable estimate.
Source: National Center for Health Statistics, Characteristics of Hospice Care Discharges and Their Length of Service: United States, 2000, Vital and Health Statistics Report, Series 13, No. 154, 2003; Internet site http://www.cdc.gov/nchs/pressroom/03facts/hospicecare.htm

Table 7.2 Hospice Care Discharges by Primary Diagnosis and Functional Status, 2000

(number and percent distribution of hospice care discharges by primary admission diagnosis and functional status, 2000)

	number	percent distribution
Total hospice discharges	**621,100**	**100.0%**
Primary admission diagnosis		
Malignant neoplasms	357,000	57.5
Large intestine and rectum	51,500	8.3
Trachea, bronchus, and lung	120,500	19.4
Dementias	39,400	6.3
Heart disease	42,500	6.8
Congestive heart failure	23,500	3.8
Cerebrovascular disease	29,600	4.8
Chronic obstructive pulmonary disease	27,600	4.4
Received help from agency with activities of daily living (ADL)		
Bathing or showering	431,800	69.5
Dressing	364,700	58.7
Eating	218,300	35.1
Transferring in or out of beds or chairs	294,900	47.5
Using the toilet room	236,400	38.1
Continence status		
Continent	181,300	29.2
Incontinent	439,800	70.8
Only bladder incontinence	126,700	20.4
Only bowel incontinence	40,700	6.6
Both bladder, bowel incontinence	272,500	43.9
Mobility status		
No mobility limitation	110,700	17.8
Mobility limitation	510,400	82.2
Mild	106,800	17.2
Moderate	89,900	14.5
Severe	313,700	50.5
Use of selected aids or devices		
No aids or devices	114,700	18.5
Aids or devices	506,400	81.5
Hospital bed	435,000	70.0
Oxygen	313,500	50.5
IV therapy equipment	46,700	7.5
Enteral feeding equipment	19,200	3.1

Source: National Center for Health Statistics, Characteristics of Hospice Care Discharges and Their Length of Service: United States, 2000, *Vital and Health Statistics Report, Series 13, No. 154, 2003; Internet site http://www.cdc.gov/nchs/pressroom/03facts/ hospicecare.htm*

Table 7.3 Hospice Care Discharges by Services Received and Type of Provider, 2000

(number, percent distribution, average and median length of service for patients discharged from hospice care, by services received and type of provider seen during the thirty days prior to discharge, 2000)

	number	percent	average length of service (days)	median length of service (days)
Total hospice discharges	**621,100**	**100.0%**	**46.9**	**15.6**
Medical and skilled nursing				
Skilled nursing	570,400	91.8	46.7	16.0
Physician	186,900	30.1	42.5	14.9
Equipment and medication				
Medications	367,100	59.1	51.0	15.4
Durable medical equip. and supplies	279,600	45.0	49.0	18.5
Personal care				
Homemaker—household or personal care	387,100	62.3	51.1	20.9
Companion or volunteer	195,300	31.4	63.6	26.9
Continuous home care	23,800	3.8	68.3	42.1
Psychosocial				
Referral or social	446,300	71.9	47.4	16.9
Pastoral or spiritual care	366,200	59.0	46.3	15.7
Counseling or psychological	194,400	31.3	49.5	20.7
Respite care	43,400	7.0	62.6	–
Type of provider seen in past 30 days				
Nurses	598,700	96.4	45.8	15.2
Social workers, mental health specialists	470,700	75.8	45.6	18.1
Home health aides, nursing aides, attendants	427,500	68.8	49.7	20.4
Chaplains	328,400	52.9	43.2	14.9
Volunteers	192,900	31.1	64.2	28.2
Physicians	153,000	24.6	37.3	–
Homemakers, personal caretakers	40,900	6.6	77.4	–
Other	116,700	18.8	40.8	–

Note: (–) means sample too small to make a reliable estimate.
Source: National Center for Health Statistics, Characteristics of Hospice Care Discharges and Their Length of Service: United States, 2000, *Vital and Health Statistics Report, Series 13, No. 154, 2003; Internet site http://www.cdc.gov/nchs/pressroom/03facts/hospicecare.htm*

Most People Believe in the "Right to Die"

Since 1990 most Americans have supported the concept.

In 1977 only 38 percent thought the incurably ill should be permitted to commit suicide. Although legalized assisted suicide is still a highly controversial issue, the majority of Americans now think those with an incurable disease should have the right to end their life. In 2002, 58 percent of respondents to the General Social Survey agreed with the "right to die," while 40 percent disagreed. Perhaps equally remarkable is the fact that only 2 percent say they "don't know," indicating relatively little ambivalence among respondents.

The share of the public in support of allowing the incurably ill to end their lives has generally increased over the years. In 1977 only 38 percent agreed. By 1986, the majority (52 percent) favored being able to end one's life if incurably ill. The share continued to rise, peaking at 62 percent in 1994. Since then, however, the share has dropped somewhat, although it rose again between 2000 and 2002. In every year since 1990, the majority has favored giving the incurably ill the "right to die."

■ Although most people think someone with an incurable illness should have the right to end his or her own life, this does not mean they support "assisted suicide."

In the 1970s, only 38 percent supported the "right to die"

(percent of people aged 18 or older who believe the incurably ill should be able to end their life, 1977 to 2002)

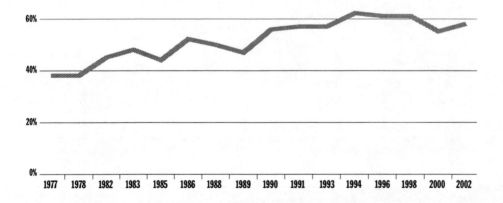

Table 7.4 Suicide If Person Has an Incurable Disease, 1977 to 2002

"Do you think a person has the right to end his or her
own life if this person has an incurable disease?"

(number of respondents aged 18 or older, and percent distribution by response, 1977–2002)

	number of respondents	total	yes	no	don't know
2002	907	100.0%	57.8%	40.1%	2.1%
2000	1,871	100.0	54.8	39.8	5.4
1998	1,867	100.0	60.6	34.5	4.9
1996	1,956	100.0	61.2	33.8	5.0
1994	1,969	100.0	61.5	33.7	4.8
1993	1,077	100.0	56.7	38.6	4.6
1991	1,022	100.0	56.7	39.9	3.4
1990	927	100.0	56.0	38.2	5.8
1989	1,004	100.0	46.7	48.6	4.7
1988	983	100.0	50.1	46.2	3.8
1986	1,467	100.0	51.7	45.1	3.2
1985	1,532	100.0	44.1	52.5	3.4
1983	1,591	100.0	47.8	48.4	3.8
1982	1,853	100.0	44.5	50.8	4.7
1978	1,532	100.0	38.4	58.4	3.2
1977	1,524	100.0	37.9	58.9	3.2

Source: General Social Surveys, National Opinion Research Center, University of Chicago; calculations by New Strategist

Leading Causes of Death Differ by Sex, Race, and Hispanic Origin

But heart disease and cancer claim the largest share regardless of demographics.

Two diseases account for the majority of deaths in the United States—heart disease and cancer. Combined, they accounted for 51 percent of all deaths in 2002. In contrast, the third leading cause of death, cerebrovascular disease, accounted for just 7 percent of the total.

Heart disease and cancer rank first and second as the cause of death for both men and women. But there are differences by sex in the percentage of deaths attributable to other causes. For men, the third-leading cause is accidents, accounting for 6 percent of total male deaths in 2002. Accidents rank seventh among causes of death for women, accounting for only 3 percent of the total.

Among blacks, Hispanics, and non-Hispanic whites, heart disease and cancer account for the largest share of deaths. Beyond that, however, differences emerge. For example, homicide is the sixth-leading cause of death among blacks and Hispanics, but among non-Hispanics whites homicide does not even rank in the top ten. Hispanics are more likely than non-Hispanic whites to die in an accident. Blacks are more likely than non-Hispanic whites to die of HIV.

■ Accidents rank high as a cause of death among males because of the large number of teen and young-adult males who die in accidents.

Most deaths among non-Hispanic whites are due to cancer or heart disease

(percent of deaths attributable to heart disease and cancer, by sex, race, and Hispanic origin, 2002)

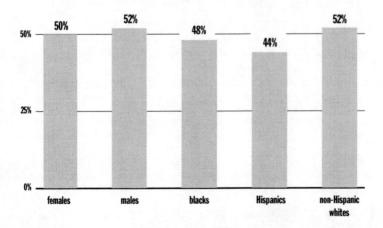

Table 7.5 Leading Causes of Death, 2002

(number and percent distribution of deaths accounted for by the fifteen leading causes of death, 2002)

		number	percent distribution
	All causes	**2,443,387**	**100.0%**
1.	Diseases of the heart	696,947	28.5
2.	Malignant neoplasms (cancer)	557,271	22.8
3.	Cerebrovascular diseases	162,672	6.7
4.	Chronic lower respiratory disease	124,816	5.1
5.	Accidents (unintentional injuries)	106,742	4.4
6.	Diabetes mellitus	73,249	3.0
7.	Influenza and pneumonia	65,681	2.7
8.	Alzheimer's disease	58,866	2.4
9.	Nephritis, nephrotic syndrome, nephrosis	40,974	1.7
10.	Septicemia	33,865	1.4
11.	Suicide	31,655	1.3
12.	Chronic liver disease and cirrhosis	27,257	1.1
13.	Essential (primary) hypertension and hypertensive renal disease	20,261	0.8
14.	Homicide	17,638	0.7
15.	Pneumonitis due to solids and liquids	17,593	0.7
	All other causes	407,900	16.7

Source: National Center for Health Statistics, Deaths: Final Data for 2002, National Vital Statistics Reports, Vol. 53, No. 5, 2004; calculations by New Strategist

Table 7.6 Leading Causes of Death among Females, 2002

(number and percent distribution of deaths to females accounted for by the ten leading causes of death among females, 2002)

		number	percent distribution
	All causes	**1,244,123**	**100.0%**
1.	Diseases of the heart (1)	356,014	28.6
2.	Malignant neoplasms (cancer) (2)	268,503	21.6
3.	Cerebrovascular diseases (3)	100,050	8.0
4.	Chronic lower respiratory disease (4)	64,103	5.2
5.	Alzheimer's disease (8)	41,877	3.4
6.	Diabetes mellitus (6)	38,948	3.1
7.	Accidents (unintentional injuries) (5)	37,485	3.0
8.	Influenza and pneumonia (7)	36,763	3.0
9.	Nephritis, nephrotic syndrome, nephrosis (9)	21,279	1.7
10.	Septicemia (10)	18,918	1.5
	All other causes	260,183	20.9

Note: Numbers in parentheses show rank for all age groups if the cause of death is among top fifteen.
Source: National Center for Health Statistics, **Deaths: Final Data** *for 2002, National Vital Statistics Reports, Vol. 53, No. 5, 2004; calculations by New Strategist*

Table 7.7 Leading Causes of Death among Males, 2002

(number and percent distribution of deaths to males accounted for by the ten leading causes of death among males, 2002)

		number	percent distribution
	All causes	**1,199,264**	**100.0%**
1.	Diseases of the heart (1)	340,933	28.4
2.	Malignant neoplasms (cancer) (2)	288,768	24.1
3.	Accidents (unintentional injuries) (5)	69,257	5.8
4.	Cerebrovascular diseases (3)	62,622	5.2
5.	Chronic lower respiratory disease (4)	60,713	5.1
6.	Influenza and pneumonia (7)	28,918	2.4
7.	Diabetes mellitus (6)	34,301	2.9
8.	Suicide (11)	25,409	2.1
9.	Chronic liver disease and cirrhosis (12)	17,401	1.5
10.	Septicemia (10)	14,947	1.2
	All other causes	255,995	21.3

Note: Numbers in parentheses show rank for all age groups if the cause of death is among top fifteen.
Source: National Center for Health Statistics, Deaths: Final Data for 2002, National Vital Statistics Reports, Vol. 53, No. 5, 2004; calculations by New Strategist

Table 7.8 Leading Causes of Death among Blacks, 2002

(number and percent distribution of deaths to blacks accounted for by the ten leading causes of death among blacks, 2002)

		number	percent distribution
	All causes	**290,051**	**100.0%**
1.	Diseases of the heart (1)	77,621	26.8
2.	Malignant neoplasms (cancer) (2)	62,617	21.6
3.	Cerebrovascular diseases (3)	18,856	6.5
4.	Diabetes mellitus (6)	12,687	4.4
5.	Accidents (unintentional injuries) (5)	12,513	4.3
6.	Homicide (14)	8,287	2.9
7.	Human immunodeficiency virus infection	7,835	2.7
8.	Chronic lower respiratory disease (4)	7,831	2.7
9.	Septicemia (10)	6,137	2.1
10.	Influenza and pneumonia (7)	5,871	2.0
	All other causes	69,796	24.1

Note: Numbers in parentheses show rank for all age groups if the cause of death is among top fifteen.
Source: National Center for Health Statistics, **Deaths: Final Data for 2002,** *National Vital Statistics Reports, Vol. 53, No. 5, 2004; calculations by New Strategist*

Table 7.9 Leading Causes of Death among Hispanics, 2002

(number and percent distribution of deaths to Hispanics accounted for by the ten leading causes of death among Hispanics, 2002)

		number	percent distribution
	All causes	**117,135**	**100.0%**
1.	Diseases of the heart (1)	27,887	23.8
2.	Malignant neoplasms (cancer) (2)	23,141	19.8
3.	Accidents (unintentional injuries) (5)	10,106	8.6
4.	Cerebrovascular diseases (3)	6,451	5.5
5.	Diabetes mellitus (6)	5,912	5.0
6.	Homicide (14)	3,129	2.7
7.	Chronic lower respiratory disease (4)	3,058	2.6
8.	Influenza and pneumonia (7)	2,824	2.4
9.	Certain conditions originating in the perinatal period	2,402	2.1
10.	Suicide (11)	1,954	1.7
	All other causes	30,271	25.8

Note: Numbers in parentheses show rank for all age groups if the cause of death is among top fifteen.
Source: National Center for Health Statistics, Deaths: Final Data for 2002, National Vital Statistics Reports, Vol. 53, No. 5, 2004; calculations by New Strategist

Table 7.10 Leading Causes of Death among Non-Hispanic Whites, 2002

(number and percent distribution of deaths to non-Hispanic whites accounted for by the ten leading causes of death among non-Hispanic whites, 2002)

		number	percent distribution
	All causes	**1,981,973**	**100.0%**
1.	Diseases of the heart (1)	577,761	29.2
2.	Malignant neoplasms (cancer) (2)	458,754	23.1
3.	Cerebrovascular diseases (3)	133,118	6.7
4.	Chronic lower respiratory disease (4)	112,128	5.7
5.	Accidents (unintentional injuries) (5)	80,605	4.1
6.	Influenza and pneumonia (7)	55,419	2.8
7.	Alzheimer's disease (8)	53,486	2.7
8.	Diabetes mellitus (6)	52,463	2.6
9.	Nephritis, nephrotic syndrome, nephrosis (9)	30,669	1.5
10.	Suicide (11)	26,691	1.3
	All other causes	400,879	20.2

Note: Numbers in parentheses show rank for all age groups if the cause of death is among top fifteen.
Source: National Center for Health Statistics, Deaths: Final Data for 2002, *National Vital Statistics Reports, Vol. 53, No. 5, 2004; calculations by New Strategist*

Heart Disease Is the Leading Killer of the Oldest Adults

Cancer claims more lives among those aged 55 to 74, however.

The majority of deaths in any given year occur among people aged 75 or older, as might be expected. In 2002, 85 percent of deaths occurred in the 55-or-older age group; 57 percent were among people aged 75 or older.

People aged 55 or older account for the great majority of deaths for most of the 15 leading causes of death. They account for 96 percent of deaths from chronic lower respiratory disease and nearly all deaths from Alzheimer's. In fact, nearly half the deaths from Alzheimer's disease are among people aged 85 or older. Only three of the leading causes of death are more likely to claim people under age 55—accidents, suicide, and homicide. Thirty-nine percent of people who die in accidents are aged 55 or older, as are 29 percent of those who commit suicide and just 9 percent of homicide victims.

As people age, the likelihood of dying from a particular disease changes. Among 55-to-64-year-olds who died in 2002, the largest share died of cancer. This was also true in the 65-to-74 age group. Among older adults, however, heart disease causes a larger share of deaths than cancer. The percentage of deaths due to cancer falls from 37 percent in the 55-to-64 age group to just 12 percent among those aged 85 or older.

■ As the baby-boom generation reaches the older age groups, leading causes of death may change thanks to advances in treatments for heart disease and cancer.

The majority of deaths occur among people aged 75 or older

(percent distribution of deaths, by age, 2002)

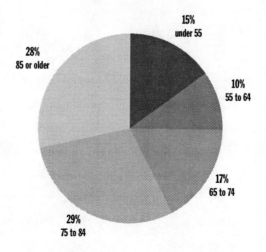

15%
under 55

10%
55 to 64

17%
65 to 74

29%
75 to 84

28%
85 or older

Table 7.11 Deaths from the Fifteen Leading Causes of Death, 2002

(number and percent distribution of deaths from the fifteen leading causes, by age, 2002; ranked by total number of deaths)

	total	total	55 to 64	65 to 74	75 to 84	85+
			aged 55 or older			
Total deaths	**2,443,387**	**2,065,062**	**253,342**	**422,990**	**707,654**	**681,076**
Diseases of the heart	696,947	640,535	64,234	112,547	213,581	250,173
Malignant neoplasms (cancer)	557,271	484,392	93,391	144,757	167,062	79,182
Cerebrovascular diseases	162,672	153,190	9,897	21,992	54,889	66,412
Chronic lower respiratory disease	124,816	119,593	11,280	29,788	49,241	29,284
Accidents (unintentional injuries)	106,742	41,986	8,345	8,086	12,904	12,651
Diabetes mellitus	73,249	64,737	10,022	16,709	23,282	14,724
Influenza and pneumonia	65,681	61,813	2,987	6,847	19,984	31,995
Alzheimer's disease	58,866	58,799	510	3,602	20,135	34,552
Nephritis, nephrotic syndrome, and nephrosis	40,974	37,771	3,455	7,164	13,896	13,256
Septicemia	33,865	30,030	3,360	6,336	11,010	9,324
Suicide	31,655	9,166	3,618	2,463	2,259	826
Chronic liver disease and cirrhosis	27,257	16,463	6,097	5,381	4,000	985
Essential (primary) hypertension and hypertensive renal disease	20,261	18,871	1,526	2,922	6,138	8,285
Homicide	17,638	1,653	841	421	296	95
Pneumonitis due to solids and liquids	17,593	16,907	671	1,793	5,900	8,543
PERCENT DISTRIBUTION BY AGE						
Total deaths	**100.0%**	**84.5%**	**10.4%**	**17.3%**	**29.0%**	**27.9%**
Diseases of the heart	100.0	91.9	9.2	16.1	30.6	35.9
Malignant neoplasms (cancer)	100.0	86.9	16.8	26.0	30.0	14.2
Cerebrovascular diseases	100.0	94.2	6.1	13.5	33.7	40.8
Chronic lower respiratory disease	100.0	95.8	9.0	23.9	39.5	23.5
Accidents (unintentional injuries)	100.0	39.3	7.8	7.6	12.1	11.9
Diabetes mellitus	100.0	88.4	13.7	22.8	31.8	20.1
Influenza and pneumonia	100.0	94.1	4.5	10.4	30.4	48.7
Alzheimer's disease	100.0	99.9	0.9	6.1	34.2	58.7
Nephritis, nephrotic syndrome, and nephrosis	100.0	92.2	8.4	17.5	33.9	32.4
Septicemia	100.0	88.7	9.9	18.7	32.5	27.5
Suicide	100.0	29.0	11.4	7.8	7.1	2.6
Chronic liver disease and cirrhosis	100.0	60.4	22.4	19.7	14.7	3.6
Essential (primary) hypertension and hypertensive renal disease	100.0	93.1	7.5	14.4	30.3	40.9
Homicide	100.0	9.4	4.8	2.4	1.7	0.5
Pneumonitis due to solids and liquids	100.0	96.1	3.8	10.2	33.5	48.6

(continued)

	total	aged 55 or older				
		total	55 to 64	65 to 74	75 to 84	85+
Percent distribution by cause of death						
Total deaths	**100.0%**	**100.0%**	**100.0%**	**100.0%**	**100.0%**	**100.0%**
Diseases of the heart	28.5	31.0	25.4	26.6	30.2	36.7
Malignant neoplasms (cancer)	22.8	23.5	36.9	34.2	23.6	11.6
Cerebrovascular diseases	6.7	7.4	3.9	5.2	7.8	9.8
Chronic lower respiratory disease	5.1	5.8	4.5	7.0	7.0	4.3
Accidents (unintentional injuries)	4.4	2.0	3.3	1.9	1.8	1.9
Diabetes mellitus	3.0	3.1	4.0	4.0	3.3	2.2
Influenza and pneumonia	2.7	3.0	1.2	1.6	2.8	4.7
Alzheimer's disease	2.4	2.8	0.2	0.9	2.8	5.1
Nephritis, nephrotic syndrome, and nephrosis	1.7	1.8	1.4	1.7	2.0	1.9
Septicemia	1.4	1.5	1.3	1.5	1.6	1.4
Suicide	1.3	0.4	1.4	0.6	0.3	0.1
Chronic liver disease and cirrhosis	1.1	0.8	2.4	1.3	0.6	0.1
Essential (primary) hypertension and hypertensive renal disease	0.8	0.9	0.6	0.7	0.9	1.2
Homicide	0.7	0.1	0.3	0.1	0.0	0.0
Pneumonitis due to solids and liquids	0.7	0.8	0.3	0.4	0.8	1.3

Note: Numbers will not add to total because age not stated is not shown.
Source: National Center for Health Statistics, **Deaths: Final Data for 2002,** *National Vital Statistics Reports, Vol. 53, No. 5, 2004*

Accidents Are the Primary Cause of Death among the Young

Homicide accounts for a sizable share of deaths.

The leading causes of death vary significantly by age. The majority of deaths among infants are the result of congenital anomalies (conditions that are present at birth), sudden infant death syndrome, or complications of pregnancy or delivery. In many cases, the deaths are due to premature delivery. In spite of extraordinary advances in this area, infants born prematurely still suffer considerable mortality.

After the first year of life, accidents become the leading cause of death among children and young adults. Accidents account for 34 percent of deaths among children aged 1 to 4, 38 percent of deaths among children aged 5 to 14, and nearly half (47 percent) of deaths among people aged 15 to 24.

One of the more disturbing facts revealed by these statistics is the relatively large number of children who are murdered or commit suicide. Homicide accounted for 9 percent of the deaths of children aged 1 to 4 in 2002 and for 5 percent of the deaths of children aged 5 to 14. Among people aged 15 to 24, homicide is the second-leading cause of death, accounting for 16 percent of deaths in the age group. Among 15-to-24-year-olds, suicide accounts for 12 percent of deaths, placing it third among causes of death.

■ Many of the deaths of children and young adults could be prevented if parents were more vigilant and teenagers more cautious.

Nearly half of deaths among 15-to-24-year-olds are due to accidents

(percent of deaths due to accidents, by age, 2002)

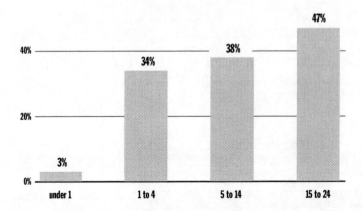

Table 7.12 Leading Causes of Death for Infants, 2002

(number and percent distribution of deaths accounted for by the ten leading causes of death for children under age 1, 2002)

		number	percent distribution
	All causes	**28,034**	**100.0%**
1.	Congenital malformations, deformations, and chromosomal abnormalities	5,623	20.1
2.	Disorders relating to short gestation and low birthweight	4,637	16.5
3.	Sudden infant death syndrome	2,295	8.2
4.	Newborn affected by maternal complications of pregnancy	1,708	6.1
5.	Newborn affected by complications of placenta, cord, and membranes	1,028	3.7
6.	Accidents (unintentional injuries) (5)	946	3.4
7.	Respiratory distress syndrome	943	3.4
8.	Bacterial sepsis of newborn	749	2.7
9.	Diseases of the circulatory system	667	2.4
10.	Intrauterine hypoxia and birth asphyxia	583	2.1
	All other causes	8,855	31.6

Note: Numbers in parentheses show rank for all age groups if the cause of death is among top fifteen.
Source: National Center for Health Statistics, Deaths: Final Data for 2002, National Vital Statistics Reports, Vol. 53, No. 5, 2004; calculations by New Strategist

Table 7.13 Leading Causes of Death for Children Aged 1 to 4, 2002

(number and percent distribution of deaths accounted for by the ten leading causes of death for children aged 1 to 4, 2002)

		number	percent distribution
	All causes	**4,858**	**100.0%**
1.	Accidents (unintentional injuries) (5)	1,641	33.8
2.	Congenital malformations, deformations, and chromosomal abnormalities	530	10.9
3.	Homicide (14)	423	8.7
4.	Malignant neoplasms (cancer) (2)	402	8.3
5.	Diseases of the heart (1)	165	3.4
6.	Influenza and pneumonia (7)	110	2.3
7.	Septicemia (10)	79	1.6
8.	Chronic lower respiratory diseases	65	1.3
9.	Certain conditions originating in the perinatal period	65	1.3
10.	Benign neoplasms	60	1.2
	All other causes	1,318	27.1

Note: Numbers in parentheses show rank for all age groups if the cause of death is among top fifteen.
Source: National Center for Health Statistics, Deaths: Final Data for 2002, *National Vital Statistics Reports, Vol. 53, No. 5, 2004; calculations by New Strategist*

Table 7.14 Leading Causes of Death for Children Aged 5 to 14, 2002

(number and percent distribution of deaths accounted for by the ten leading causes of death for children aged 5 to 14, 2002)

		number	percent distribution
	All causes	**7,150**	**100.0%**
1.	Accidents (unintentional injuries) (5)	2,718	38.0
2.	Malignant neoplasms (cancer) (2)	1,072	15.0
3.	Congenital malformations, deformations	417	5.8
4.	Homicide (14)	356	5.0
5.	Suicide (11)	264	3.7
6.	Diseases of the heart (1)	255	3.6
7.	Chronic lower respiratory disease (4)	136	1.9
8.	Septicemia (10)	95	1.3
9.	Cerebrovascular diseases (3)	91	1.3
10.	Influenza and pneumonia (7)	91	1.3
	All other causes	1,655	23.1

Note: Numbers in parentheses show rank for all age groups if the cause of death is among top fifteen.
Source: National Center for Health Statistics, Deaths: Final Data for 2002, National Vital Statistics Reports, Vol. 53, No. 5, 2004; calculations by New Strategist

Table 7.15 Leading Causes of Death for People Aged 15 to 24, 2002

(number and percent distribution of deaths accounted for by the ten leading causes of death for people aged 15 to 24, 2002)

		number	percent distribution
	All causes	**33,046**	**100.0%**
1.	Accidents (unintentional injuries) (5)	15,412	46.6
2.	Homicide (14)	5,219	15.8
3.	Suicide (11)	4,010	12.1
4.	Malignant neoplasms (cancer) (2)	1,730	5.2
5.	Diseases of the heart (1)	1,022	3.1
6.	Congenital malformations, deformations	492	1.5
7.	Chronic lower respiratory disease (4)	192	0.6
8.	Human immunodeficiency virus infection	178	0.5
9.	Diabetes mellitus (6)	171	0.5
10.	Cerebrovascular diseases (3)	171	0.5
	All other causes	4,449	13.5

Note: Numbers in parentheses show rank for all age groups if the cause of death is among top fifteen.
Source: National Center for Health Statistics, **Deaths: Final Data for 2002,** *National Vital Statistics Reports, Vol. 53, No. 5, 2004; calculations by New Strategist*

Accidental Deaths Become Less Common with Age

Cancer and heart disease claim a larger share as people get older.

Among people aged 25 to 44, accidents are the leading cause of death. There are two reasons for this. One, people aged 25 to 44 often still engage in activities that put them at risk—although they are generally not as reckless as teenagers and young adults. Two, accidents are an important cause of death simply because diseases, such as cancer and heart disease, are relatively rare.

Accidents drop to third place as a cause of death among people aged 45 to 54, and they fall to sixth place among people aged 55 to 64. Not only are people more careful at these ages, but they are also more vulnerable to life-threatening illnesses. Among people aged 45 to 64, cancer is the leading cause of death followed by heart disease. The growing importance of cancer as a cause of death can be seen as early as the 35-to-44 age group. Among people aged 35 to 44, cancer causes almost as many deaths as accidents.

■ As a cause of death, homicide ranks second among 25-to-34-year-olds, but does not even make the top-ten list among 45-to-54-year-olds.

Among people aged 45 to 64, accidents cause fewer than 10 percent of deaths

(percent of deaths due to accidents, by age, 2002)

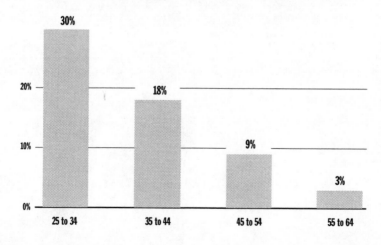

Table 7.16 Leading Causes of Death for People Aged 25 to 34, 2002

(number and percent distribution of deaths accounted for by the ten leading causes of death for people aged 25 to 34, 2002)

		number	percent distribution
	All causes	**41,355**	**100.0%**
1.	Accidents (unintentional injuries) (5)	12,569	30.4
2.	Suicide (2)	5,046	12.2
3.	Homicide (3)	4,489	10.9
4.	Malignant neoplasms (cancer) (2)	3,872	9.4
5.	Diseases of the heart (1)	3,165	7.7
6.	Human immunodeficiency virus infection	1,839	4.4
7.	Diabetes mellitus (6)	642	1.6
8.	Cerebrovascular diseases (3)	567	1.4
9.	Congenital malformations, deformations	475	1.1
10.	Chronic liver disease and cirrhosis (12)	374	0.9
	All other causes	8,317	20.1

Note: Numbers in parentheses show rank for all age groups if the cause of death is among top fifteen.
Source: National Center for Health Statistics, Deaths: Final Data for 2002, *National Vital Statistics Reports, Vol. 53, No. 5, 2004;*

Table 7.17   Leading Causes of Death for People Aged 35 to 44, 2002

(number and percent distribution of deaths accounted for by the ten leading causes of death for people aged 35 to 44, 2002)

		number	percent distribution
	All causes	**91,140**	**100.0%**
1.	Accidents (unintentional injuries) (5)	16,710	18.3
2.	Malignant neoplasms (cancer) (2)	16,085	17.6
3.	Diseases of the heart (1)	13,688	15.0
4.	Suicide (11)	6,851	7.5
5.	Human immunodeficiency virus infection	5,707	6.3
6.	Homicide (14)	3,239	3.6
7.	Chronic liver disease and cirrhosis (12)	3,154	3.5
8.	Cerebrovascular diseases (3)	2,425	2.7
9.	Diabetes mellitus (6)	2,164	2.4
10.	Chronic lower respiratory disease (4)	1,008	1.1
	All other causes	20,109	22.1

Note: Numbers in parentheses show rank for all age groups if the cause of death is among top fifteen.
Source: National Center for Health Statistics, Deaths: Final Data for 2002, National Vital Statistics Reports, Vol. 53, No. 5, 2004;

Table 7.18 Leading Causes of Death for People Aged 45 to 54, 2002

(number and percent distribution of deaths accounted for by the ten leading causes of death for people aged 45 to 54, 2002)

		number	percent distribution
	All causes	**172,385**	**100.0%**
1.	Malignant neoplasms (cancer) (2)	49,637	28.8
2.	Diseases of heart (1)	37,570	21.8
3.	Accidents (unintentional injuries) (5)	14,675	8.5
4.	Chronic liver disease and cirrhosis (12)	7,216	4.2
5.	Suicide (11)	6,308	3.7
6.	Cerebrovascular diseases (3)	6,055	3.5
7.	Diabetes mellitus (6)	5,496	3.2
8.	Human immunodeficiency virus infection	4,474	2.6
9.	Chronic lower respiratory disease (4)	3,475	2.0
10.	Viral hepatitis	2,331	1.4
	All other causes	35,148	20.4

Note: Numbers in parentheses show rank for all age groups if the cause of death is among top fifteen.
Source: National Center for Health Statistics, **Deaths: Final Data for 2002,** *National Vital Statistics Reports, Vol. 53, No. 5, 2004;*

Table 7.19 Leading Causes of Death for People Aged 55 to 64, 2002

(number and percent distribution of deaths accounted for by the ten leading causes of death for people aged 55 to 64, 2002)

		number	percent distribution
	All causes	**253,342**	**100.0%**
1.	Malignant neoplasms (cancer) (2)	93,391	36.9
2.	Diseases of heart (1)	64,234	25.4
3.	Chronic lower respiratory disease (4)	11,280	4.5
4.	Diabetes mellitus (6)	10,022	4.0
5.	Cerebrovascular diseases (3)	9,897	3.9
6.	Accidents (unintentional injuries) (5)	8,345	3.3
7.	Chronic liver disease and cirrhosis (12)	6,097	2.4
8.	Suicide (11)	3,618	1.4
9.	Nephritis, nephrotic syndrome, nephrosis (9)	3,455	1.4
10.	Septicemia (10)	3,360	1.3
	All other causes	39,643	15.6

Note: Numbers in parentheses show rank for all age groups if the cause of death is among top fifteen.
Source: National Center for Health Statistics, Deaths: Final Data for 2002, National Vital Statistics Reports, Vol. 53, No. 5, 2004;

The Oldest Adults Die from a Wide Variety of Causes

Most of those aged 65 to 84 die from cancer or heart disease.

Although medical research and lifestyle changes have reduced the death rates from cancer and heart disease, these two causes still account for the majority of deaths among people aged 65 to 84, and for nearly half the deaths among those aged 85 or older. If both cancer and heart disease were eradicated, however, something else would emerge to take their place since there is no means for prolonging life indefinitely.

In fact, this is what happens among those aged 85 or older. This group might be considered "survivors" in that they have not yet succumbed to any of the myriad causes of death among younger people. While heart disease and cancer remain the most common causes of death in this group, other diseases claim a larger share of the oldest adults. For example, 10 percent of people aged 85 or older die of cerebrovascular disease compared with only 5 percent of those aged 65 to 74. Twenty percent of the oldest adults die from a variety of causes that do not make it into the nation's top ten list.

■ Medical research has focused heavily on lengthening life, but it is equally important to insure a good quality of life in the later years.

Cancer accounts for only 12 percent of deaths among people aged 85 or older

(percent of deaths from heart disease and cancer, by age, 2002)

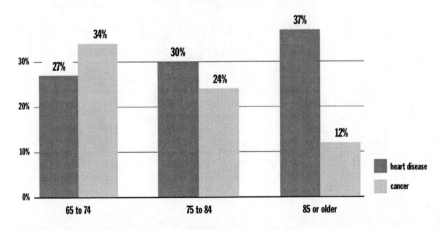

Table 7.20 Leading Causes of Death for People Aged 65 to 74, 2002

(number and percent distribution of deaths accounted for by the ten leading causes of death for people aged 65 to 74, 2002)

		number	percent distribution
	All causes	**422,990**	**100.0%**
1.	Malignant neoplasms (cancer) (2)	144,757	34.2
2.	Diseases of the heart (1)	112,547	26.6
3.	Chronic lower respiratory disease (4)	29,788	7.0
4.	Cerebrovascular diseases (3)	21,992	5.2
5.	Diabetes mellitus (6)	16,709	4.0
6.	Accidents (unintentional injuries) (5)	8,086	1.9
7.	Nephritis, nephrotic syndrome, nephrosis (9)	7,164	1.7
8.	Influenza and pneumonia (7)	6,847	1.6
9.	Septicemia (10)	6,336	1.5
10.	Chronic liver disease and cirrhosis (12)	5,381	1.3
	All other causes	63,383	15.0

Note: Numbers in parentheses show rank for all age groups if the cause of death is among top fifteen.
Source: National Center for Health Statistics, Deaths: Final Data for 2002, National Vital Statistics Reports, Vol. 53, No. 5, 2004;

Table 7.21 Leading Causes of Death for People Aged 75 to 84, 2002

(number and percent distribution of deaths accounted for by the ten leading causes of death for people aged 75 to 84, 2002)

		number	percent distribution
	All causes	**707,654**	**100.0%**
1.	Diseases of the heart (1)	213,581	30.2
2.	Malignant neoplasms (cancer) (2)	167,062	23.6
3.	Cerebrovascular diseases (3)	54,889	7.8
4.	Chronic lower respiratory disease (4)	49,241	7.0
5.	Diabetes mellitus (6)	23,282	3.3
6.	Alzheimer's disease (8)	20,135	2.8
7.	Influenza and pneumonia (7)	19,984	2.8
8.	Nephritis, nephrotic syndrome, nephrosis (9)	13,896	2.0
9.	Accidents (unintentional injuries) (5)	12,904	1.8
10.	Septicemia (10)	11,010	1.6
	All other causes	121,670	17.2

Note: Numbers in parentheses show rank for all age groups if the cause of death is among top fifteen.
Source: National Center for Health Statistics, Deaths: Final Data for 2002, National Vital Statistics Reports, Vol. 53, No. 5, 2004;

Table 7.22 Leading Causes of Death for People Aged 85 or Older, 2002

(number and percent distribution of deaths accounted for by the ten leading causes of death for people aged 85 or older, 2002)

		number	percent distribution
	All causes	**681,076**	**100.0%**
1.	Diseases of the heart (1)	250,173	36.7
2.	Malignant neoplasms (cancer) (2)	79,182	11.6
3.	Cerebrovascular diseases (3)	66,412	9.8
4.	Alzheimer's disease (8)	34,552	5.1
5.	Influenza and pneumonia (7)	31,995	4.7
6.	Chronic lower respiratory disease (4)	29,284	4.3
7.	Diabetes mellitus (6)	14,724	2.2
8.	Nephritis, nephrotic syndrome, nephrosis (9)	13,256	1.9
9.	Accidents (unintentional injuries) (5)	12,651	1.9
10.	Septicemia (10)	9,324	1.4
	All other causes	139,523	20.5

Note: Numbers in parentheses show rank for all age groups if the cause of death is among top fifteen.
Source: National Center for Health Statistics, Deaths: Final Data for 2002, National Vital Statistics Reports, Vol. 53, No. 5, 2004;

Americans Are Living Longer

Life expectancy continues to increase.

Life expectancy rose considerably in the second half of the twentieth century. In 1950, a newborn could expect to live 68.2 years, on average. By 2002, life expectancy had increased to 77.3 years, a gain of 9.1 years. Much of the increase resulted from reduced infant mortality, but some was attributable to lower mortality among older adults. Between 1950 and 2002, life expectancy at age 65 increased 4.3 years.

Life expectancy changes with age. The older you get, the longer you can expect to live. A child born in 2002 could expect to live 77.3 years, on average. But a person reaching age 65 in 2002 could expect to live another 18.2 years, on average, to 83.2. Someone aged 85 in 2002 could expect to live another 6.5 years, on average.

Women have longer life expectancies than men at every age. A girl born in 2002 could expect to live to age 79.9. Her male counterpart could expect to live to age 74.5. At age 65, women could expect to live an additional 19.5 years compared with 16.6 years for men. By age 90, however, the difference in life expectancy between men and women is measured in months rather than years.

■ Although life expectancy has increased substantially, the United States ranks well below many other developed nations in expected length of life.

Life expectancy at birth reached 77.3 years in 2002

(years of life remaining at birth for selected years, 2002)

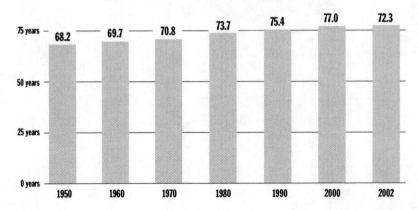

Table 7.23 Life Expectancy by Age, 1950 to 2002

(years of life remaining at birth and age 65, 1950 to 2002; change in years of life remaining for selected years)

	at birth	age 65
2002	77.3	18.2
2001	77.2	18.1
2000	77.0	17.9
1999	76.7	17.7
1998	76.7	17.8
1997	76.5	17.7
1996	76.1	17.5
1995	75.8	17.4
1994	75.7	17.4
1993	75.5	17.3
1992	75.8	17.5
1991	75.5	17.4
1990	75.4	17.2
1980	73.7	16.4
1970	70.8	15.2
1960	69.7	14.3
1950	68.2	13.9
Change (years)		
1990–2002	1.9	1.0
1950–2002	9.1	4.3

Source: National Center for Health Statistics, Health, United States, 2004; *and Deaths: Final Data for 2002, National Vital Statistics Report, Vol. 53, No. 5, 2004; calculations by New Strategist*

Table 7.24 Life Expectancy by Age and Sex, 2002

(years of life remaining at selected ages, by sex, 2002)

	total	females	males
At birth	77.3	79.9	74.5
Aged 1	76.8	79.4	74.1
Aged 5	72.9	75.4	70.2
Aged 10	67.9	70.5	65.3
Aged 15	63.0	65.5	60.3
Aged 20	58.2	60.7	55.6
Aged 25	53.5	55.8	51.0
Aged 30	48.7	51.0	46.3
Aged 35	44.0	46.1	41.6
Aged 40	39.3	41.4	37.0
Aged 45	34.8	36.7	32.6
Aged 50	30.3	32.2	28.3
Aged 55	26.1	27.7	24.1
Aged 60	22.0	23.5	20.2
Aged 65	18.2	19.5	16.6
Aged 70	14.7	15.8	13.2
Aged 75	11.5	12.4	10.3
Aged 80	8.8	9.4	7.8
Aged 85	6.5	6.9	5.7
Aged 90	4.8	5.0	4.2
Aged 95	3.6	3.7	3.2
Aged 100	2.7	2.8	2.5

Source: National Center for Health Statistics, **Deaths: Final Data for 2002,** *National Vital Statistics Report, Vol. 53, No. 5, 2004; calculations by New Strategist*

8

Disability

■ **Nearly one in five Americans is disabled.**

People aged 65 or older are most likely to be disabled, with 42 percent reporting some kind of limitation.

■ **Disability rates vary by demographic characteristic.**

The rate declines with increasing education, from 28 percent of people who did not graduate from high school to just 7 percent of college graduates.

■ **Seventeen percent of people aged 65 or older rely on special equipment.**

Most commonly, the special equipment is mobility aids, such as canes, walkers, or wheelchairs.

■ **More than 4 million children participate in special education or early intervention services.**

Boys are more likely than girls to be in special programs, as are children from low-income families and those on Medicaid.

■ **Work limitations are common among those with low incomes.**

Among people with household incomes below $20,000, 18 percent cannot work due to a disability. One-third of Medicaid recipients cannot work.

Older Women Are Most Likely to Be Disabled

Among people under age 65, men have higher disability rates.

The 2000 Census counted almost 50 million people—19 percent of the population—with a disability of some type. Most likely to be disabled are those aged 65 or older, 42 percent of whom have some form of disability. In contrast, a much smaller 19 percent of people aged 16 to 64 have a disability.

Among older adults, the most common forms of disability are physical problems—usually mobility impairments such as difficulty walking or climbing stairs. A substantial share also reports having difficulty going outside the home, a condition often related to other disabilities such as having difficulty walking.

Older women are slightly more likely than older men to report being disabled, but among people aged 16 to 64 the disability rate is slightly higher for men. The gender difference is probably the result of conditions present at birth as well as a greater tendency for young men to have accidents that impair them. Among older adults, the larger share of women with disabilities is the result of their older age relative to men, since women live longer.

■ As the older population grows, the number of disabled Americans will increase.

Disability rises sharply with age

(percent of people with any disability, by age and sex, 2000)

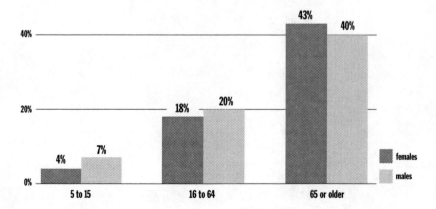

Table 8.1 Disability Status of People by Age, 2000 Census

(total number of people aged 5 or older and number and percent with disabilities, by age and type of disability, 2000)

	total		female		male	
	number	percent distribution	number	percent distribution	number	percent distribution
TOTAL PEOPLE	**257,167,527**	**100.0%**	**132,530,702**	**100.0%**	**124,636,825**	**100.0%**
With any disability	**49,746,248**	**19.3**	**25,306,717**	**19.1**	**24,439,531**	**19.6**
TOTAL PEOPLE						
AGED 5 TO 15	**45,133,667**	**100.0**	**22,008,343**	**100.0**	**23,125,324**	**100.0**
With any disability	**2,614,919**	**5.8**	**948,689**	**4.3**	**1,666,230**	**7.2**
Sensory	442,894	1.0	200,689	0.9	242,706	1.0
Physical	455,461	1.0	203,609	0.9	251,852	1.1
Mental	2,078,502	4.6	691,109	3.1	1,387,393	6.0
Self care	419,018	0.9	174,194	0.8	244,824	1.1
TOTAL PEOPLE						
AGED 16 TO 64	**178,687,234**	**100.0**	**91,116,651**	**100.0**	**87,570,583**	**100.0**
With any disability	**33,153,211**	**18.6**	**16,014,192**	**17.6**	**17,139,019**	**19.6**
Sensory	4,123,902	2.3	1,735,781	1.9	2,388,121	2.7
Physical	11,150,365	6.2	5,870,634	6.4	5,279,731	6.0
Mental	6,764,439	3.8	3,329,808	3.7	3,434,631	3.9
Self care	3,149,875	1.8	1,686,691	1.9	1,463,184	1.7
Difficulty going outside the home	11,414,508	6.4	5,845,146	6.4	5,569,362	6.4
Employment disability	21,287,570	11.9	9,913,784	10.9	11,373,786	13.0
TOTAL PEOPLE						
AGED 65 OR OLDER	**33,346,626**	**100.0**	**19,405,708**	**100.0**	**13,940,918**	**100.0**
With any disability	**13,978,118**	**41.9**	**8,343,836**	**43.0**	**5,634,282**	**40.4**
Sensory	4,738,479	14.2	2,561,263	13.2	2,177,216	15.6
Physical	9,545,680	28.6	5,955,541	30.7	3,590,139	25.8
Mental	3,592,912	10.8	2,212,852	11.4	1,380,060	9.9
Self care	3,183,840	9.5	2,138,930	11.0	1,044,910	7.5
Difficulty going outside the home	6,795,517	20.4	4,456,389	23.0	2,339,128	16.8

Note: Sensory disabilities are long-lasting impairments of vision and hearing; physical disabilities are limitations such as difficulty walking or climbing stairs; mental disabilities are difficulty with cognitive tasks such as learning, remembering, and concentrating; self-care disabilities are difficulty taking care of personal needs like dressing and bathing; employment disabilities are physical, mental, or emotional conditions making it difficult for people to work at a job; difficulty going outside the home is difficulty shopping or visiting the doctor
Source: Bureau of the Census, Disability Status: 2000, *Census 2000 Brief, 2003; Internet site http://www.census.gov/population/www/cen2000/briefs.html*

Disability Rates Vary by Demographic Characteristic

There are differences not only by age and sex, but also by race, income, and education.

Disability is a concept with as many different definitions as there are surveys to measure it. A 2002 survey by the National Center for Health Statistics found 14 percent of adults having some type of physical difficulty. The rate rises with age from 5 percent of those aged 18 to 44 to 44 percent of those aged 75 or older. The oldest adults account for about one-quarter of all people with physical difficulties. The most commonly reported conditions are difficulties walking a quarter mile; climbing stairs; stooping, bending, or kneeling; and pushing or pulling large objects.

Women make up 52 percent of all adults with disabilities, similar to their share of the total population. But they account for a larger share of people with certain types of disabilities. They account for 71 percent of people with difficulty lifting or carrying ten pounds, for example, and women are 69 percent of those who find it difficult to push or pull large objects.

The share of people with physical difficulties also varies by race and Hispanic origin, income, and education. Non-Hispanic whites and blacks are more likely than Asians and Hispanics to have physical difficulties. The share of people with disabilities declines with income, from 26 percent of those with the lowest incomes to 6 percent of those with the highest incomes. And the more education people have, the less likely they are to be disabled.

■ As the baby-boom generation enters the older age groups, the share of the elderly with disabilities may decline because of boomers' high level of education.

Physical difficulties are less common among the educated

(percent of people aged 18 or older with any type of difficulty in physical functioning, by education, 2002)

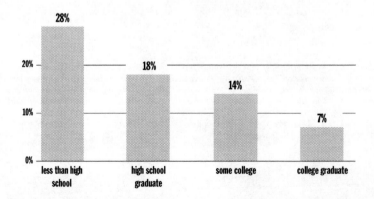

Table 8.2 Difficulties in Physical Functioning among Adults by Age, 2002

(number of people aged 18 or older with difficulties in physical functioning, by type of difficulty and age, 2002; numbers in thousands)

				aged 65 or older		
	total	18 to 44	45 to 64	total	65 to 74	75 or older
TOTAL PEOPLE	**205,825**	**108,114**	**64,650**	**33,061**	**17,809**	**15,252**
Total with any physical difficulty	**28,319**	**5,599**	**11,272**	**11,447**	**4,750**	**6,697**
Walk quarter of a mile	12,437	1,719	4,488	6,230	2,280	3,950
Climb up ten steps without resting	9,621	1,288	3,742	4,590	1,624	2,966
Stand for two hours	16,455	2,761	6,470	7,224	2,666	4,558
Sit for two hours	6,309	1,687	2,927	1,696	716	980
Stoop, bend, or kneel	16,265	2,659	6,605	7,001	2,930	4,071
Reach over head	4,797	668	2,198	1,931	673	1,258
Grasp or handle small objects	3,475	466	1,414	1,595	560	1,035
Lift or carry ten pounds	7,772	1,159	3,057	3,556	1,248	2,308
Push or pull large objects	11,516	2,108	4,617	4,791	1,812	2,979

PERCENT WITH PHYSICAL DIFFICULTY BY AGE

TOTAL PEOPLE	**100.0%**	**100.0%**	**100.0%**	**100.0%**	**100.0%**	**100.0%**
Total with any physical difficulty	**13.8**	**5.2**	**17.4**	**34.6**	**26.7**	**43.9**
Walk quarter of a mile	6.0	1.6	6.9	18.8	12.8	25.9
Climb up ten steps without resting	4.7	1.2	5.8	13.9	9.1	19.4
Stand for two hours	8.0	2.6	10.0	21.9	15.0	29.9
Sit for two hours	3.1	1.6	4.5	5.1	4.0	6.4
Stoop, bend, or kneel	7.9	2.5	10.2	21.2	16.5	26.7
Reach over head	2.3	0.6	3.4	5.8	3.8	8.2
Grasp or handle small objects	1.7	0.4	2.2	4.8	3.1	6.8
Lift or carry ten pounds	3.8	1.1	4.7	10.8	7.0	15.1
Push or pull large objects	5.6	1.9	7.1	14.5	10.2	19.5

PERCENT DISTRIBUTION OF THOSE WITH PHYSICAL DIFFICULTIES BY AGE

TOTAL PEOPLE	**100.0%**	**52.5%**	**31.4%**	**16.1%**	**8.7%**	**7.4%**
Total with any physical difficulty	**100.0**	**19.8**	**39.8**	**40.4**	**16.8**	**23.6**
Walk quarter of a mile	100.0	13.8	36.1	50.1	18.3	31.8
Climb up ten steps without resting	100.0	13.4	38.9	47.7	16.9	30.8
Stand for two hours	100.0	16.8	39.3	43.9	16.2	27.7
Sit for two hours	100.0	26.7	46.4	26.9	11.3	15.5
Stoop, bend, or kneel	100.0	16.3	40.6	43.0	18.0	25.0
Reach over head	100.0	13.9	45.8	40.3	14.0	26.2
Grasp or handle small objects	100.0	13.4	40.7	45.9	16.1	29.8
Lift or carry ten pounds	100.0	14.9	39.3	45.8	16.1	29.7
Push or pull large objects	100.0	18.3	40.1	41.6	15.7	25.9

Note: Respondents were classified as having difficulties if they responded "very difficult" or "can't do at all."
Source: National Center for Health Statistics, Summary Health Statistics for U.S. Adults: National Health Interview Survey, 2002, Series 10, No. 222, 2004; Internet site http://www.cdc.gov/nchs/nhis.htm

Table 8.3 Difficulties in Physical Functioning among Adults by Sex, 2002

(number of people aged 18 or older with difficulties in physical functioning, by type of difficulty and sex, 2002; numbers in thousands)

	total	men	women
TOTAL PEOPLE	**205,825**	**98,749**	**107,076**
Total with any physical difficulty	**28,319**	**10,097**	**18,222**
Walk quarter of a mile	12,437	4,581	7,856
Climb up ten steps without resting	9,621	3,282	6,339
Stand for two hours	16,455	5,949	10,506
Sit for two hours	6,309	2,214	4,095
Stoop, bend, or kneel	16,265	5,898	10,367
Reach over head	4,797	1,598	3,199
Grasp or handle small objects	3,475	1,290	2,185
Lift or carry ten pounds	7,772	2,284	5,488
Push or pull large objects	11,516	3,550	7,966
PERCENT WITH PHYSICAL DIFFICULTY BY SEX			
TOTAL PEOPLE	**100.0%**	**100.0%**	**100.0%**
Total with any physical difficulty	**13.8**	**10.2**	**17.0**
Walk quarter of a mile	6.0	4.6	7.3
Climb up ten steps without resting	4.7	3.3	5.9
Stand for two hours	8.0	6.0	9.8
Sit for two hours	3.1	2.2	3.8
Stoop, bend, or kneel	7.9	6.0	9.7
Reach over head	2.3	1.6	3.0
Grasp or handle small objects	1.7	1.3	2.0
Lift or carry ten pounds	3.8	2.3	5.1
Push or pull large objects	5.6	3.6	7.4
PERCENT DISTRIBUTION OF THOSE WITH PHYSICAL DIFFICULTIES BY SEX			
TOTAL PEOPLE	**100.0%**	**48.0%**	**52.0%**
Total with any physical difficulty	**100.0**	**35.7**	**64.3**
Walk quarter of a mile	100.0	36.8	63.2
Climb up ten steps without resting	100.0	34.1	65.9
Stand for two hours	100.0	36.2	63.8
Sit for two hours	100.0	35.1	64.9
Stoop, bend, or kneel	100.0	36.3	63.7
Reach over head	100.0	33.3	66.7
Grasp or handle small objects	100.0	37.1	62.9
Lift or carry ten pounds	100.0	29.4	70.6
Push or pull large objects	100.0	30.8	69.2

Note: Respondents were classified as having difficulties if they responded "very difficult" or "can't do at all."
Source: National Center for Health Statistics, Summary Health Statistics for U.S. Adults: National Health Interview Survey, 2002, *Series 10, No. 222, 2004; Internet site http://www.cdc.gov/nchs/nhis.htm*

Table 8.4 Difficulties in Physical Functioning among Adults by Race and Hispanic Origin, 2002

(number of people aged 18 or older with difficulties in physical functioning, by type of difficulty, race, and Hispanic origin, 2002; numbers in thousands)

	total	Asian	black	Hispanic	non-Hispanic white
TOTAL PEOPLE	**205,825**	**7,270**	**23,499**	**22,691**	**149,584**
Total with any physical difficulty	**28,319**	**469**	**3,472**	**2,105**	**21,675**
Walk quarter of a mile	12,437	183	1,710	855	9,427
Climb up ten steps without resting	9,621	108	1,576	826	6,909
Stand for two hours	16,455	335	2,142	1,143	12,537
Sit for two hours	6,309	129	861	524	4,673
Stoop, bend, or kneel	16,265	225	1,990	1,238	12,484
Reach over head	4,797	43	601	372	3,650
Grasp or handle small objects	3,475	30	528	356	2,482
Lift or carry ten pounds	7,772	193	1,199	809	5,403
Push or pull large objects	11,516	223	1,599	1,047	8,423

PERCENT WITH PHYSICAL DIFFICULTY BY RACE AND HISPANIC ORIGIN

	total	Asian	black	Hispanic	non-Hispanic white
TOTAL PEOPLE	**100.0%**	**100.0%**	**100.0%**	**100.0%**	**100.0%**
Total with any physical difficulty	**13.8**	**6.5**	**14.8**	**9.3**	**14.5**
Walk quarter of a mile	6.0	2.5	7.3	3.8	6.3
Climb up ten steps without resting	4.7	1.5	6.7	3.6	4.6
Stand for two hours	8.0	4.6	9.1	5.0	8.4
Sit for two hours	3.1	1.8	3.7	2.3	3.1
Stoop, bend, or kneel	7.9	3.1	8.5	5.5	8.3
Reach over head	2.3	0.6	2.6	1.6	2.4
Grasp or handle small objects	1.7	0.4	2.2	1.6	1.7
Lift or carry ten pounds	3.8	2.7	5.1	3.6	3.6
Push or pull large objects	5.6	3.1	6.8	4.6	5.6

PERCENT DISTRIBUTION OF THOSE WITH PHYSICAL DIFFICULTIES BY RACE AND HISPANIC ORIGIN

	total	Asian	black	Hispanic	non-Hispanic white
TOTAL PEOPLE	**100.0%**	**3.5%**	**11.4%**	**11.0%**	**72.7%**
Total with any physical difficulty	**100.0**	**1.7**	**12.3**	**7.4**	**76.5**
Walk quarter of a mile	100.0	1.5	13.7	6.9	75.8
Climb up ten steps without resting	100.0	1.1	16.4	8.6	71.8
Stand for two hours	100.0	2.0	13.0	6.9	76.2
Sit for two hours	100.0	2.0	13.6	8.3	74.1
Stoop, bend, or kneel	100.0	1.4	12.2	7.6	76.8
Reach over head	100.0	0.9	12.5	7.8	76.1
Grasp or handle small objects	100.0	0.9	15.2	10.2	71.4
Lift or carry ten pounds	100.0	2.5	15.4	10.4	69.5
Push or pull large objects	100.0	1.9	13.9	9.1	73.1

Note: Respondents were classified as having difficulties if they responded "very difficult" or "can't do at all." Numbers by race and Hispanic origin may not sum to total because not all races are shown and Hispanics may be of any race.
Source: National Center for Health Statistics, Summary Health Statistics for U.S. Adults: National Health Interview Survey, 2002, *Series 10, No. 222, 2004; Internet site http://www.cdc.gov/nchs/nhis.htm*

Table 8.5 Difficulties in Physical Functioning among Adults by Household Income, 2002

(number of people aged 18 or older with difficulties in physical functioning, by type of difficulty and household income, 2002; numbers in thousands)

	total	under $20,000	$20,000–$34,999	$35,000–$54,999	$55,000–$74,999	$75,000 or more
TOTAL PEOPLE	**205,825**	**37,369**	**29,671**	**31,814**	**23,984**	**41,572**
Total with any physical difficulty	**28,319**	**9,602**	**4,816**	**3,740**	**2,007**	**2,659**
Walk quarter of a mile	12,437	4,989	2,185	1,375	637	805
Climb up ten steps without resting	9,621	4,261	1,597	980	509	371
Stand for two hours	16,455	6,301	2,636	2,014	998	1,234
Sit for two hours	6,309	2,489	1,068	699	417	492
Stoop, bend, or kneel	16,265	5,968	2,693	1,955	993	1,459
Reach over head	4,797	2,065	749	484	290	281
Grasp or handle small objects	3,475	1,581	499	296	169	228
Lift or carry ten pounds	7,772	3,327	1,135	746	424	599
Push or pull large objects	11,516	4,640	1,831	1,211	767	951

PERCENT WITH PHYSICAL DIFFICULTY BY HOUSEHOLD INCOME

TOTAL PEOPLE	**100.0%**	**100.0%**	**100.0%**	**100.0%**	**100.0%**	**100.0%**
Total with any physical difficulty	**13.8**	**25.7**	**16.2**	**11.8**	**8.4**	**6.4**
Walk quarter of a mile	6.0	13.4	7.4	4.3	2.7	1.9
Climb up ten steps without resting	4.7	11.4	5.4	3.1	2.1	0.9
Stand for two hours	8.0	16.9	8.9	6.3	4.2	3.0
Sit for two hours	3.1	6.7	3.6	2.2	1.7	1.2
Stoop, bend, or kneel	7.9	16.0	9.1	6.1	4.1	3.5
Reach over head	2.3	5.5	2.5	1.5	1.2	0.7
Grasp or handle small objects	1.7	4.2	1.7	0.9	0.7	0.5
Lift or carry ten pounds	3.8	8.9	3.8	2.3	1.8	1.4
Push or pull large objects	5.6	12.4	6.2	3.8	3.2	2.3

PERCENT DISTRIBUTION OF THOSE WITH PHYSICAL DIFFICULTIES BY HOUSEHOLD INCOME

TOTAL PEOPLE	**100.0%**	**18.2%**	**14.4%**	**15.5%**	**11.7%**	**20.2%**
Total with any physical difficulty	**100.0**	**33.9**	**17.0**	**13.2**	**7.1**	**9.4**
Walk quarter of a mile	100.0	40.1	17.6	11.1	5.1	6.5
Climb up ten steps without resting	100.0	44.3	16.6	10.2	5.3	3.9
Stand for two hours	100.0	38.3	16.0	12.2	6.1	7.5
Sit for two hours	100.0	39.5	16.9	11.1	6.6	7.8
Stoop, bend, or kneel	100.0	36.7	16.6	12.0	6.1	9.0
Reach over head	100.0	43.0	15.6	10.1	6.0	5.9
Grasp or handle small objects	100.0	45.5	14.4	8.5	4.9	6.6
Lift or carry ten pounds	100.0	42.8	14.6	9.6	5.5	7.7
Push or pull large objects	100.0	40.3	15.9	10.5	6.7	8.3

Note: Respondents were classified as having difficulties if they responded "very difficult" or "can't do at all."
Source: National Center for Health Statistics, Summary Health Statistics for U.S. Adults: National Health Interview Survey, 2002, *Series 10, No. 222, 2004; Internet site http://www.cdc.gov/nchs/nhis.htm*

Table 8.6 Difficulties in Physical Functioning among Adults by Educational Attainment, 2002

(number of people aged 18 or older with difficulties in physical functioning, by type of difficulty and educational attainment, 2002; numbers in thousands)

	total	less than high school	high school graduate	some college	college graduate
TOTAL PEOPLE	205,825	28,248	52,556	48,091	47,197
Total with any physical difficulty	**28,319**	**7,883**	**9,216**	**6,566**	**3,407**
Walk quarter of a mile	12,437	4,315	4,206	2,364	1,150
Climb up ten steps without resting	9,621	3,544	3,143	1,910	696
Stand for two hours	16,455	4,952	5,474	3,582	1,797
Sit for two hours	6,309	1,808	2,059	1,600	576
Stoop, bend, or kneel	16,265	4,802	5,385	3,590	1,905
Reach over head	4,797	1,481	1,782	1,052	394
Grasp or handle small objects	3,475	1,146	1,121	768	314
Lift or carry ten pounds	7,772	2,539	2,641	1,717	622
Push or pull large objects	11,516	3,594	3,850	2,480	1,211
PERCENT WITH PHYSICAL DIFFICULTY BY EDUCATION					
TOTAL PEOPLE	100.0%	100.0%	100.0%	100.0%	100.0%
Total with any physical difficulty	**13.8**	**27.9**	**17.5**	**13.7**	**7.2**
Walk quarter of a mile	6.0	15.3	8.0	4.9	2.4
Climb up ten steps without resting	4.7	12.5	6.0	4.0	1.5
Stand for two hours	8.0	17.5	10.4	7.4	3.8
Sit for two hours	3.1	6.4	3.9	3.3	1.2
Stoop, bend, or kneel	7.9	17.0	10.2	7.5	4.0
Reach over head	2.3	5.2	3.4	2.2	0.8
Grasp or handle small objects	1.7	4.1	2.1	1.6	0.7
Lift or carry ten pounds	3.8	9.0	5.0	3.6	1.3
Push or pull large objects	5.6	12.7	7.3	5.2	2.6
PERCENT DISTRIBUTION OF THOSE WITH PHYSICAL DIFFICULTIES BY EDUCATION					
TOTAL PEOPLE	100.0%	13.7%	25.5%	23.4%	22.9%
Total with any physical difficulty	**100.0**	**27.8**	**32.5**	**23.2**	**12.0**
Walk quarter of a mile	100.0	34.7	33.8	19.0	9.2
Climb up ten steps without resting	100.0	36.8	32.7	19.9	7.2
Stand for two hours	100.0	30.1	33.3	21.8	10.9
Sit for two hours	100.0	28.7	32.6	25.4	9.1
Stoop, bend, or kneel	100.0	29.5	33.1	22.1	11.7
Reach over head	100.0	30.9	37.1	21.9	8.2
Grasp or handle small objects	100.0	33.0	32.3	22.1	9.0
Lift or carry ten pounds	100.0	32.7	34.0	22.1	8.0
Push or pull large objects	100.0	31.2	33.4	21.5	10.5

Note: Respondents were classified as having difficulties if they responded "very difficult" or "can't do at all."
Source: National Center for Health Statistics, Summary Health Statistics for U.S. Adults: National Health Interview Survey, 2002, *Series 10, No. 222, 2004; Internet site http://www.cdc.gov/nchs/nhis.htm*

Chronic Health Conditions Often Limit Activities

Older adults are especially likely to be limited in their usual activities.

A sizable 13 percent of the population has some kind of activity limitation because of health problems. Most have one or more chronic conditions that limit what they can do.

The incidence of activity limitations due to health problems increases sharply beginning in the 45-to-64 age group. From 6 to 9 percent of people under age 45 have activity limitations, but among those aged 45 to 64 the share is 17 percent. Twenty-six percent of people aged 65 to 74 and 46 percent of those aged 75 or older have activity limitations because of health problems.

Some people need special equipment to help overcome limitations that result from health problems. Most likely to use some type of equipment are people aged 65 or older, 17 percent of whom do so. Most commonly, these are mobility aids such as canes, walkers, or wheelchairs.

Many children need assistance as well, due to learning difficulties or other conditions. About 6 percent of children under age 18 receive special education or early intervention services. Boys are considerably more likely than girls to receive these services. By race and Hispanic origin, black children are more likely than whites or Hispanics to receive special education services.

■ As the number of older adults rises in the coming years, there will be an increasing need for special assistance and aids to help overcome activity limitations.

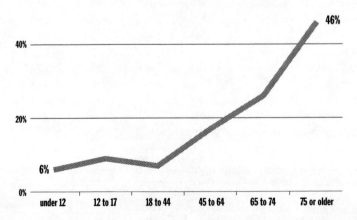

Nearly half of the oldest adults are limited

(percent of people with activity limitations due to health problems, 2002)

Table 8.7 Limitations in Usual Activities Due to Health Problems, 2002

(total number of people, and percent distribution by limitation status in usual activities, by selected characteristics, 2002; numbers in thousands)

	total		no	limitations	
	number	percent	limitations	total	due to chronic conditions
Total people	**278,789**	**100.0%**	**87.0%**	**12.6%**	**12.1%**
Sex					
Female	142,731	100.0	86.5	13.1	12.6
Male	136,058	100.0	87.5	12.1	11.6
Age					
Under age 12	48,356	100.0	93.2	6.4	6.2
Aged 12 to 17	24,612	100.0	90.6	8.9	8.7
Aged 18 to 44	108,111	100.0	93.1	6.6	6.2
Aged 45 to 64	64,650	100.0	82.6	17.1	16.5
Aged 65 to 74	17,752	100.0	73.6	25.8	24.9
Aged 75 or older	15,308	100.0	53.4	46.1	44.3
Race and Hispanic origin					
Asian	10,740	100.0	94.6	5.0	4.8
Black	34,037	100.0	86.2	13.4	12.8
Hispanic	35,254	100.0	91.5	8.2	7.9
Non-Hispanic white	193,860	100.0	86.1	13.6	13.0
Household income					
Under $20,000	46,934	100.0	74.8	25.0	24.3
$20,000 to $34,999	36,568	100.0	83.6	16.2	15.7
$35,000 to $54,999	40,451	100.0	89.4	10.5	10.3
$55,000 to $74,999	31,344	100.0	92.2	7.6	7.4
$75,000 or more	55,653	100.0	93.9	5.9	5.7
Education					
Not a high school graduate	27,467	100.0	70.6	29.2	28.4
High school graduate	52,064	100.0	82.2	17.6	17.1
Some college	46,703	100.0	85.3	14.4	13.9
College graduate	45,541	100.0	91.7	8.0	7.7
Health insurance coverage among people under age 65					
Private	169,418	100.0	92.7	7.0	6.7
Medicaid	27,538	100.0	77.1	22.6	21.8
Other	5,883	100.0	64.8	34.9	34.3
Uninsured	40,127	100.0	91.5	8.0	7.7

Note: Assessment of limitation in usual activities is based on a series of questions concerning limitations in a person's ability to engage in work, school, play, or other activities for health reasons, the specific conditions causing the limitation, and the duration of the conditions. Conditions lasting more than three months are classified as chronic. Selected conditions (such as arthritis, diabetes, cancer, heart conditions, etc.) are considered chronic regardless of duration. Numbers by race and Hispanic origin will not sum to total because not all races are shown and Hispanics may be of any race.
Source: National Center for Health Statistics, Summary Health Statistics for the U.S. Population: National Health Interview Survey, 2002, Vital and Health Statistics, Series 10, No. 220, 2004; Internet site http://www.cdc.gov/nchs/nhis.htm

Table 8.8 Use of Special Equipment Due to Health Problems, 2003

(percent distribution of people aged 18 or older by whether they use special equipment because of health problems, by selected characteristics, 2003)

	yes	no
Total people	**5.9%**	**94.1%**
Sex		
Men	6.7	93.3
Women	5.4	94.6
Age		
Aged 18 to 24	1.0	99.0
Aged 25 to 34	1.5	98.5
Aged 35 to 44	3.2	96.8
Aged 45 to 54	5.6	94.4
Aged 55 to 64	8.2	91.8
Aged 65 or older	16.6	83.4
Race and Hispanic origin		
Black	8.2	91.9
Hispanic	4.1	95.9
White	6.0	94.0
Multiracial	8.6	91.7
Other	4.6	95.4
Household income		
Under $15,000	15.4	84.6
$15,000 to $24,999	8.8	91.2
$25,000 to $34,999	5.1	94.9
$35,000 to $49,999	3.7	96.3
$50,000 or more	2.5	97.5
Education		
Not a high school graduate	11.3	88.7
High school graduate	6.2	93.8
Some college	5.7	94.3
College graduate	3.9	96.1

Source: Centers for Disease Control and Prevention, Behavioral Risk Factor Surveillance System, Prevalence Data, Internet site http://apps.nccd.cdc.gov/brfss/; calculations by New Strategist

Table 8.9 Children Receiving Special Education or Early Intervention Services, 2002

(total number of people under age 18, and percent receiving special education or early intervention services, by selected characteristics, 2002; numbers in thousands)

| | total | receiving services | |
		number	percent
Total children	**72,968**	**4,313**	**5.9%**
Sex			
Female	35,658	1,476	4.1
Male	37,310	2,837	7.6
Age			
Under age 12	48,356	2,524	5.2
Aged 12 to 17	24,612	1,789	7.3
Race and Hispanic origin			
Asian	2,716	68	2.5
Black	10,601	769	7.3
Hispanic	12,563	595	4.7
Non-Hispanic white	45,120	2,752	6.1
Household income			
Less than $20,000	12,086	967	8.0
$20,000 to $34,999	9,688	763	8.0
$35,000 to $54,999	11,116	653	5.9
$55,000 to $74,999	9,088	506	5.6
$75,000 or more	15,548	753	4.8
Health insurance coverage			
Private	46,278	2,326	5.0
Medicaid/other public	17,004	1,561	9.5
Other	1,384	73	5.3
Uninsured	7,782	335	4.3

Source: National Center for Health Statistics, Summary Health Statistics for the U.S. Population: National Health Interview Survey, 2002, *Vital and Health Statistics, Series 10, No. 220, 2004; Internet site http://www.cdc.gov/nchs/nhis.htm*

Many Medicaid Recipients Cannot Work

A substantial portion of the working-age population has a work limitation due to health problems.

Nine percent of people aged 18 to 69 have some kind of limitation in work activity because of a health condition, with 6 percent being unable to work. The share of people with a work limitation rises with age, from 5 percent of those aged 18 to 44 to 19 percent of people aged 65 to 69.

People with the lowest household incomes (under $20,000) are most likely to have a work limitation, with 23 percent falling into this category. For most, their inability to work is the cause of their low income. Similarly, 39 percent of Medicaid recipients are limited in their work. Their disabilities are the reason they must rely on Medicaid.

The lower the level of education, the greater the chances of a work disability. Among people aged 16 to 64, only 5 percent of college graduates have a work disability compared with 15 percent of people who did not complete high school.

■ The Americans with Disabilities Act has helped many of the disabled lead more productive lives.

Nearly one-quarter of people with household incomes below $20,000 have a work limitation

(percent of people aged 16 to 69 who are limited or unable to work, by household income, 2002)

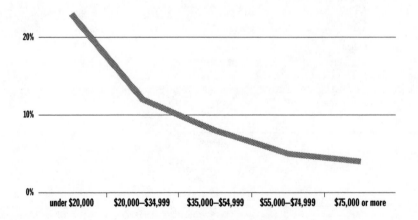

Table 8.10 Limitations in Work Activity Due to Health Problems, 2002

(total number of people aged 18 to 69, and percent distribution by work limitation status, by selected characteristics, 2002; numbers in thousands)

	total		not limited in work	limited in work	unable to work
	number	percent		total	
Total people	**182,017**	**100.0%**	**91.0%**	**9.0%**	**5.7%**
Sex					
Female	93,025	100.0	90.7	9.3	5.9
Male	88,992	100.0	91.4	8.6	5.4
Age					
Aged 18 to 44	108,111	100.0	94.8	5.2	3.2
Aged 45 to 64	64,650	100.0	85.9	14.1	9.4
Aged 65 to 69	9,256	100.0	80.8	19.3	10.7
Race and Hispanic origin					
Asian	7,494	100.0	96.5	3.5	2.0
Black	21,572	100.0	88.8	11.2	8.3
Hispanic	21,331	100.0	92.9	7.1	5.3
Non-Hispanic white	128,847	100.0	91.0	9.0	5.4
Household income					
Under $20,000	27,438	100.0	77.1	22.9	17.5
$20,000 to $34,999	22,705	100.0	87.4	12.5	7.3
$35,000 to $54,999	26,979	100.0	92.2	7.8	4.2
$55,000 to $74,999	21,415	100.0	94.6	5.3	2.7
$75,000 or more	38,750	100.0	96.4	3.7	1.8
Education					
Not a high school graduate	20,527	100.0	81.2	18.9	14.4
High school graduate	44,302	100.0	88.6	11.4	7.2
Some college	42,342	100.0	90.0	9.9	5.9
College graduate	41,975	100.0	95.6	4.4	2.0
Health insurance coverage among people under age 65					
Private	123,140	100.0	95.0	5.1	2.6
Medicaid	10,535	100.0	60.9	39.1	32.8
Other	4,498	100.0	67.1	32.9	26.2
Uninsured	32,345	100.0	91.8	8.1	4.7

Note: Assessment of ability to work is based on the question, "Does a physical, mental, or emotional problem now keep (respondent or family member aged 18 or older) from working at a job or business?" Assessment of limitation to work is based on the question, "Is (respondent or family member aged 18 or older) limited in the kind or amount of work they can do because of a physical, mental, or emotional problem?" Numbers by race and Hispanic origin will not sum to total because not all races are shown and Hispanics may be of any race.
Source: National Center for Health Statistics, Summary Health Statistics for the U.S. Population: National Health Interview Survey, 2002, Vital and Health Statistics, Series 10, No. 220, 2004; Internet site http://www.cdc.gov/nchs/nhis.htm

Table 8.11 People with a Work Disability by Age and Educational Attainment, 2004

(number and percent of people aged 16 to 64 with a work disability and percent in the labor force, by age and educational attainment, 2004; numbers in thousands)

		with a work disability		
	total	number	percent of total	percent in labor force
Aged 16 to 64	**187,850**	**19,016**	**10.1%**	**26.1%**
Less than high school	33,077	4,915	14.9	14.2
High school graduate	55,584	7,157	12.9	24.4
Some college	51,838	4,702	9.1	33.2
College graduate	47,350	2,241	4.7	43.1
Aged 16 to 24	**36,338**	**1,504**	**4.1**	**33.5**
Less than high school	14,680	666	4.5	22.8
High school graduate	8,373	515	6.2	38.9
Some college	10,938	279	2.5	44.0
College graduate	2,347	43	1.8	–
Aged 25 to 34	**38,884**	**2,331**	**6.0**	**33.1**
Less than high school	5,068	524	10.3	22.8
High school graduate	11,178	983	8.8	28.0
Some college	10,885	617	5.7	42.7
College graduate	11,754	208	1.8	55.3
Aged 35 to 44	**43,270**	**3,741**	**8.6**	**30.9**
Less than high school	5,230	916	17.5	17.6
High school graduate	13,697	1,448	10.6	27.8
Some college	11,607	976	8.4	40.6
College graduate	12,736	401	3.1	48.8
Aged 45 to 54	**41,003**	**5,320**	**13.0**	**26.2**
Less than high school	4,246	1,207	28.4	11.9
High school graduate	12,902	1,903	14.8	24.5
Some college	11,349	1,424	12.5	30.5
College graduate	12,506	786	6.3	44.4
Aged 55 to 64	**28,355**	**6,120**	**21.6**	**18.7**
Less than high school	3,855	1,601	41.5	7.7
High school graduate	9,435	2,308	24.5	17.4
Some college	7,058	1,407	19.9	24.5
College graduate	8,007	803	10.0	34.6

Note: (–) means sample is too small to make a reliable estimate.
Source: Bureau of the Census, Disability Data from the March 2004 Current Population Survey, Internet site http://www.census
.gov/hhes/www/disable/disabcps.html

9

Diseases and Conditions

■ **Twenty-three million Americans have heart disease.**

Among people with heart disease, 45 percent are aged 65 or older.

■ **Blacks are most likely to have been diagnosed with asthma.**

Twelve percent of blacks aged 18 or older have had asthma compared with only 7 percent of Hispanics.

■ **Thirty percent of adults have high blood pressure.**

The proportion of the population with high blood pressure is rising, thanks in part to increased monitoring of the condition.

■ **Cholesterol levels are declining.**

Diet changes and cholesterol-lowering medications are helping to combat high cholesterol.

■ **Eight percent of adults have diabetes.**

The proportion of people with diabetes is rising as obesity becomes a growing problem.

■ **Forty-three percent of adults have taken at least one prescription drug in the past month.**

In 2002, 10 million children took a prescription medication regularly for at least three months.

■ **Some health conditions are more costly than others.**

The four most expensive health conditions are heart disease, trauma, cancer, and mental illness.

The Most Serious Diseases Are More Common among the Elderly

The incidence of heart disease rises sharply with age.

Almost 23 million adults have some form of heart disease. Many more are at risk of developing heart disease because of other conditions. For example, 43 million adults have high blood pressure (hypertension) and 13 million have diabetes—both of which can contribute to heart disease.

Among people with heart disease, 45 percent are aged 65 or older. The 65-or-older age group accounts for about half of adults with cancer and 39 percent of those with diabetes. People aged 18 to 44 account for the largest share of those with some health conditions, however. More than half of adults with asthma or hay fever are in the 18-to-44 age group, as are 61 percent of people with migraines.

In general, serious conditions tend to develop later in life. While the share of people who have sinusitis, a relatively benign condition, peaks among those aged 45 to 64, the likelihood of having heart disease, hypertension, diabetes, or cancer increases with age. Only 4 percent of people aged 18 to 44 have some type of heart disease, compared with more than one-third of those aged 75 or older.

■ Medical advances in treating heart disease have reduced death rates and increased life expectancy.

More than one-third of people aged 75 or older have heart disease

(percent of people aged 18 or older with heart disease, by age, 2002)

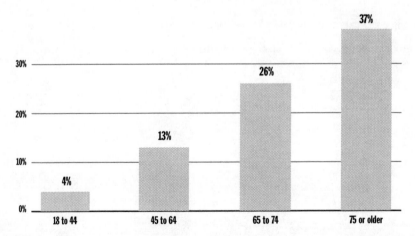

Table 9.1 Number of Health Conditions among Adults by Age, 2002

(number of people aged 18 or older with selected health conditions, by type of condition and age, 2002; numbers in thousands)

	total	18 to 44	45 to 64	65 to 74	75 or older
TOTAL PEOPLE	**205,825**	**108,114**	**64,650**	**17,809**	**15,252**
Selected circulatory diseases					
Heart disease, all types	22,719	4,322	8,186	4,664	5,547
Coronary	12,527	966	4,548	3,312	3,701
Hypertension	43,330	7,995	18,704	8,792	7,838
Stroke	4,836	422	1,598	1,126	1,690
Selected respiratory conditions					
Emphysema	3,131	287	1,272	862	710
Asthma					
Ever	21,927	12,454	6,836	1,487	1,150
Still	13,963	7,438	4,592	1,141	793
Hay fever	18,225	9,211	7,007	1,249	759
Sinusitis	29,222	13,420	11,487	2,505	1,810
Chronic bronchitis	9,114	3,761	3,563	978	811
Selected type of cancer					
Any cancer	14,381	2,140	5,096	3,516	3,629
Breast cancer	2,186	159	803	507	717
Cervical cancer	1,243	652	467	71	54
Prostate cancer	1,501	0	295	613	593
Other selected diseases and conditions					
Diabetes	13,391	2,080	6,030	3,029	2,252
Ulcers	15,632	5,598	5,850	2,189	1,995
Kidney disease	2,609	658	944	417	590
Liver disease	2,426	821	1,237	236	132
Arthritis	42,704	8,469	18,523	7,948	7,765
Chronic joint symptoms	51,416	17,090	20,807	6,972	6,548
Migraines or severe headaches	31,066	19,051	9,836	1,396	784
Pain in neck	28,401	12,872	10,892	2,514	2,123
Pain in lower back	54,325	25,628	19,225	5,120	4,353
Pain in face or jaw	9,535	5,056	3,353	658	468
Selected sensory problems					
Hearing	30,826	7,222	11,324	5,282	6,999
Vision	19,069	6,151	7,135	2,578	3,205
Absence of all natural teeth	17,177	2,517	5,472	4,253	4,935

Note: The conditions shown are those that have ever been diagnosed by a doctor, except as noted. Hay fever, sinusitis, and chronic bronchitis have been diagnosed in the past twelve months. Kidney and liver disease have been diagnosed in the past twelve months and exclude kidney stones, bladder infections, and incontinence. Chronic joint symptoms are shown if respondent had pain, aching, or stiffness in or around a joint (excluding back and neck) and the condition began more than three months ago. Migraines, pain in neck, lower back, face, or jaw are shown only if pain lasted a whole day or more.
Source: National Center for Health Statistics, Summary Health Statistics for U.S. Adults: National Health Interview Survey, 2002, Series 10, No. 222, 2004; Internet site http://www.cdc.gov/nchs/nhis.htm

Table 9.2 Percent Distribution of Health Conditions among Adults by Age, 2002

(percent distribution of people aged 18 or older with selected health conditions, by type of condition and age, 2002)

	total	18 to 44	45 to 64	65 to 74	75 or older
TOTAL PEOPLE	**100.0%**	**52.5%**	**31.4%**	**8.7%**	**7.4%**
Selected circulatory diseases					
Heart disease, all types	100.0	19.0	36.0	20.5	24.4
Coronary	100.0	7.7	36.3	26.4	29.5
Hypertension	100.0	18.5	43.2	20.3	18.1
Stroke	100.0	8.7	33.0	23.3	34.9
Selected respiratory conditions					
Emphysema	100.0	9.2	40.6	27.5	22.7
Asthma					
Ever	100.0	56.8	31.2	6.8	5.2
Still	100.0	53.3	32.9	8.2	5.7
Hay fever	100.0	50.5	38.4	6.9	4.2
Sinusitis	100.0	45.9	39.3	8.6	6.2
Chronic bronchitis	100.0	41.3	39.1	10.7	8.9
Selected type of cancer					
Any cancer	100.0	14.9	35.4	24.4	25.2
Breast cancer	100.0	7.3	36.7	23.2	32.8
Cervical cancer	100.0	52.5	37.6	5.7	4.3
Prostate cancer	100.0	0	19.7	40.8	39.5
Other selected diseases and conditions					
Diabetes	100.0	15.5	45.0	22.6	16.8
Ulcers	100.0	35.8	37.4	14.0	12.8
Kidney disease	100.0	25.2	36.2	16.0	22.6
Liver disease	100.0	33.8	51.0	9.7	5.4
Arthritis	100.0	19.8	43.4	18.6	18.2
Chronic joint symptoms	100.0	33.2	40.5	13.6	12.7
Migraines or severe headaches	100.0	61.3	31.7	4.5	2.5
Pain in neck	100.0	45.3	38.4	8.9	7.5
Pain in lower back	100.0	47.2	35.4	9.4	8.0
Pain in face or jaw	100.0	53.0	35.2	6.9	4.9
Selected sensory problems					
Hearing	100.0	23.4	36.7	17.1	22.7
Vision	100.0	32.3	37.4	13.5	16.8
Absence of all natural teeth	100.0	14.7	31.9	24.8	28.7

Note: The conditions shown are those that have ever been diagnosed by a doctor, except as noted. Hay fever, sinusitis, and chronic bronchitis have been diagnosed in the past twelve months. Kidney and liver disease have been diagnosed in the past twelve months and exclude kidney stones, bladder infections, and incontinence. Chronic joint symptoms are shown if respondent had pain, aching, or stiffness in or around a joint (excluding back and neck) and the condition began more than three months ago. Migraines, pain in neck, lower back, face, or jaw are shown only if pain lasted a whole day or more.
Source: National Center for Health Statistics, Summary Health Statistics for U.S. Adults: National Health Interview Survey, 2002, *Series 10, No. 222, 2004; Internet site http://www.cdc.gov/nchs/nhis.htm*

Table 9.3 Percent of Adults with Health Conditions by Age, 2002

(percent of people aged 18 or older with selected health conditions, by type of condition and age, 2002)

	total	18 to 44	45 to 64	65 to 74	75 or older
TOTAL PEOPLE	100.0%	100.0%	100.0%	100.0%	100.0%
Selected circulatory diseases					
Heart disease, all types	11.1	4.0	12.7	26.3	36.6
Coronary	6.1	0.9	7.1	18.7	24.5
Hypertension	21.1	7.4	29.0	49.6	51.8
Stroke	2.4	0.4	2.5	6.4	11.1
Selected respiratory conditions					
Emphysema	1.5	0.3	2.0	4.9	4.7
Asthma					
Ever	10.7	11.5	10.6	8.4	7.6
Still	6.8	6.9	7.1	6.4	5.2
Hay fever	8.9	8.5	10.9	7.1	5.0
Sinusitis	14.2	12.4	17.8	14.1	11.9
Chronic bronchitis	4.4	3.5	5.5	5.5	5.3
Selected type of cancer					
Any cancer	7.0	2.0	7.9	19.8	23.9
Breast cancer	1.1	0.1	1.2	2.9	4.7
Cervical cancer	1.2	1.2	1.4	0.7	0.6
Prostate cancer	1.5	0	0.9	7.5	9.9
Other selected diseases and conditions					
Diabetes	6.6	1.9	9.5	17.3	15.0
Ulcers	7.6	5.2	9.1	12.3	13.1
Kidney disease	1.3	0.6	1.5	2.3	3.9
Liver disease	1.2	0.8	1.9	1.3	0.9
Arthritis	20.8	7.8	28.8	44.9	51.2
Chronic joint symptoms	25.1	15.8	32.3	39.5	43.3
Migraines or severe headaches	15.1	17.6	15.3	7.9	5.2
Pain in neck	13.8	11.9	16.9	14.2	14.0
Pain in lower back	26.5	23.7	29.8	28.8	28.7
Pain in face or jaw	4.6	4.7	5.2	3.7	3.1
Selected sensory problems					
Hearing	15.0	6.7	17.5	29.7	46.0
Vision	9.3	5.7	11.0	14.5	21.1
Absence of all natural teeth	8.4	2.3	8.5	24.0	32.5

Note: The conditions shown are those that have ever been diagnosed by a doctor, except as noted. Hay fever, sinusitis, and chronic bronchitis have been diagnosed in the past twelve months. Kidney and liver disease have been diagnosed in the past twelve months and exclude kidney stones, bladder infections, and incontinence. Chronic joint symptoms are shown if respondent had pain, aching, or stiffness in or around a joint (excluding back and neck) and the condition began more than three months ago. Migraines, pain in neck, lower back, face, or jaw are shown only if pain lasted a whole day or more.
Source: National Center for Health Statistics, Summary Health Statistics for U.S. Adults: National Health Interview Survey, 2002, Series 10, No. 222, 2004; Internet site http://www.cdc.gov/nchs/nhis.htm

Biological Differences between Men and Women Are behind Disease Patterns

The incidence of many conditions differs by sex.

There are more women than men in the American population. This imbalance means that if the prevalence of a health condition is roughly the same for men and women, women will account for a larger number of sufferers. Evidence can be seen in hypertension statistics. Twenty-three million women have high blood pressure compared with 20 million men, but the prevalence rate is 21 percent for either sex.

For some health conditions, there can be sizable differences by sex in disease prevalence. Men are more likely than women to have coronary heart disease, for example, while women are more likely than men to have arthritis. Women are far more likely to suffer from migraines and sinusitis.

Some differences in the prevalence of health problems are believed to be rooted in biology. Age differences between the male and female populations also contribute to differences in disease patterns. The female population is older, on average, than the male population. The older age of women means a higher incidence of conditions related to aging, such as arthritis.

■ As medical researchers develop a better understanding of the differences between men and women, individualized treatments that take gender into consideration are likely to become more common.

Women are more likely than men to have arthritis

(percent of people aged 18 or older with selected health conditions, by sex, 2002)

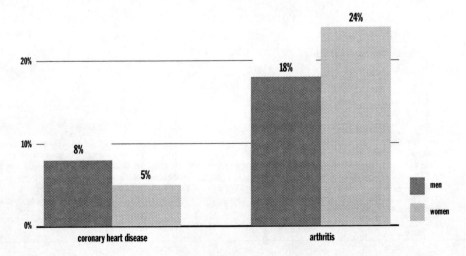

Table 9.4 Number of Health Conditions among Adults by Sex, 2002

(number of people aged 18 or older with selected health conditions, by type of condition and sex, 2002; numbers in thousands)

	total	men	women
TOTAL PEOPLE	**205,825**	**98,749**	**107,076**
Selected circulatory diseases			
Heart disease, all types	22,719	11,279	11,439
Coronary	12,527	7,115	5,412
Hypertension	43,330	19,948	23,381
Stroke	4,836	2,364	2,472
Selected respiratory conditions			
Emphysema	3,131	1,822	1,310
Asthma			
Ever	21,927	9,151	12,776
Still	13,963	4,940	9,022
Hay fever	18,225	7,971	10,254
Sinusitis	29,222	10,251	18,971
Chronic bronchitis	9,114	2,892	6,222
Selected type of cancer			
Any cancer	14,381	6,195	8,186
Breast cancer	2,186	29	2,157
Cervical cancer	1,243	0	1,243
Prostate cancer	1,501	1,501	0
Other selected diseases and conditions			
Diabetes	13,391	6,826	6,565
Ulcers	15,632	7,199	8,432
Kidney disease	2,609	1,104	1,505
Liver disease	2,426	1,187	1,239
Arthritis	42,704	16,835	25,869
Chronic joint symptoms	51,416	23,016	28,400
Migraines or severe headaches	31,066	9,235	21,831
Pain in neck	28,401	11,556	16,845
Pain in lower back	54,325	23,991	30,334
Pain in face or jaw	9,535	2,774	6,761
Selected sensory problems			
Hearing	30,826	17,904	12,922
Vision	19,069	7,742	11,327
Absence of all natural teeth	17,177	7,432	9,745

Note: The conditions shown are those that have ever been diagnosed by a doctor, except as noted. Hay fever, sinusitis, and chronic bronchitis have been diagnosed in the past twelve months. Kidney and liver disease have been diagnosed in the past twelve months and exclude kidney stones, bladder infections, and incontinence. Chronic joint symptoms are shown if respondent had pain, aching, or stiffness in or around a joint (excluding back and neck) and the condition began more than three months ago. Migraines, pain in neck, lower back, face, or jaw are shown only if pain lasted a whole day or more.
Source: National Center for Health Statistics, Summary Health Statistics for U.S. Adults: National Health Interview Survey, 2002, Series 10, No. 222, 2004; Internet site http://www.cdc.gov/nchs/nhis.htm

Table 9.5 Percent Distribution of Health Conditions among Adults by Sex, 2002

(percent distribution of people aged 18 or older with selected health conditions, by type of condition and sex, 2002)

	total	men	women
TOTAL PEOPLE	**100.0%**	**48.0%**	**52.0%**
Selected circulatory diseases			
Heart disease, all types	100.0	49.6	50.3
Coronary	100.0	56.8	43.2
Hypertension	100.0	46.0	54.0
Stroke	100.0	48.9	51.1
Selected respiratory conditions			
Emphysema	100.0	58.2	41.8
Asthma			
Ever	100.0	41.7	58.3
Still	100.0	35.4	64.6
Hay fever	100.0	43.7	56.3
Sinusitis	100.0	35.1	64.9
Chronic bronchitis	100.0	31.7	68.3
Selected type of cancer			
Any cancer	100.0	43.1	56.9
Breast cancer	100.0	1.3	98.7
Cervical cancer	100.0	0.0	100.0
Prostate cancer	100.0	100.0	0.0
Other selected diseases and conditions			
Diabetes	100.0	51.0	49.0
Ulcers	100.0	46.1	53.9
Kidney disease	100.0	42.3	57.7
Liver disease	100.0	48.9	51.1
Arthritis	100.0	39.4	60.6
Chronic joint symptoms	100.0	44.8	55.2
Migraines or severe headaches	100.0	29.7	70.3
Pain in neck	100.0	40.7	59.3
Pain in lower back	100.0	44.2	55.8
Pain in face or jaw	100.0	29.1	70.9
Selected sensory problems			
Hearing	100.0	58.1	41.9
Vision	100.0	40.6	59.4
Absence of all natural teeth	100.0	43.3	56.7

Note: The conditions shown are those that have ever been diagnosed by a doctor, except as noted. Hay fever, sinusitis, and chronic bronchitis have been diagnosed in the past twelve months. Kidney and liver disease have been diagnosed in the past twelve months and exclude kidney stones, bladder infections, and incontinence. Chronic joint symptoms are shown if respondent had pain, aching, or stiffness in or around a joint (excluding back and neck) and the condition began more than three months ago. Migraines, pain in neck, lower back, face, or jaw are shown only if pain lasted a whole day or more.
Source: National Center for Health Statistics, Summary Health Statistics for U.S. Adults: National Health Interview Survey, 2002, *Series 10, No. 222, 2004; Internet site http://www.cdc.gov/nchs/nhis.htm*

Table 9.6 Percent of Adults with Health Conditions by Sex, 2002

(percent of people aged 18 or older with selected health conditions, by type of condition and sex, 2002)

	total	men	women
TOTAL PEOPLE	100.0%	100.0%	100.0%
Selected circulatory diseases			
Heart disease, all types	11.1	12.2	10.5
Coronary	6.1	7.8	4.9
Hypertension	21.1	20.9	21.4
Stroke	2.4	2.6	2.2
Selected respiratory conditions			
Emphysema	1.5	2.0	1.2
Asthma			
Ever	10.7	9.2	12.0
Still	6.8	5.0	8.4
Hay fever	8.9	8.0	9.6
Sinusitis	14.2	10.4	17.7
Chronic bronchitis	4.4	3.0	5.8
Selected type of cancer			
Any cancer	7.0	6.9	7.5
Breast cancer	1.1	0	2.0
Cervical cancer	1.2	0	1.2
Prostate cancer	1.5	1.8	0
Other selected diseases and conditions			
Diabetes	6.6	7.3	6.1
Ulcers	7.6	7.5	7.8
Kidney disease	1.3	1.2	1.4
Liver disease	1.2	1.2	1.1
Arthritis	20.8	17.8	23.7
Chronic joint symptoms	25.1	23.8	26.3
Migraines or severe headaches	15.1	9.2	20.6
Pain in neck	13.8	11.7	15.7
Pain in lower back	26.5	24.3	28.3
Pain in face or jaw	4.6	2.8	6.3
Selected sensory problems			
Hearing	15.0	19.1	11.8
Vision	9.3	8.1	10.4
Absence of all natural teeth	8.4	8.1	8.9

Note: The conditions shown are those that have ever been diagnosed by a doctor, except as noted. Hay fever, sinusitis, and chronic bronchitis have been diagnosed in the past twelve months. Kidney and liver disease have been diagnosed in the past twelve months and exclude kidney stones, bladder infections, and incontinence. Chronic joint symptoms are shown if respondent had pain, aching, or stiffness in or around a joint (excluding back and neck) and the condition began more than three months ago. Migraines, pain in neck, lower back, face, or jaw are shown only if pain lasted a whole day or more.

Source: National Center for Health Statistics, Summary Health Statistics for U.S. Adults: National Health Interview Survey, 2002, Series 10, No. 222, 2004; Internet site http://www.cdc.gov/nchs/nhis.htm

Disease Prevalence Is Higher among Non-Hispanic Whites and Blacks

Asians have particularly low prevalence rates for many health problems.

Non-Hispanic whites are the largest segment of the U.S. population, which is the primary reason they account for the largest share of adults with various health problems. Thirty-three million non-Hispanic whites have hypertension, for example, accounting for three-quarters of all those with hypertension. But non-Hispanic whites are actually less likely than blacks to have hypertension.

For most of the health conditions considered here, blacks and non-Hispanic whites have higher prevalence rates than Asians and Hispanics. A large proportion of Asians and Hispanics are immigrants, while nearly all non-Hispanic whites and blacks are native-born. This distribution suggests that cultural differences could be a factor in the prevalence of many health problems. Differences in diet, for example, can affect the likelihood of developing high blood pressure.

Population characteristics also influence disease prevalence. In general, Asians and Hispanics are younger than non-Hispanic whites and blacks. With fewer older adults, the prevalence of age-related health conditions among Hispanics and Asians is often below average.

■ Many immigrants adhere to traditional diets that are healthier than the average American diet of fast food and soft drinks. As immigrants become more acculturated, the prevalence of health problems may rise.

Blacks are most likely to have problems with asthma

(percent of people aged 18 or older with asthma, by race and Hispanic origin, 2002)

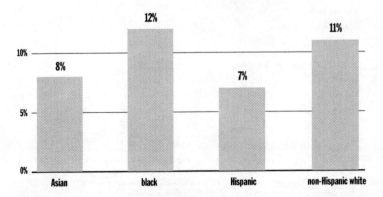

Table 9.7 Number of Health Conditions among Adults by Race and Hispanic Origin, 2002

(number of people aged 18 or older with selected health conditions, by type of condition, race, and Hispanic origin, 2002; numbers in thousands)

	total	Asian	black	Hispanic	non-Hispanic white
TOTAL PEOPLE	**205,825**	**7,270**	**23,499**	**22,691**	**149,584**
Selected circulatory diseases					
Heart disease, all types	22,719	518	2,000	1,294	18,540
Coronary	12,527	256	1,093	771	10,195
Hypertension	43,330	941	6,186	3,149	32,551
Stroke	4,836	139	566	367	3,634
Selected respiratory conditions					
Emphysema	3,131	5	192	79	2,753
Asthma					
Ever	21,927	573	2,839	1,652	16,331
Still	13,963	294	1,914	933	10,459
Hay fever	18,225	604	1,658	1,425	14,311
Sinusitis	29,222	499	3,323	1,860	23,134
Chronic bronchitis	9,114	125	1,065	630	7,060
Selected type of cancer					
Any cancer	14,381	98	644	479	12,886
Breast cancer	2,186	50	120	78	1,902
Cervical cancer	1,243	0	71	50	1,035
Prostate cancer	1,501	17	134	40	1,313
Other selected diseases and conditions					
Diabetes	13,391	363	2,080	1,542	9,153
Ulcers	15,632	409	1,550	1,077	12,204
Kidney disease	2,609	12	314	445	1,791
Liver disease	2,426	127	216	330	1,706
Arthritis	42,704	531	4,509	2,648	34,325
Chronic joint symptoms	51,416	876	5,529	3,648	40,413
Migraines or severe headaches	31,066	652	3,622	3,143	22,893
Pain in neck	28,401	569	2,700	2,907	21,621
Pain in lower back	54,325	1,353	5,541	5,331	41,135
Pain in face or jaw	9,535	131	917	936	7,254
Selected sensory problems					
Hearing	30,826	553	1,759	1,522	26,358
Vision	19,069	461	2,514	1,690	14,021
Absence of all natural teeth	17,177	252	1,833	1,314	13,530

Note: The conditions shown are those that have ever been diagnosed by a doctor, except as noted. Hay fever, sinusitis, and chronic bronchitis have been diagnosed in the past twelve months. Kidney and liver disease have been diagnosed in the past twelve months and exclude kidney stones, bladder infections, and incontinence. Chronic joint symptoms are shown if respondent had pain, aching, or stiffness in or around a joint (excluding back and neck) and the condition began more than three months ago. Migraines, pain in neck, lower back, face, or jaw are shown only if pain lasted a whole day or more.
Source: National Center for Health Statistics, Summary Health Statistics for U.S. Adults: National Health Interview Survey, 2002, Series 10, No. 222, 2004; Internet site http://www.cdc.gov/nchs/nhis.htm

Table 9.8 Percent Distribution of Health Conditions among Adults by Race and Hispanic Origin, 2002

(percent distribution of people aged 18 or older with selected health conditions, by type of condition, race, and Hispanic origin, 2002)

	total	Asian	black	Hispanic	non-Hispanic white
TOTAL PEOPLE	100.0%	3.5%	11.4%	11.0%	72.7%
Selected circulatory diseases					
Heart disease, all types	100.0	2.3	8.8	5.7	81.6
Coronary	100.0	2.0	8.7	6.2	81.4
Hypertension	100.0	2.2	14.3	7.3	75.1
Stroke	100.0	2.9	11.7	7.6	75.1
Selected respiratory conditions					
Emphysema	100.0	0.2	6.1	2.5	87.9
Asthma					
Ever	100.0	2.6	12.9	7.5	74.5
Still	100.0	2.1	13.7	6.7	74.9
Hay fever	100.0	3.3	9.1	7.8	78.5
Sinusitis	100.0	1.7	11.4	6.4	79.2
Chronic bronchitis	100.0	1.4	11.7	6.9	77.5
Selected type of cancer					
Any cancer	100.0	0.7	4.5	3.3	89.6
Breast cancer	100.0	2.3	5.5	3.6	87.0
Cervical cancer	100.0	0	5.7	4.0	83.3
Prostate cancer	100.0	1.1	8.9	2.7	87.5
Other selected diseases and conditions					
Diabetes	100.0	2.7	15.5	11.5	68.4
Ulcers	100.0	2.6	9.9	6.9	78.1
Kidney disease	100.0	0.5	12.0	17.1	68.6
Liver disease	100.0	5.2	8.9	13.6	70.3
Arthritis	100.0	1.2	10.6	6.2	80.4
Chronic joint symptoms	100.0	1.7	10.8	7.1	78.6
Migraines or severe headaches	100.0	2.1	11.7	10.1	73.7
Pain in neck	100.0	2.0	9.5	10.2	76.1
Pain in lower back	100.0	2.5	10.2	9.8	75.7
Pain in face or jaw	100.0	1.4	9.6	9.8	76.1
Selected sensory problems					
Hearing	100.0	1.8	5.7	4.9	85.5
Vision	100.0	2.4	13.2	8.9	73.5
Absence of all natural teeth	100.0	1.5	10.7	7.6	78.8

Note: The conditions shown are those that have ever been diagnosed by a doctor, except as noted. Hay fever, sinusitis, and chronic bronchitis have been diagnosed in the past twelve months. Kidney and liver disease have been diagnosed in the past twelve months and exclude kidney stones, bladder infections, and incontinence. Chronic joint symptoms are shown if respondent had pain, aching, or stiffness in or around a joint (excluding back and neck) and the condition began more than three months ago. Migraines, pain in neck, lower back, face, or jaw are shown only if pain lasted a whole day or more.

Source: National Center for Health Statistics, Summary Health Statistics for U.S. Adults: National Health Interview Survey, 2002, Series 10, No. 222, 2004; Internet site http://www.cdc.gov/nchs/nhis.htm

Table 9.9 Percent of Adults with Health Conditions by Race and Hispanic Origin, 2002

(percent of people aged 18 or older with selected health conditions, by type of condition, race, and Hispanic origin, 2002)

	total	Asian	black	Hispanic	non-Hispanic white
TOTAL PEOPLE	100.0%	100.0%	100.0%	100.0%	100.0%
Selected circulatory diseases					
Heart disease, all types	11.1	9.0	9.9	7.7	11.8
Coronary	6.1	5.0	5.6	4.8	6.4
Hypertension	21.1	16.7	29.8	18.2	20.7
Stroke	2.4	2.4	2.9	2.4	2.3
Selected respiratory conditions					
Emphysema	1.5	0.1	1.1	0.5	1.7
Asthma					
Ever	10.7	7.8	11.9	7.4	11.0
Still	6.8	4.2	8.0	4.2	7.0
Hay fever	8.9	8.2	7.0	6.8	9.6
Sinusitis	14.2	6.8	14.5	8.7	15.4
Chronic bronchitis	4.4	1.7	4.5	3.1	4.6
Selected type of cancer					
Any cancer	7.0	2.2	3.4	3.0	8.2
Breast cancer	1.1	1.3	0.6	0.6	1.2
Cervical cancer	1.2	0	0.6	0.5	1.4
Prostate cancer	1.5	1.1	2.0	0.8	1.9
Other selected diseases and conditions					
Diabetes	6.6	6.3	10.1	9.4	5.8
Ulcers	7.6	6.3	7.1	5.7	8.0
Kidney disease	1.3	0.2	1.5	2.4	1.2
Liver disease	1.2	1.7	1.0	1.7	1.1
Arthritis	20.8	9.5	22.2	15.8	21.9
Chronic joint symptoms	25.1	14.0	25.5	19.2	26.4
Migraines or severe headaches	15.1	8.4	14.9	13.6	15.6
Pain in neck	13.8	8.0	11.7	13.6	14.3
Pain in lower back	26.5	19.0	24.0	24.3	27.4
Pain in face or jaw	4.6	1.7	3.8	4.4	4.9
Selected sensory problems					
Hearing	15.0	10.4	8.8	8.7	16.9
Vision	9.3	7.1	11.7	9.0	9.1
Absence of all natural teeth	8.4	5.6	10.0	8.3	8.6

Note: The conditions shown are those that have ever been diagnosed by a doctor, except as noted. Hay fever, sinusitis, and chronic bronchitis have been diagnosed in the past twelve months. Kidney and liver disease have been diagnosed in the past twelve months and exclude kidney stones, bladder infections, and incontinence. Chronic joint symptoms are shown if respondent had pain, aching, or stiffness in or around a joint (excluding back and neck) and the condition began more than three months ago. Migraines, pain in neck, lower back, face, or jaw are shown only if pain lasted a whole day or more.
Source: National Center for Health Statistics, Summary Health Statistics for U.S. Adults: National Health Interview Survey, 2002, *Series 10, No. 222, 2004; Internet site http://www.cdc.gov/nchs/nhis.htm*

Low Incomes Are Related to Health Problems

But other factors also play a role in differences.

Income is linked to many health problems. There is both a direct and an indirect relationship between income and health. People with lower incomes generally have less access to health care, and poor health can make it difficult for people to earn a good living. But people with lower incomes are also more likely to be older, and aging leads to more health problems.

People with household incomes below $20,000 are more likely to suffer from most of the health problems examined here. One-third of those suffering from a stroke, for example, had household incomes below $20,000, although this income group accounts for only 18 percent of the adult population.

Health differences are also apparent in the percentage of adults with various health problems by income. While 1.5 percent of all adults have been diagnosed with emphysema, among those with incomes below $20,000 the figure is more than twice as large at 3.1 percent.

■ Because older adults are likely to have low incomes, many health differences by income are related to aging rather than economics.

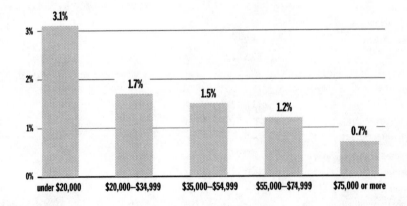

Emphysema becomes less likely as household income rises

(percent of people aged 18 or older with emphysema, by household income, 2002)

Table 9.10 Number of Health Conditions among Adults by Household Income, 2002

(number of people aged 18 or older with selected health conditions, by type of condition and household income, 2002; numbers in thousands)

	total	under $20,000	$20,000–$34,999	$35,000–$54,999	$55,000–$74,999	$75,000 or more
TOTAL PEOPLE	205,825	37,369	29,671	31,814	23,984	41,572
Selected circulatory diseases						
Heart disease, all types	22,719	5,747	3,837	3,260	1,881	3,509
Coronary	12,527	3589	2,389	1,862	874	1,342
Hypertension	43,330	10,356	6,802	6,159	4,228	6,602
Stroke	4,836	1,619	941	655	231	445
Selected respiratory conditions						
Emphysema	3,131	1,191	519	393	234	155
Asthma						
Ever	21,927	4,907	3,160	3,585	2,278	4,420
Still	13,963	3,320	2,089	2,107	1,423	2,751
Hay fever	18,225	2,903	2,370	2,893	2,573	4,274
Sinusitis	29,222	5,430	4,339	4,670	3,618	6,251
Chronic bronchitis	9,114	2,492	1,630	1,378	1,073	1,080
Selected type of cancer						
Any cancer	14,381	3,017	2,490	2,168	1,284	2,106
Breast cancer	2,186	574	428	235	210	280
Cervical cancer	1,243	301	194	187	166	212
Prostate cancer	1,501	256	324	281	57	118
Other selected diseases and conditions						
Diabetes	13,391	3,422	2,588	1,819	1,254	1,543
Ulcers	15,632	3,733	2,732	2,546	1,604	2,155
Kidney disease	2,609	1,101	437	302	132	131
Liver disease	2,426	715	432	370	246	360
Arthritis	42,704	9,894	6,835	6,363	4,272	6,683
Chronic joint symptoms	51,416	10,978	7,975	8,370	5,549	9,005
Migraines or severe headaches	31,066	6,934	5,032	5,299	3,493	5,267
Pain in neck	28,401	6,149	4,539	4,577	3,091	5,090
Pain in lower back	54,325	11,697	8,794	8,370	5,994	9,822
Pain in face or jaw	9,535	2,270	1,598	1,409	1,181	1,571
Selected sensory problems						
Hearing	30,826	6,912	5,201	4,657	3,188	4,814
Vision	19,069	5,389	3,365	2,955	1,695	2,466
Absence of all natural teeth	17,177	6,151	3,344	2,141	1,048	1,215

Note: The conditions shown are those that have ever been diagnosed by a doctor, except as noted. Hay fever, sinusitis, and chronic bronchitis have been diagnosed in the past twelve months. Kidney and liver disease have been diagnosed in the past twelve months and exclude kidney stones, bladder infections, and incontinence. Chronic joint symptoms are shown if respondent had pain, aching, or stiffness in or around a joint (excluding back and neck) and the condition began more than three months ago. Migraines, pain in neck, lower back, face, or jaw are shown only if pain lasted a whole day or more.
Source: National Center for Health Statistics, Summary Health Statistics for U.S. Adults: National Health Interview Survey, 2002, Series 10, No. 222, 2004; Internet site http://www.cdc.gov/nchs/nhis.htm

Table 9.11 Percent Distribution of Health Conditions among Adults by Household Income, 2002

(percent distribution of people aged 18 or older with selected health conditions, by type of condition and household income, 2002)

	total	under $20,000	$20,000–$34,999	$35,000–$54,999	$55,000–$74,999	$75,000 or more
TOTAL PEOPLE	100.0%	18.2%	14.4%	15.5%	11.7%	20.2%
Selected circulatory diseases						
Heart disease, all types	100.0	25.3	16.9	14.4	8.3	15.4
Coronary	100.0	28.7	19.1	14.9	7.0	10.7
Hypertension	100.0	23.9	15.7	14.2	9.8	15.2
Stroke	100.0	33.5	19.5	13.5	4.8	9.2
Selected respiratory conditions						
Emphysema	100.0	38.0	16.6	12.6	7.5	5.0
Asthma						
Ever	100.0	22.4	14.4	16.3	10.4	20.2
Still	100.0	23.8	15.0	15.1	10.2	19.7
Hay fever	100.0	15.9	13.0	15.9	14.1	23.5
Sinusitis	100.0	18.6	14.8	16.0	12.4	21.4
Chronic bronchitis	100.0	27.3	17.9	15.1	11.8	11.8
Selected type of cancer						
Any cancer	100.0	21.0	17.3	15.1	8.9	14.6
Breast cancer	100.0	26.3	19.6	10.8	9.6	12.8
Cervical cancer	100.0	24.2	15.6	15.0	13.4	17.1
Prostate cancer	100.0	17.1	21.6	18.7	3.8	7.9
Other selected diseases and conditions						
Diabetes	100.0	25.6	19.3	13.6	9.4	11.5
Ulcers	100.0	23.9	17.5	16.3	10.3	13.8
Kidney disease	100.0	42.2	16.8	11.6	5.1	5.0
Liver disease	100.0	29.5	17.8	15.3	10.1	14.8
Arthritis	100.0	23.2	16.0	14.9	10.0	15.6
Chronic joint symptoms	100.0	21.4	15.5	16.3	10.8	17.5
Migraines or severe headaches	100.0	22.3	16.2	17.1	11.2	17.0
Pain in neck	100.0	21.7	16.0	16.1	10.9	17.9
Pain in lower back	100.0	21.5	16.2	15.4	11.0	18.1
Pain in face or jaw	100.0	23.8	16.8	14.8	12.4	16.5
Selected sensory problems						
Hearing	100.0	22.4	16.9	15.1	10.3	15.6
Vision	100.0	28.3	17.6	15.5	8.9	12.9
Absence of all natural teeth	100.0	35.8	19.5	12.5	6.1	7.1

Note: The conditions shown are those that have ever been diagnosed by a doctor, except as noted. Hay fever, sinusitis, and chronic bronchitis have been diagnosed in the past twelve months. Kidney and liver disease have been diagnosed in the past twelve months and exclude kidney stones, bladder infections, and incontinence. Chronic joint symptoms are shown if respondent had pain, aching, or stiffness in or around a joint (excluding back and neck) and the condition began more than three months ago. Migraines, pain in neck, lower back, face, or jaw are shown only if pain lasted a whole day or more.
Source: National Center for Health Statistics, Summary Health Statistics for U.S. Adults: National Health Interview Survey, 2002, Series 10, No. 222, 2004; Internet site http://www.cdc.gov/nchs/nhis.htm

Table 9.12 Percent of Adults with Health Conditions by Household Income, 2002

(percent of people aged 18 or older with selected health conditions, by type of condition and household income, 2002)

	total	under $20,000	$20,000– $34,999	$35,000– $54,999	$55,000– $74,999	$75,000 or more
TOTAL PEOPLE	100.0%	100.0%	100.0%	100.0%	100.0%	100.0%
Selected circulatory diseases						
Heart disease, all types	11.1	13.4	12.3	11.9	10.1	11.2
Coronary	6.1	8.2	7.5	7.1	5.2	5.6
Hypertension	21.1	25.2	22.4	21.2	21.4	18.9
Stroke	2.4	3.8	3.0	2.5	1.4	2.3
Selected respiratory conditions						
Emphysema	1.5	3.1	1.7	1.5	1.2	0.7
Asthma						
Ever	10.7	13.7	10.7	11.0	9.2	10.1
Still	6.8	9.2	7.1	6.5	5.8	6.3
Hay fever	8.9	8.1	8.2	8.9	10.2	9.5
Sinusitis	14.2	14.8	14.8	14.5	15.0	13.9
Chronic bronchitis	4.4	6.9	5.6	4.4	4.9	2.9
Selected type of cancer						
Any cancer	7.0	6.8	7.7	8.1	6.8	6.9
Breast cancer	1.1	1.2	1.3	0.9	1.1	0.8
Cervical cancer	1.2	1.5	1.3	1.1	1.5	0.9
Prostate cancer	1.5	1.4	1.9	2.2	0.9	1.5
Other selected diseases and conditions						
Diabetes	6.6	8.7	8.8	6.5	6.5	4.6
Ulcers	7.6	9.9	9.2	8.5	7.1	5.9
Kidney disease	1.3	2.9	1.5	1.2	0.6	0.5
Liver disease	1.2	2.1	1.5	1.2	1.0	0.9
Arthritis	20.8	24.2	22.5	22.0	20.6	19.2
Chronic joint symptoms	25.1	28.3	26.8	27.4	24.9	23.2
Migraines or severe headaches	15.1	20.3	17.4	16.0	13.2	11.6
Pain in neck	13.8	17.1	15.5	14.4	12.9	11.9
Pain in lower back	26.5	31.8	29.9	26.4	25.0	23.3
Pain in face or jaw	4.6	6.4	5.5	4.3	4.7	3.6
Selected sensory problems						
Hearing	15.0	16.2	16.9	16.5	16.3	14.3
Vision	9.3	13.9	11.3	9.7	8.3	7.5
Absence of all natural teeth	8.4	13.8	10.7	7.6	5.6	4.7

Note: The conditions shown are those that have ever been diagnosed by a doctor, except as noted. Hay fever, sinusitis, and chronic bronchitis have been diagnosed in the past twelve months. Kidney and liver disease have been diagnosed in the past twelve months and exclude kidney stones, bladder infections, and incontinence. Chronic joint symptoms are shown if respondent had pain, aching, or stiffness in or around a joint (excluding back and neck) and the condition began more than three months ago. Migraines, pain in neck, lower back, face, or jaw are shown only if pain lasted a whole day or more.
Source: National Center for Health Statistics, Summary Health Statistics for U.S. Adults: National Health Interview Survey, 2002, Series 10, No. 222, 2004; Internet site http://www.cdc.gov/nchs/nhis.htm

Higher Education Is Linked to Better Health

But the relationship is complicated by other factors.

People with higher levels of education tend to be in better health. The relationship between education and health is complicated, however. Older adults, who have the most health problems, also have the least education. The higher prevalence of heart disease among people without a high school diploma, then, is mostly a consequence of the older age of high school dropouts.

People with more education also have higher incomes, on average, and are more likely to have health insurance coverage and greater access to medical care. Greater access to care generally results in better health. The poor and the uninsured are less likely to seek health care until their condition has become serious—and the prognosis poor.

Education also directly affects health. The educated are more likely to seek information about health conditions and use that information to improve their health. They are more likely to make lifestyle changes, for example, to reduce the likelihood of getting certain diseases.

■ The rising educational level of the population suggests that the incidence of some health problems may decline in the future.

Many health problems vary by educational attainment

(percent of people aged 18 or older with hypertension, by educational attainment, 2002)

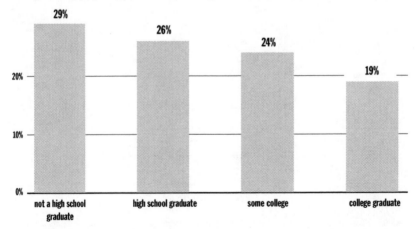

Table 9.13 Number of Health Conditions among Adults by Education, 2002

(number of people aged 18 or older with selected health conditions, by type of condition and educational attainment, 2002; numbers in thousands)

	total	not a high school graduate	high school graduate	some college	college graduate
TOTAL PEOPLE	205,825	28,248	52,556	48,091	47,197
Selected circulatory diseases					
Heart disease, all types	22,719	5,120	6,782	5,480	4,214
Coronary	12,527	3,524	3,938	2,871	1,964
Hypertension	43,330	9,514	14,345	10,471	7,785
Stroke	4,836	1,582	1,576	1,001	527
Selected respiratory conditions					
Emphysema	3,131	1,159	1,008	630	250
Asthma					
Ever	21,927	2,704	4,904	5,416	4,663
Still	13,963	1,903	3,240	3,536	2,886
Hay fever	18,225	1,769	4,248	4,859	5,538
Sinusitis	29,222	3,747	7,728	7,827	7,508
Chronic bronchitis	9,114	1,809	2,857	2,420	1,225
Selected type of cancer					
Any cancer	14,381	2,542	4,419	3,786	3,252
Breast cancer	2,186	397	747	625	391
Cervical cancer	1,243	258	349	382	184
Prostate cancer	1,501	342	477	350	329
Other selected diseases and conditions					
Diabetes	13,391	3,642	4,341	3,134	1,880
Ulcers	15,632	3,426	4,386	4,297	2,580
Kidney disease	2,609	897	761	549	294
Liver disease	2,426	532	727	710	329
Arthritis	42,704	8,464	13,428	11,214	8,192
Chronic joint symptoms	51,416	8,930	15,234	13,222	10,572
Migraines or severe headaches	31,066	4,671	8,173	7,768	5,530
Pain in neck	28,401	4,758	7,958	7,921	5,469
Pain in lower back	54,325	9,063	15,042	13,891	10,299
Pain in face or jaw	9,535	1,404	2,519	2,638	1,674
Selected sensory problems					
Hearing	30,826	6,005	9,651	7,765	6,011
Vision	19,069	4,573	5,537	4,499	3,085
Absence of all natural teeth	17,177	6,388	5,724	2,886	1,391

Note: The conditions shown are those that have ever been diagnosed by a doctor, except as noted. Hay fever, sinusitis, and chronic bronchitis have been diagnosed in the past twelve months. Kidney and liver disease have been diagnosed in the past twelve months and exclude kidney stones, bladder infections, and incontinence. Chronic joint symptoms are shown if respondent had pain, aching, or stiffness in or around a joint (excluding back and neck) and the condition began more than three months ago. Migraines, pain in neck, lower back, face, or jaw are shown only if pain lasted a whole day or more.
Source: National Center for Health Statistics, Summary Health Statistics for U.S. Adults: National Health Interview Survey, 2002, Series 10, No. 222, 2004; Internet site http://www.cdc.gov/nchs/nhis.htm

Table 9.14 Percent Distribution of Health Conditions among Adults by Education, 2002

(percent distribution of people aged 18 or older with selected health conditions, by type of condition and educational attainment, 2002)

	total	not a high school graduate	high school graduate	some college	college graduate
TOTAL PEOPLE	100.0%	13.7%	25.5%	23.4%	22.9%
Selected circulatory diseases					
Heart disease, all types	100.0	22.5	29.9	24.1	18.5
Coronary	100.0	28.1	31.4	22.9	15.7
Hypertension	100.0	22.0	33.1	24.2	18.0
Stroke	100.0	32.7	32.6	20.7	10.9
Selected respiratory conditions					
Emphysema	100.0	37.0	32.2	20.1	8.0
Asthma					
Ever	100.0	12.3	22.4	24.7	21.3
Still	100.0	13.6	23.2	25.3	20.7
Hay fever	100.0	9.7	23.3	26.7	30.4
Sinusitis	100.0	12.8	26.4	26.8	25.7
Chronic bronchitis	100.0	19.8	31.3	26.6	13.4
Selected type of cancer					
Any cancer	100.0	17.7	30.7	26.3	22.6
Breast cancer	100.0	18.2	34.2	28.6	17.9
Cervical cancer	100.0	20.8	28.1	30.7	14.8
Prostate cancer	100.0	22.8	31.8	23.3	21.9
Other selected diseases and conditions					
Diabetes	100.0	27.2	32.4	23.4	14.0
Ulcers	100.0	21.9	28.1	27.5	16.5
Kidney disease	100.0	34.4	29.2	21.0	11.3
Liver disease	100.0	21.9	30.0	29.3	13.6
Arthritis	100.0	19.8	31.4	26.3	19.2
Chronic joint symptoms	100.0	17.4	29.6	25.7	20.6
Migraines or severe headaches	100.0	15.0	26.3	25.0	17.8
Pain in neck	100.0	16.8	28.0	27.9	19.3
Pain in lower back	100.0	16.7	27.7	25.6	19.0
Pain in face or jaw	100.0	14.7	26.4	27.7	17.6
Selected sensory problems					
Hearing	100.0	19.5	31.3	25.2	19.5
Vision	100.0	24.0	29.0	23.6	16.2
Absence of all natural teeth	100.0	37.2	33.3	16.8	8.1

Note: The conditions shown are those that have ever been diagnosed by a doctor, except as noted. Hay fever, sinusitis, and chronic bronchitis have been diagnosed in the past twelve months. Kidney and liver disease have been diagnosed in the past twelve months and exclude kidney stones, bladder infections, and incontinence. Chronic joint symptoms are shown if respondent had pain, aching, or stiffness in or around a joint (excluding back and neck) and the condition began more than three months ago. Migraines, pain in neck, lower back, face, or jaw are shown only if pain lasted a whole day or more.
Source: National Center for Health Statistics, Summary Health Statistics for U.S. Adults: National Health Interview Survey, 2002, Series 10, No. 222, 2004; Internet site http://www.cdc.gov/nchs/nhis.htm

Table 9.15 Percent of Adults with Health Conditions by Education, 2002

(percent of people aged 18 or older with selected health conditions, by type of condition and educational attainment, 2002)

	total	not a high school graduate	high school graduate	some college	college graduate
TOTAL PEOPLE	100.0%	100.0%	100.0%	100.0%	100.0%
Selected circulatory diseases					
Heart disease, all types	11.1	14.3	12.3	12.9	11.2
Coronary	6.1	9.9	7.1	7.1	5.9
Hypertension	21.1	28.9	26.1	23.8	19.2
Stroke	2.4	4.4	2.8	2.5	1.6
Selected respiratory conditions					
Emphysema	1.5	3.5	1.8	1.5	0.8
Asthma					
Ever	10.7	9.7	9.4	11.0	9.8
Still	6.8	6.7	6.2	7.3	6.1
Hay fever	8.9	6.3	8.1	9.9	11.2
Sinusitis	14.2	12.8	14.6	16.1	15.4
Chronic bronchitis	4.4	6.3	5.4	5.1	2.7
Selected type of cancer					
Any cancer	7.0	6.9	8.0	9.2	8.7
Breast cancer	1.1	1.0	1.3	1.6	1.0
Cervical cancer	1.2	1.9	1.3	1.4	0.7
Prostate cancer	1.5	1.9	2.2	2.3	1.8
Other selected diseases and conditions					
Diabetes	6.6	11.4	8.0	7.2	4.8
Ulcers	7.6	11.2	8.2	9.3	6.0
Kidney disease	1.3	2.9	1.4	1.3	0.8
Liver disease	1.2	2.0	1.4	1.5	0.8
Arthritis	20.8	25.2	24.4	25.3	20.1
Chronic joint symptoms	25.1	28.9	28.3	28.8	24.2
Migraines or severe headaches	15.1	18.0	15.9	15.5	11.0
Pain in neck	13.8	16.6	15.1	16.3	11.7
Pain in lower back	26.5	31.8	28.6	28.9	22.2
Pain in face or jaw	4.6	5.0	4.8	5.4	3.3
Selected sensory problems					
Hearing	15.0	21.3	18.4	16.1	12.7
Vision	9.3	16.2	10.5	9.4	6.6
Absence of all natural teeth	8.4	17.5	10.3	7.0	3.6

Note: The conditions shown are those that have ever been diagnosed by a doctor, except as noted. Hay fever, sinusitis, and chronic bronchitis have been diagnosed in the past twelve months. Kidney and liver disease have been diagnosed in the past twelve months and exclude kidney stones, bladder infections, and incontinence. Chronic joint symptoms are shown if respondent had pain, aching, or stiffness in or around a joint (excluding back and neck) and the condition began more than three months ago. Migraines, pain in neck, lower back, face, or jaw are shown only if pain lasted a whole day or more.
Source: National Center for Health Statistics, Summary Health Statistics for U.S. Adults: National Health Interview Survey, 2002, *Series 10, No. 222, 2004; Internet site http://www.cdc.gov/nchs/nhis.htm*

Hypertension Rate Has Risen

Increased monitoring may be behind the rise.

There has been considerable progress against many health conditions in recent years. Nevertheless, the hypertension rate increased between 1988–94 and 1999–02—perhaps because of increased monitoring for the disease. Overall, the share of adults with high blood pressure rose from 24 to 30 percent. The biggest percentage point increase has been among older women.

Mexican Americans are much less likely than non-Hispanic whites or blacks to have hypertension. They also experienced the smallest percentage point increase in the prevalence of hypertension between 1988–94 and 1999–02. Age structure may explain this difference. Many Mexican Americans are young adults who have migrated to the United States in search of jobs.

The prevalence of high blood pressure falls as education rises. Only 20 percent of college graduates have high blood pressure versus 34 percent of high school dropouts. The older age of the less educated explains much of this difference.

■ As more Americans become aware of having high blood pressure, the rate of heart disease may decline.

Women are more likely than men to have hypertension

(percent of people aged 20 or older who have hypertension, by sex, 1988–94 and 1999–02)

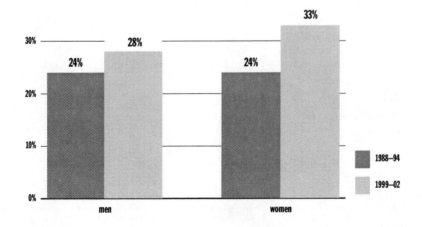

Table 9.16 High Blood Pressure by Sex and Age, 1988–94 and 1999–02

(percent of people aged 20 or older who have hypertension, by sex and age, 1988–94 and 1999–02; percentage point change, 1988–94 to 1999–02)

	1999–02	1988–94	percentage point change
TOTAL PEOPLE	**30.1%**	**24.1%**	**6.0**
Total men	**27.5**	**23.8**	**3.7**
Aged 20 to 34	8.1	7.1	1.0
Aged 35 to 44	17.1	17.1	0.0
Aged 45 to 54	30.9	29.2	1.7
Aged 55 to 64	44.9	40.6	4.3
Aged 65 to 74	58.9	54.4	4.5
Aged 75 or older	68.4	60.4	8.0
Total women	**32.7**	**24.4**	**8.3**
Aged 20 to 34	2.7	2.9	–0.2
Aged 35 to 44	15.1	11.2	3.9
Aged 45 to 54	31.7	23.9	7.8
Aged 55 to 64	53.9	42.5	11.4
Aged 65 to 74	72.5	56.1	16.4
Aged 75 or older	82.8	73.5	9.3

Note: Hypertension is indicated if a person has a systolic pressure of at least 140 mmHg or a diastolic pressure of at least 90 mmHg, or takes antihypertensive medication.
Source: National Center for Health Statistics, Health, United States, 2004; Internet site http://www.cdc.gov/nchs/hus.htm; calculations by New Strategist

Table 9.17 High Blood Pressure by Race, Hispanic Origin, and Sex, 1988—94 and 1999—02

(percent of people aged 20 or older who have hypertension, by sex, race, and Hispanic origin, 1988–94 and 1999–02; percentage point change, 1988–94 to 1999–02)

	1999–02	1988–94	percentage point change
TOTAL PEOPLE	30.1%	24.1%	6.0
Black, non-Hispanic			
Female	42.0	32.3	9.7
Male	35.8	31.1	4.7
White, non-Hispanic			
Female	32.8	24.6	8.2
Male	28.1	24.3	3.8
Hispanic, Mexican			
Female	18.8	15.9	2.9
Male	16.5	16.4	0.1

Note: Hypertension is indicated if a person has a systolic pressure of at least 140 mmHg or a diastolic pressure of at least 90 mmHg, or takes antihypertensive medication.
Source: National Center for Health Statistics, Health, United States, 2004; *Internet site http://www.cdc.gov/nchs/hus.htm; calculations by New Strategist*

Table 9.18 People with High Blood Pressure by Selected Characteristics, 2003

(percent distribution of people aged 18 or older by whether they have been told by a doctor that they have high blood pressure, by selected characteristics, 2003)

	yes	no
TOTAL PEOPLE	**24.8%**	**75.2%**
Sex		
Men	25.0	75.0
Women	24.9	75.1
Age		
Aged 18 to 24	5.2	94.8
Aged 25 to 34	8.3	91.7
Aged 35 to 44	15.3	84.7
Aged 45 to 54	26.8	73.2
Aged 55 to 64	41.9	58.1
Aged 65 or older	54.1	45.9
Race and Hispanic origin		
Black	31.4	68.6
Hispanic	17.9	82.1
White	25.8	74.2
Multiracial	26.4	73.7
Other	18.5	81.5
Household income		
Under $15,000	33.9	66.1
$15,000 to $24,999	30.5	69.5
$25,000 to $34,999	26.5	73.5
$35,000 to $49,999	24.0	76.0
$50,000 or more	20.1	79.9
Education		
Not a high school graduate	34.3	65.7
High school graduate	28.1	71.9
Some college	24.3	75.7
College graduate	20.7	79.3

Source: Centers for Disease Control and Prevention, Behavioral Risk Factor Surveillance System, Prevalence Data, Internet site http://apps.nccd.cdc.gov/brfss/; calculations by New Strategist

Prevalence of High Cholesterol Is Declining

Greater awareness of potential health problems encourages people to seek treatment.

The prevalence of high cholesterol fell between 1988-94 and 1999-02. The largest percentage point decline was among older adults. Among people aged 75 or older, the incidence of high cholesterol fell 10 percentage points among men and 12 percentage points among women. There were also declines for men and women aged 45 to 74. The percentage of people aged 20 to 44 with high cholesterol increased slightly, however.

High cholesterol rates also fell within racial and ethnic groups during those years. The decline was greatest for Mexican American and non-Hispanic white women, while their male counterparts saw the smallest drop.

Cholesterol levels may be declining because more people are having their cholesterol checked. Seventy-three percent of people aged 18 or older had their cholesterol checked in the past five years.

■ The rise in the prevalence of high cholesterol among people aged 20 to 44, coupled with their smaller-than-average likelihood of having had their cholesterol tested in the past five years, suggests a greater need for education about the dangers of the condition.

Older men and women have seen cholesterol levels decline

(percent of people aged 75 or older with high cholesterol, by sex, 1988–94 and 1999–02)

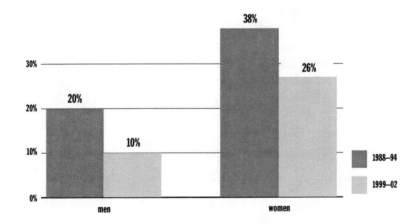

Table 9.19 High Cholesterol by Sex and Age, 1988–94 and 1999–02

(percent of people aged 20 or older who have high serum cholesterol, by sex and age, 1988–94 and 1999–02; percentage point change, 1988–94 to 1999–02)

	1999–02	1988–94	percentage point change
TOTAL PEOPLE	**17.3%**	**19.6%**	**−2.3**
Total men	**16.6**	**17.7**	**−1.1**
Aged 20 to 34	9.8	8.2	1.6
Aged 35 to 44	19.8	19.4	0.4
Aged 45 to 54	23.6	26.6	−3.0
Aged 55 to 64	19.9	28.0	−8.1
Aged 65 to 74	13.7	21.9	−8.2
Aged 75 or older	10.2	20.4	−10.2
Total women	**18.0**	**21.3**	**−3.3**
Aged 20 to 34	8.9	7.3	1.6
Aged 35 to 44	12.4	12.3	0.1
Aged 45 to 54	21.4	26.7	−5.3
Aged 55 to 64	25.6	40.9	−15.3
Aged 65 to 74	32.3	41.3	−9.0
Aged 75 or older	26.5	38.2	−11.7

Note: High cholesterol is defined as greater than or equal to 240 mg/dL.
Source: National Center for Health Statistics, Health, United States, 2004; Internet site http://www.cdc.gov/nchs/hus.htm; calculations by New Strategist

Table 9.20 High Cholesterol by Sex, Race, and Hispanic Origin, 1988–94 and 1999–02

(percent of people aged 20 or older who have high serum cholesterol, by sex race, and Hispanic origin, 1988–94 and 1999–02; percentage point change, 1988–94 to 1999–02)

	1999–02	1988–94	percentage point change
TOTAL PEOPLE	17.3%	19.6%	–2.3
Black, non-Hispanic			
Female	16.1	18.2	–2.1
Male	12.2	14.7	–2.5
White, non-Hispanic			
Female	19.1	22.5	–3.4
Male	16.9	18.0	–1.1
Hispanic, Mexican			
Female	10.7	14.3	–3.6
Male	15.0	15.4	–0.4

Note: High cholesterol is defined as greater than or equal to 240 mg/dL.
Source: National Center for Health Statistics, Health, United States, 2004; Internet site http://www.cdc.gov/nchs/hus.htm; calculations by New Strategist

Table 9.21 Cholesterol Status by Selected Characteristics, 2003

(percent distribution of people aged 18 or older by whether they have had their blood cholesterol checked in the past five years, and whether they have been told by a doctor that their cholesterol is high, by selected characteristics, 2003)

	checked in past five years	not checked in past five years	never checked	cholesterol is high
TOTAL PEOPLE	**72.9%**	**4.0%**	**23.4%**	**33.1%**
Sex				
Men	71.0	4.1	24.9	33.8
Women	74.9	3.9	21.2	32.1
Age				
Aged 18 to 24	40.1	1.6	58.2	8.4
Aged 25 to 34	56.9	4.7	39.2	15.5
Aged 35 to 44	71.6	5.6	22.9	25.4
Aged 45 to 54	82.9	4.7	12.5	35.0
Aged 55 to 64	90.4	3.2	6.2	46.4
Aged 65 or older	92.2	2.1	5.9	47.9
Race and Hispanic origin				
Black	71.6	2.5	26.0	28.3
Hispanic	62.9	2.5	34.6	28.0
White	75.8	4.7	19.7	34.4
Multiracial	72.0	3.9	25.2	32.3
Other	65.9	2.9	30.7	26.9
Household income				
Under $15,000	65.9	3.2	31.2	37.8
$15,000 to $24,999	66.9	3.4	30.0	35.0
$25,000 to $34,999	71.2	3.7	24.9	33.4
$35,000 to $49,999	74.2	4.1	22.1	31.4
$50,000 or more	80.7	4.4	14.5	29.8
Education				
Not a high school graduate	65.8	2.4	31.2	39.6
High school graduate	70.0	3.5	26.3	35.6
Some college	73.8	4.1	22.1	31.5
College graduate	80.9	4.7	13.9	29.0

Source: Centers for Disease Control and Prevention, Behavioral Risk Factor Surveillance System, Prevalence Data, Internet site http://apps.nccd.cdc.gov/brfss/; calculations by New Strategist

Diabetes Is Increasingly Common

Rate is likely to rise as the ranks of the obese grow.

Less than 10 percent of the population has been diagnosed with diabetes. But the long-term health consequences of diabetes make it one of the nation's more important health problems—particularly because the disease is on the rise.

Between 1988–94 and 1999–00 the share of people aged 20 or older with diabetes increased from 7.8 to 8.3 percent. Among non-Hispanic blacks, the percentage rose from 10.4 to 12.4 percent. Of great concern is the fact that these figures include only people who have been diagnosed by a doctor. The National Center for Health Statistics estimates that as many as 30 percent of diabetics have not yet been diagnosed.

The likelihood of having diabetes rises with age. In 2003, fewer than 1 percent of people aged 18 to 24 had diabetes. Among those aged 65 or older, the proportion is a much higher 16 percent. People with low incomes and levels of education are also more likely to have diabetes—in large part because older adults are over-represented in these groups.

■ The prevalence of diabetes has grown in recent years. The rise is likely to accelerate as Americans continue to put on weight.

One in six Americans has diabetes

(percent of people aged 18 or older who have been diagnosed with diabetes, by age, 2003)

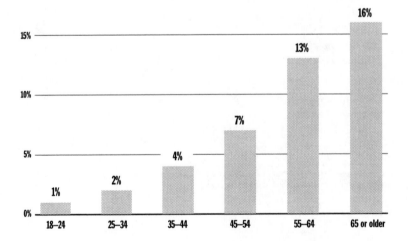

Table 9.22 Diabetes by Selected Characteristics, 1988–94 and 1999–00

(percent of people aged 20 or older with diabetes, by sex, race, Hispanic origin, and age, 1988–94 and 1999–00, and percentage point change 1988–94 to 1999–00)

	1999–00	1988–94	percentage point change
TOTAL PEOPLE	**8.3%**	**7.8%**	**0.5**
Sex			
Female	8.0	7.8	0.2
Male	8.6	7.9	0.7
Race and Hispanic origin			
Black, non-Hispanic	12.4	10.4	2.0
White, non-Hispanic	7.7	7.5	0.2
Hispanic, Mexican	7.7	9.0	–1.3
Age			
Aged 20 to 39	2.2	1.6	0.6
Aged 40 to 59	9.1	8.9	0.2
Aged 60 or older	19.2	18.9	0.3

Note: People with diabetes include those diagnosed by a physician and those who have not been diagnosed but who have a fasting blood glucose of at least 126 mg/dL.
Source: National Center for Health Statistics, Health, United States, 2004; *Internet site http://www.cdc.gov/nchs/hus.htm; calculations by New Strategist*

Table 9.23 People with Diabetes by Selected Characteristics, 2003

(percent distribution of people aged 18 or older by whether they have been told by a doctor that they have diabetes, by selected characteristics, 2003)

	yes	yes, pregnancy related	no
Total people	**7.2%**	**0.7%**	**92.0%**
Sex			
Men	7.3	–	92.7
Women	7.0	1.4	91.7
Age			
Aged 18 to 24	0.7	0.5	98.9
Aged 25 to 34	1.7	1.3	96.9
Aged 35 to 44	3.6	1.2	95.1
Aged 45 to 54	7.4	0.5	92.0
Aged 55 to 64	13.1	0.3	86.7
Aged 65 or older	16.3	0.2	83.5
Race and Hispanic origin			
Black	10.2	0.7	89.7
Hispanic	6.4	1.4	92.2
White	6.6	0.7	92.9
Multiracial	7.9	1.8	91.3
Other	6.2	1.3	92.2
Household income			
Under $15,000	12.8	0.8	86.0
$15,000 to $24,999	9.9	0.7	89.2
$25,000 to $34,999	7.2	0.8	92.1
$35,000 to $49,999	6.1	0.7	93.2
$50,000 or more	4.5	0.7	94.8
Education			
Not a high school graduate	13.0	0.7	86.5
High school graduate	7.8	0.6	91.5
Some college	6.7	0.7	92.5
College graduate	4.9	0.7	94.3

Note: (–) means not applicable.
Source: Centers for Disease Control and Prevention, Behavioral Risk Factor Surveillance System, Prevalence Data, Internet site http://apps.nccd.cdc.gov/brfss

AIDS Hits Minorities Hard

Among women with AIDS, most are black.

The emergence of AIDS in the 1980s presented a new and serious challenge to medical science. Since then, deaths from AIDS (or HIV disease as it is now known) have been dramatically reduced by the development of new treatments, primarily pharmaceuticals. None of the treatments are a cure, however.

Sexual contact or needle sharing are the primary HIV transmission routes. This is why most AIDS cases are diagnosed among people who are relatively young; they are at the age when people are most likely to have multiple sex partners or to use intravenous drugs. By the end of 2003, of the more than 874,000 Americans diagnosed with AIDS, a substantial 44 percent were aged 30 to 39 at the time of diagnosis. Taking into account the lag time between infection and diagnosis means that they were considerably younger when they became infected with the virus.

Most AIDS cases are among men (81 percent), primarily because HIV infection was at first confined to the homosexual male population. The number of blacks with AIDS is nearly equal to the number of non-Hispanic whites with the disease.

■ The development of drugs that can arrest the progression of HIV disease and allow people to live relatively normal lives is one of the great medical successes of the past century.

Among AIDS victims, blacks and non-Hispanic whites are nearly equal in number

(percent distribution of AIDS cases among people aged 13 or older, by race and Hispanic origin, through 2003)

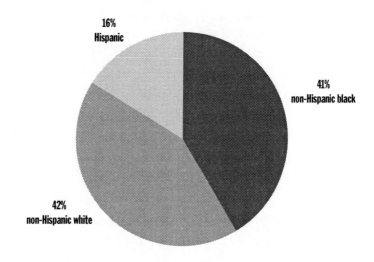

16%
Hispanic

41%
non-Hispanic black

42%
non-Hispanic white

Table 9.24 AIDS Cases by Sex and Age, through December 2003

(cumulative number and percent distribution of AIDS cases by age at diagnosis and sex for those aged 13 or older, through December 2003)

	number	percent of total cases
Total cases	**874,230**	**100.0%**
Under age 5	6,812	0.8
Aged 5 to 12	2,127	0.2
Aged 13 to 19	5,038	0.6
Aged 20 to 29	139,399	15.9
Aged 30 to 39	381,747	43.7
Aged 40 to 49	237,933	27.2
Aged 50 to 59	74,388	8.5
Aged 60 or older	26,784	3.1
Females		
Aged 13 or older	**156,837**	**17.9**
Aged 13 to 19	2,177	0.2
Aged 20 to 29	31,748	3.6
Aged 30 to 39	67,523	7.7
Aged 40 to 49	38,685	4.4
Aged 50 to 59	11,483	1.3
Aged 60 or older	5,221	0.6
Males		
Aged 13 or older	**708,452**	**81.0**
Aged 13 to 19	2,861	0.3
Aged 20 to 29	107,651	12.3
Aged 30 to 39	314,224	35.9
Aged 40 to 49	199,248	22.8
Aged 50 to 59	62,905	7.2
Aged 60 or older	21,563	2.5

Source: National Center for Health Statistics, Health, United States, 2004; *Internet site http://www.cdc.gov/nchs/hus.htm*

Table 9.25 AIDS Cases by Sex, Race, and Hispanic Origin, through December 2003

(cumulative number and percent distribution of AIDS cases by sex, race, and Hispanic origin, through December 2003)

	number	percent distribution
Total cases	**874,230**	**100.0%**
Non-Hispanic		
American Indian	2,946	0.3
Asian	6,837	0.8
Black	354,920	40.6
White	369,252	42.2
Hispanic	138,812	15.9
Total females aged 13 or older	**156,837**	**100.0**
Non-Hispanic		
American Indian	562	0.4
Asian	905	0.6
Black	96,338	61.4
White	33,766	21.5
Hispanic	24,997	15.9
Total males aged 13 or older	**708,452**	**100.0**
Non-Hispanic		
American Indian	2,353	0.3
Asian	5,875	0.8
Black	253,078	35.7
White	333,873	47.1
Hispanic	112,101	15.8
Children under age 13	**8,939**	**100.0**
Non-Hispanic		
American Indian	31	0.3
Asian	57	0.6
Black	5,504	61.6
White	1,613	18.0
Hispanic	1,714	19.2

Source: National Center for Health Statistics, Health, United States, 2004; Internet site http://www.cdc.gov/nchs/hus.htm

Most Children Receive Recommended Vaccinations

But some racial and ethnic groups have lower vaccination rates.

More than 90 percent of children between the ages of 19 and 35 months had received polio; measles, mumps, and rubella; haemophilus influenza type b; and hepatitis B vaccines. The high rate of vaccinations is the result of concerted efforts by health care professionals to reach children not only through physician's offices, but in schools and communities.

There are some differences by race and Hispanic origin in the percentage of children who receive various vaccines. While 71 percent of non-Hispanic white and Asian children receive the pneumococcal conjugate vaccine, for example, American Indian, black, and Hispanic children are less likely to get the vaccination. In general, non-Hispanic whites and Asians are more likely to be vaccinated.

■ Concerns are occasionally raised about side effects of particular vaccines. These concerns have not prevented most parents from having their children vaccinated.

American Indian children have a lower vaccination rate

(percent of children aged 19 to 35 months who have received the pneumococcal conjugate vaccine, by race and Hispanic origin, 2003)

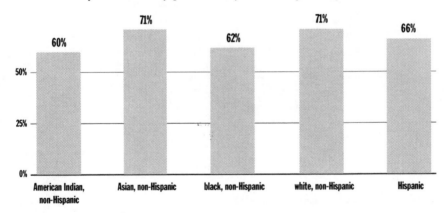

Table 9.26   Vaccinations of Children Aged 19 to 35 Months by Race and Hispanic Origin, 2003

(percent of children aged 19 to 35 months who have received vaccinations, by type of vaccine, race, and Hispanic origin, 2003)

		non-Hispanic				
	total	American Indian	Asian	black	white	Hispanic
Combined series (4:3:1:3)	**81%**	**77%**	**81%**	**75%**	**84%**	**79%**
Diphtheria tetanus, pertussis vaccine (DTP/DT/DTaP, four doses or more)	85	80	89	80	88	82
Polio (three doses or more)	92	91	91	89	93	90
Measles, mumps, rubella	93	92	96	92	93	93
Haemophilus influenza type b vaccine (Hib, three doses or more)	94	89	91	92	95	93
Hepatitis B (three doses or more)	92	90	94	92	93	91
Varicella	85	81	91	85	84	86
Pneumococcal conjugate vaccine (PCV, three doses or more)	68	60	71	62	71	66

Note: The combined series consists of four or more doses of DTP/DT/DTaP, three or more doses of polio virus, one or more doses of measles vaccine, and three or more doses of Hib.
Source: National Center for Health Statistics, Health, United States, 2004; Internet site http://www.cdc.gov/nchs/hus.htm

Children's Health Problems Vary by Age, Sex, Race

Boys are more likely than girls to have problems.

Prescription drugs are popular among children as well as adults. In 2002, nearly 10 million children under age 18 had been taking prescription medication for at least three months. Among children taking medication, the majority (57 percent) were boys.

Among the health conditions considered here, the most common are asthma and respiratory allergies, with 12 percent of children experiencing one of these conditions in the past year. Other types of allergies are almost as common (11 percent). Boys are more likely than girls to have various health problems.

The prevalence of some health conditions increases with the age of the child. Only 7 percent of children under age 5 have been diagnosed with asthma, for example, but the share rises to 15 percent among those aged 12 to 17. There are also differences by race, as black and non-Hispanic white children are more likely than Asian or Hispanic children to have various health problems.

■ The percentage of children with asthma has been increasing for years, but the reason for the increase is not known.

Non-Hispanic white children are most likely to be taking a prescription medication

(percent of children taking prescription medication regularly for at least three months, by race and Hispanic origin, 2002)

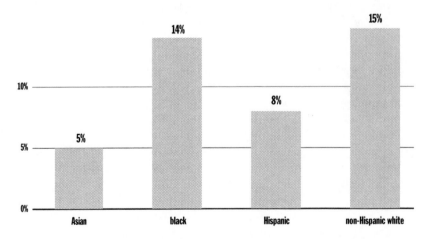

Table 9.27 Health Conditions among Children by Selected Characteristics, 2002

(number of people under age 18 with selected health conditions, by selected characteristics and type of condition, 2002; numbers in thousands)

| | total children | diagnosed with asthma | experienced in last 12 months | | | | ever told had * | | prescription medication taken regularly for at least 3 months |
			asthma attack	hay fever	respiratory allergies	other allergies	learning disability	attention deficit hyperactivity disorder	
Total children	**72,970**	**8,894**	**4,197**	**7,503**	**8,905**	**8,253**	**4,942**	**4,365**	**9,847**
Sex									
Female	35,659	3,704	1,679	3,453	3,993	4,169	1,791	1,175	4,253
Male	37,311	5,190	2,518	4,050	4,912	4,084	3,151	3,190	5,594
Age									
Aged 0 to 4	19,827	1,452	958	771	1,236	2,246	81	77	1,542
Aged 5 to 11	28,780	3,801	1,801	3,144	4,126	3,614	2,297	1,952	4,089
Aged 12 to 17	24,363	3,641	1,438	3,588	3,544	2,392	2,563	2,336	4,217
Race and Hispanic origin									
Asian	2,554	272	111	243	171	330	23	–	138
Black	10,578	1,873	910	838	1,257	1,449	915	696	1,504
Hispanic	12,563	1,273	558	937	1,077	1,035	589	378	1,038
Non-Hispanic white	45,253	5,214	2,478	5,275	6,161	5,150	3,245	3,185	6,957
Family structure									
Mother and father	52,588	5,644	2,568	5,562	6,301	5,818	2,880	2,499	6,537
Mother, no father	16,175	2,684	1,381	1,576	2,137	2,024	1,666	1,468	2,805
Father, no mother	2,124	229	93	193	239	225	162	159	202
Neither mother nor father	2,081	338	155	172	229	186	234	239	303
Parent's education									
Less than high school diploma	9,438	1,092	460	586	774	708	782	476	973
High school diploma	16,411	2,035	1,022	1,421	1,878	1,663	1,338	1,246	2,295
More than high school	44,560	5,407	2,546	5,303	6,017	5,685	2,567	2,389	6,251
Household income									
Less than $20,000	12,299	1,956	996	966	1,403	1,212	1,268	920	1,944
$20,000 to $34,999	10,174	1,231	556	892	1,228	1,329	870	741	1,393
$35,000 to $54,999	11,667	1,274	601	1,248	1,383	1,366	664	668	1,500
$55,000 to $74,999	9,565	1,155	565	1,066	1,277	1,092	635	607	1,272
$75,000 or more	16,223	1,868	829	2,159	2,251	2,198	805	822	2,292

* *"Ever told" by a school representative or health professional. Data exclude children under age 3.*
Note: "Mother and father" can include biological, adoptive, step, in-law, or foster relationships. Legal guardians are classified as "neither mother nor father." Parent's education is the education level of the parent with the higher level of education. Other allergies include food or digestive allergies, eczema, and other skin allergies. (–) means data not available.
Source: National Center for Health Statistics, Summary Health Statistics for U.S. Children: National Health Interview Survey, *2002, Series 10, No. 221, 2004; Internet site http://www.cdc.gov/nchs/nhis.htm*

Table 9.28 Distribution of Health Conditions by Selected Characteristics of Children, 2002

(percent distribution of people under age 18 with health condition by selected characteristics, 2002)

	total children	diagnosed with asthma	asthma attack	hay fever	respiratory allergies	other allergies	learning disability	attention deficit hyperactivity disorder	prescription medication taken regularly for at least 3 months
			experienced in last 12 months					*ever told had*	
Total children	100.0%	100.0%	100.0%	100.0%	100.0%	100.0%	100.0%	100.0%	100.0%
Sex									
Female	48.9	41.6	40.0	46.0	44.8	50.5	36.2	26.9	43.2
Male	51.1	58.4	60.0	54.0	55.2	49.5	63.8	73.1	56.8
Age									
Aged 0 to 4	27.2	16.3	22.8	10.3	13.9	27.2	1.6	1.8	15.7
Aged 5 to 11	39.4	42.7	42.9	41.9	46.3	43.8	46.5	44.7	41.5
Aged 12 to 17	33.4	40.9	34.3	47.8	39.8	29.0	51.9	53.5	42.8
Race and Hispanic origin									
Asian	3.5	3.1	2.6	3.2	1.9	4.0	0.5	–	1.4
Black	14.5	21.1	21.7	11.2	14.1	17.6	18.5	15.9	15.3
Hispanic	17.2	14.3	13.3	12.5	12.1	12.5	11.9	8.7	10.5
Non-Hispanic white	62.0	58.6	59.0	70.3	69.2	62.4	65.7	73.0	70.7
Family structure									
Mother and father	72.1	63.5	61.2	74.1	70.8	70.5	58.3	57.3	66.4
Mother, no father	22.2	30.2	32.9	21.0	24.0	24.5	33.7	33.6	28.5
Father, no mother	2.9	2.6	2.2	2.6	2.7	2.7	3.3	3.6	2.1
Neither mother nor father	2.9	3.8	3.7	2.3	2.6	2.3	4.7	5.5	3.1
Parent's education									
Less than high school diploma	12.9	12.3	11.0	7.8	8.7	8.6	15.8	10.9	9.9
High school diploma	22.5	22.9	24.4	18.9	21.1	20.2	27.1	28.5	23.3
More than high school	61.1	60.8	60.7	70.7	67.6	68.9	51.9	54.7	63.5
Household income									
Less than $20,000	16.9	22.0	23.7	12.9	15.8	14.7	25.7	21.1	19.7
$20,000 to $34,999	13.9	13.8	13.2	11.9	13.8	16.1	17.6	17.0	14.1
$35,000 to $54,999	16.0	14.3	14.3	16.6	15.5	16.6	13.4	15.3	15.2
$55,000 to $74,999	13.1	13.0	13.5	14.2	14.3	13.2	12.9	13.9	12.9
$75,000 or more	22.2	21.0	19.8	28.8	25.3	26.6	16.3	18.8	23.3

* *"Ever told" by a school representative or health professional. Data exclude children under age 3.*
Note: "Mother and father" can include biological, adoptive, step, in-law, or foster relationships. Legal guardians are classified as "neither mother nor father." Parent's education is the education level of the parent with the higher level of education. Other allergies include food or digestive allergies, eczema, and other skin allergies. (–) means data not available.
Source: National Center for Health Statistics, Summary Health Statistics for U.S. Children: National Health Interview Survey, 2002, Series 10, No. 221, 2004; Internet site http://www.cdc.gov/nchs/nhis.htm

Table 9.29 Percent of Children with Health Conditions by Selected Characteristics, 2002

(percent of people under age 18 with selected health conditions, by type of condition and selected characteristics, 2002)

			experienced in last 12 months				ever told had *		prescription medication
	total children	diagnosed with asthma	asthma attack	hay fever	respiratory allergies	other allergies	learning disability	attention deficit hyperactivity disorder	taken regularly for at least 3 months
Total children	100.0%	12.2%	5.8%	10.3%	12.2%	11.3%	8.1%	7.2%	13.5%
Sex									
Female	100.0	10.4	4.7	9.7	11.3	11.7	6.0	4.0	12.0
Male	100.0	14.0	6.8	10.9	13.3	11.0	10.1	10.3	15.0
Age									
Aged 0 to 4	100.0	7.3	4.8	3.9	6.3	11.3	1.0	1.0	7.8
Aged 5 to 11	100.0	13.2	6.3	11.0	14.4	12.6	8.0	6.8	14.2
Aged 12 to 17	100.0	15.0	5.9	14.8	14.6	9.8	10.5	9.6	17.3
Race and Hispanic origin									
Asian	100.0	10.6	4.2	9.7	6.7	12.8	1.1	–	5.3
Black	100.0	17.7	8.6	7.9	11.9	13.8	10.2	7.8	14.2
Hispanic	100.0	10.3	4.4	7.7	8.8	8.2	5.9	3.8	8.4
Non-Hispanic white	100.0	11.4	5.5	11.6	13.6	11.4	8.4	8.3	15.3
Family structure									
Mother and father	100.0	11.0	4.9	10.9	12.2	11.1	6.8	5.9	12.6
Mother, no father	100.0	16.6	8.6	9.5	13.1	12.6	11.8	10.4	17.2
Father, no mother	100.0	9.9	4.4	8.0	10.2	10.8	7.8	7.3	8.5
Neither mother nor father	100.0	16.4	7.6	7.8	10.5	9.0	12.1	12.4	13.4
Parent's education									
Less than high school diploma	100.0	11.7	4.7	6.4	8.4	7.5	10.6	6.5	10.4
High school diploma	100.0	12.4	6.2	8.6	11.5	10.2	9.6	9.0	13.9
More than high school	100.0	12.2	5.7	12.0	13.6	12.8	6.9	6.4	14.1
Household income									
Less than $20,000	100.0	16.2	8.1	8.1	11.7	9.9	13.0	9.5	16.1
$20,000 to $34,999	100.0	12.2	5.4	9.0	12.3	12.9	10.5	9.0	14.0
$35,000 to $54,999	100.0	11.1	5.2	10.9	12.0	11.7	7.0	7.1	13.0
$55,000 to $74,999	100.0	12.0	5.9	11.1	13.3	11.4	7.9	7.5	13.2
$75,000 or more	100.0	11.3	5.1	13.0	13.7	13.6	5.7	5.8	13.8

* *"Ever told" by a school representative or health professional. Data exclude children under age 3.*

Note: "Mother and father" can include biological, adoptive, step, in-law, or foster relationships. Legal guardians are classified as "neither mother nor father." Parent's education is the education level of the parent with the higher level of education. Other allergies include food or digestive allergies, eczema, and other skin allergies. (–) means data not available.

Source: National Center for Health Statistics, Summary Health Statistics for U.S. Children: National Health Interview Survey, *2002, Series 10, No. 221, 2004; Internet site http://www.cdc.gov/nchs/nhis.htm*

Prescription Drug Use Is Increasing

More Americans are using a growing number of prescriptions.

The use of prescription drugs to treat a variety of illnesses, particularly chronic conditions, increased between 1988–94 and 1999–00. The percentage of people who took at least one drug in the past month rose from 38 to 43 percent during those years. The percentage of those who used three or more prescription drugs in the past month climbed from 11 to 16 percent.

The increase in prescription drug use was greatest among people aged 65 or older. The share of people aged 65 or older who took at least one prescription drug in the past month rose from 74 to 84 percent between 1988–94 and 1999–00. The percentage of those who used three or more drugs grew from 35 to 48 percent.

Women are more likely than men to have taken at least one prescription medication in the past month (49 versus 37 percent). Non-Hispanic whites and blacks are more likely to have used prescription drugs in the past month than Mexican Americans are (48 and 35 percent, respectively, versus 24 percent).

■ Behind the increase in the use of prescriptions is the introduction and marketing of new drugs to treat chronic health problems.

Half of older women took three or more prescription drugs in the past month

(percent of people aged 65 or older who took three or more prescription drugs in the past month, by sex, 1988–94 and 1999–00)

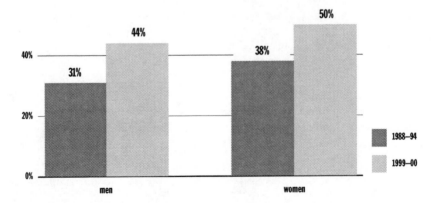

Table 9.30 Prescription Drug Use by Sex and Age, 1988–94 and 1999–00

(percent of people aged 18 or older taking at least one or three or more prescription drugs in the past month, by sex and age, 1988–94 and 1999–00; percentage point change, 1988–94 to 1999–00)

	at least one			three or more		
	1999–00	1988–94	percentage point change	1999–00	1988–94	percentage point change
Total people	**43.0%**	**37.8%**	**5.2**	**15.5%**	**11.0%**	**4.5**
Under age 18	24.1	20.5	3.6	3.7	2.4	1.3
Aged 18 to 44	34.7	31.3	3.4	7.5	5.7	1.8
Aged 45 to 64	62.1	54.8	7.3	29.5	20.0	9.5
Aged 65 or older	83.9	73.6	10.3	47.6	35.3	12.3
Female	**49.2**	**44.6**	**4.6**	**19.2**	**13.6**	**5.6**
Under age 18	22.2	20.6	1.6	4.3	2.3	2.0
Aged 18 to 44	43.8	40.7	3.1	10.1	7.6	2.5
Aged 45 to 64	69.8	62.0	7.8	35.9	24.7	11.2
Aged 65 or older	86.0	78.3	7.7	50.3	38.2	12.1
Male	**36.7**	**30.6**	**6.1**	**11.8**	**8.3**	**3.5**
Under age 18	25.8	20.4	5.4	3.1	2.6	0.5
Aged 18 to 44	25.4	21.5	3.9	4.9	3.6	1.3
Aged 45 to 64	53.6	47.2	6.4	22.4	15.1	7.3
Aged 65 or older	81.1	67.2	13.9	43.9	31.3	12.6

Source: National Center for Health Statistics, Health, United States, 2004; *Internet site http://www.cdc.gov/nchs/hus.htm; calculations by New Strategist*

Table 9.31 Prescription Drug Use by Race, Hispanic Origin, Age, and Sex, 1999–00

(percent of people aged 18 or older who took at least one or three or more prescription drugs in the past month, by race, Hispanic origin, age, and sex, 1999–00)

	total		female		male	
	at least one	three or more	at least one	three or more	at least one	three or more
Total people	**43.0%**	**15.5%**	**49.2%**	**19.2%**	**36.7%**	**11.8%**
Under age 18	24.1	3.7	22.2	4.3	25.8	3.1
Aged 18 to 44	34.7	7.5	43.8	10.1	25.4	4.9
Aged 45 to 64	62.1	29.5	69.8	35.9	53.6	22.4
Aged 65 or older	83.9	47.6	86.0	50.3	81.1	43.9
Black, non-Hispanic, total	**34.6**	**12.1**	**40.2**	**13.6**	**28.3**	**10.4**
Under age 18	19.2	2.5	17.9	–	20.4	–
Aged 18 to 44	26.5	5.0	33.8	–	17.9	–
Aged 45 to 64	61.7	29.9	70.4	32.0	50.6	27.1
Aged 65 or older	86.7	55.4	89.4	54.5	83.1	56.6
White, non-Hispanic, total	**48.2**	**18.0**	**54.8**	**22.0**	**41.5**	**13.9**
Under age 18	27.2	4.1	24.8	4.8	29.5	3.5
Aged 18 to 44	39.6	9.4	49.6	12.4	29.4	6.3
Aged 45 to 64	63.5	30.1	72.0	36.9	55.0	23.4
Aged 65 or older	84.5	47.4	86.6	50.6	81.6	43.0
Hispanic, Mexican, total	**24.1**	**5.6**	**28.8**	**6.7**	**19.7**	**4.5**
Under age 18	16.4	2.0	15.7	1.6	17.2	2.4
Aged 18 to 44	19.4	–	25.7	–	13.7	–
Aged 45 to 64	51.2	19.5	60.7	21.3	40.2	17.4
Aged 65 or older	69.1	37.1	74.7	41.6	62.3	31.5

Note: (–) means data not available.
Source: National Center for Health Statistics, Health, United States, 2004; *Internet site http://www.cdc.gov/nchs/hus.htm*

Some Health Conditions Are More Costly than Others

The top four are heart disease, trauma, cancer, and mental illness.

Trauma resulted in the largest number of visits to emergency rooms and to outpatient and office-based health care providers in 2002. Heart conditions and childbirth produced the largest number of hospital stays, while chronic obstructive pulmonary disease and asthma were responsible for the largest number of prescriptions written that year.

Heart conditions and trauma-related disorders are the most expensive conditions to treat. The nation spent almost $68 billion on the treatment of heart disease in 2002 and nearly $56 billion on trauma-related health problems. On a per event basis, though, the highest average expenditure is for the treatment of perinatal conditions ($4,075 per event), followed by appendicitis ($2,168)—which almost always requires surgery. Perinatal conditions also rank first in expenditures on a per-person basis, costing $23,811 per person with the condition (mostly premature infants) in 2002.

■ Reducing the incidence of just a few conditions—such as premature births, trauma, and heart disease—would have a noticeable impact on health care spending in the United States.

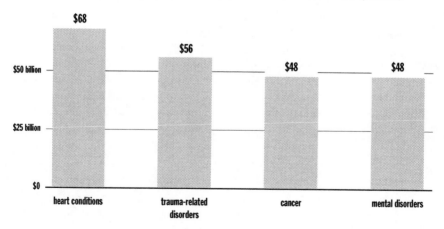

Heart problems are the most expensive health condition

(total amount spent on selected health conditions, 2002; in billions of dollars)

Table 9.32 Number of Health Events by Condition and Type of Service, 2002

(number of health events by condition and type of service, 2002; numbers in thousands; ranked by total number of events)

	total health events	visits to outpatient and office-based medical providers	hospital inpatient stays	visits to emergency rooms	prescriptions	home health care visits
Chronic obstructive pulmonary disease, asthma	237,385	102,470	1,395	4,206	125,478	3,836
Mental disorders	215,520	127,541	1,364	1,708	74,891	10,016
Hypertension	193,792	66,462	467	837	122,097	3,929
Trauma-related disorders	187,948	138,376	2,134	15,312	27,087	5,038
Back problems	140,229	114,556	568	1,432	21,784	1,888
Heart conditions	132,151	64,558	3,851	4,078	53,337	6,326
Osteoarthritis, other nontraumatic joint disorders	124,651	75,956	715	875	40,351	6,754
Diabetes mellitus	118,989	52,795	816	743	59,771	4,865
Other care and screening	96,948	37,750	133	142	57,769	1,154
Acute bronchitis and upper respiratory infections	96,740	46,154	195	1,725	48,420	246
Skin disorders	82,219	45,001	543	980	33,903	1,791
Systemic lupus and connective tissue disorders	79,589	58,080	275	884	18,138	2,212
Cancer	78,017	65,981	1,811	652	7,985	1,588
Hyperlipidemia	68,781	29,186	61	39	39,036	459
Other central nervous system disorders	60,991	45,262	381	1,171	12,078	2,099
Kidney disease	60,440	52,271	766	1,358	5,250	795
Disorders of the upper gastrointestinal tract	56,172	20,060	538	1,204	33,600	769
Normal birth, live born	51,888	42,343	3,319	1,031	5,045	151
Female genital disorders and contraception	50,735	18,801	471	560	30,766	138
Infectious diseases	50,105	28,210	757	1,402	19,149	587
Residual codes	50,098	20,067	626	566	26,471	2,368
Other endocrine, nutritional, immune disorders	42,632	18,255	524	729	22,088	1,036
Thyroid disease	42,219	16,444	57	85	25,279	353
Otitis media	39,792	21,365	47	1,186	17,180	14
Other eye disorders	38,368	26,473	107	434	9,600	1,754
Other circulatory conditions of arteries, veins, and lymphatics	35,804	22,779	1,020	726	9,584	1,695
Headache	32,867	18,018	100	1,123	13,479	146
Other bone and musculoskeletal disease	32,413	19,610	84	228	10,972	1,519
Other gastrointestinal disorders	23,135	11,323	558	867	9,926	461
Allergic reactions	20,224	10,581	10	551	9,057	24
Urinary tract infections	19,808	9,194	234	1,006	8,678	697
Symptoms	19,686	11,630	481	1,530	5,582	463
Cataract	19,025	15,101	29	19	3,575	301
Cerebrovascular disease	18,194	9,939	857	707	3,633	3,059
Pneumonia	16,792	6,978	1,395	1,481	6,218	720
Glaucoma	16,528	8,203	6	3	8,107	209
Intestinal infection	15,566	8,057	148	1,065	6,276	19
Disorders of teeth and jaw	14,854	2,768	66	287	11,733	–

(continued)

	total health events	visits to outpatient and office-based medical providers	hospital inpatient stays	visits to emergency rooms	prescriptions	home health care visits
Epilepsy and convulsions	14,040	5,378	339	705	6,785	834
Gall bladder, pancreatic, and liver disease	12,976	8,218	1,018	809	2,275	655
Other urinary disorders	12,886	6,210	96	231	5,961	388
Anemia and other deficiencies	12,507	9,217	194	130	2,607	360
Hereditary, degenerative, and other nervous system disorders	12,331	6,091	136	72	4,110	1,923
Male genital disorders	11,444	6,466	147	139	4,599	93
Nonmalignant neoplasm	11,247	9,495	226	133	1,384	8
Congenital anomalies	10,841	8,693	214	57	1,126	751
Influenza	8,793	4,268	67	369	4,082	7
Hernias	8,535	5,269	263	123	2,633	247
Other stomach and intestinal disorders	7,802	4,170	443	344	2,606	240
Nonmalignant breast disease	7,295	6,600	56	40	538	62
Poisoning by medical and nonmedical substances	6,287	3,247	285	890	1,702	162
Hemorrhagic, coagulation, and disorders of white blood cells	5,790	4,221	239	149	1,098	83
Paralysis	5,783	3,956	17	10	259	1,541
Tonsillitis	4,182	2,352	14	144	1,673	–
Complications of pregnancy and birth	3,922	2,213	218	245	1,209	35
Complications of surgery or device	2,817	1,452	164	198	900	102
Disorders of mouth and esophagus	2,202	891	–	96	1,215	–
Appendicitis	1,563	598	334	297	334	–
Perinatal conditions	1,379	1,131	79	16	73	80
Central nervous system infection	1,219	593	122	136	222	146
Coma, brain damage	278	120	18	3	4	133

Note: (–) means sample is too small to make a reliable estimate.
Source: Center for Financing, Access and Cost Trends, Agency for Healthcare Research and Quality: Medical Expenditure Panel Survey, 2002; Internet site http://www.meps.ahrq.gov/CompendiumTables/TC_TOC.htm

Table 9.33 Number of People Experiencing Health Events by Condition and Type of Service, 2002

(number of people experiencing health events by condition and type of service, 2002; people in thousands; ranked by total experiencing event)

	total people experiencing event	visits to outpatient and office-based medical providers	hospital inpatient stays	visits to emergency rooms	prescriptions	home health care visits
Chronic obstructive pulmonary disease, asthma	50,236	29,485	1,121	3,233	44,586	715
Hypertension	37,086	21,179	415	698	35,676	661
Trauma-related disorders	35,768	27,182	1,870	13,152	15,939	1,119
Acute bronchitis and upper respiratory infections	34,877	28,700	171	1,574	27,941	82
Mental disorders	31,205	18,825	966	1,210	26,580	1,604
Other care and screening	27,507	12,419	125	115	22,141	270
Skin disorders	24,990	18,680	458	862	17,202	344
Osteoarthritis, other nontraumatic joint disorders	23,479	16,830	521	665	17,233	1,166
Heart conditions	19,693	14,445	2,892	3,166	14,308	1,180
Hyperlipidemia	19,433	11,084	53	39	17,324	114
Disorders of the upper gastrointestinal tract	18,751	8,362	441	1,020	16,427	194
Female genital disorders and contraception	18,389	7,126	458	479	15,393	28
Back problems	18,185	15,562	536	1,177	9,260	390
Infectious diseases	17,828	12,934	574	1,214	11,154	194
Residual codes	15,922	6,015	473	381	13,188	441
Systemic lupus and connective tissue disorders	15,166	12,168	259	650	8,618	310
Other eye disorders	14,742	12,949	100	345	6,272	269
Other central nervous system disorders	14,091	11,812	322	1,002	6,643	490
Diabetes mellitus	14,019	11,041	587	546	13,169	867
Other endocrine, nutritional, immune disorders	12,100	5,185	467	686	9,654	259
Otitis media	11,956	9,940	47	1,044	10,594	8
Thyroid disease	11,617	5,751	45	72	10,816	73
Cancer	10,852	10,351	1,348	369	3,519	549
Headache	8,382	4,998	100	776	6,153	34
Disorders of teeth and jaw	8,337	1,343	66	235	7,615	–
Other gastrointestinal disorders	8,212	4,488	468	710	5,442	123
Other bone and musculoskeletal diseases	7,807	4,890	78	141	5,127	340
Symptoms	7,765	5,225	395	1,305	3,734	110
Intestinal infection	7,710	6,026	148	1,008	4,468	16
Other circulatory conditions of arteries, veins, and lymphatics	7,098	5,331	822	576	4,200	333
Urinary tract infections	7,064	5,249	227	836	5,970	120
Allergic reactions	6,209	4,354	10	500	4,995	6
Normal birth, live born	6,158	5,743	3,101	819	3,227	96
Nonmalignant neoplasm	4,863	4,759	226	92	851	8
Pneumonia	4,480	3,182	1,144	1,312	3,393	205
Other urinary disorders	4,327	2,314	85	161	3,265	63
Cataract	4,255	4,147	29	19	1,789	88
Influenza	4,022	3,154	59	365	2,802	7

(continued)

	total people experiencing event	visits to outpatient and office-based medical providers	hospital inpatient stays	visits to emergency rooms	prescriptions	home health care visits
Kidney disease	3,546	2,844	607	1,034	2,104	193
Glaucoma	3,545	3,038	6	3	2,660	75
Male genital disorders	3,385	2,287	121	134	2,329	62
Gall bladder, pancreatic, and liver disease	2,865	2,292	890	635	1,188	80
Anemia and other deficiencies	2,739	1,766	159	114	1,583	91
Nonmalignant breast disease	2,577	2,499	56	37	441	31
Epilepsy and convulsions	2,455	1,401	301	515	2,203	168
Cerebrovascular disease	2,446	1,713	697	598	1,331	427
Hernias	2,427	1,712	254	108	1,507	47
Poisoning by medical and nonmedical substances	2,274	1,427	252	869	1,043	25
Other stomach and intestinal disorders	1,908	1,434	386	305	1,140	77
Hereditary, degenerative, and other nervous system disorders	1,533	1,140	95	61	1,226	204
Congenital anomalies	1,444	1,261	183	48	478	102
Tonsillitis	1,340	1,150	14	125	1,021	–
Complications of pregnancy and birth	1,292	713	191	189	830	9
Disorders of mouth and esophagus	1,144	473	–	77	934	–
Complications of surgery or device	967	466	154	179	568	45
Hemorrhagic, coagulation, and disorders of white blood cells	914	684	101	108	513	27
Appendicitis	421	302	327	259	231	–
Paralysis	400	287	17	10	139	148
Perinatal conditions	236	186	78	16	50	34
Central nervous system infection	235	127	91	79	129	36
Coma, brain damage	44	18	15	3	4	22

Note: (–) means sample is too small to make a reliable estimate.
Source: Center for Financing, Access and Cost Trends, Agency for Healthcare Research and Quality: Medical Expenditure Panel Survey, 2002; Internet site http://www.meps.ahrq.gov/CompendiumTables/TC_TOC.htm

Table 9.34 Cost of Health Events by Condition and Type of Service, 2002

(amount spent on health events by condition and type of service, 2002; in millions of dollars; ranked by total amount spent)

	total spent on health events	visits to outpatient and office-based medical providers	hospital inpatient stays	visits to emergency rooms	prescriptions	home health care visits
Heart conditions	$67,621.38	$12,494.33	$41,167.88	$2,730.44	$6,519.62	$4,709.12
Trauma-related disorders	55,833.77	19,266.32	21,094.72	7,439.78	1,988.89	6,044.07
Cancer	48,425.36	21,281.99	23,609.40	323.20	1,543.20	1,667.57
Mental disorders	47,507.52	13,414.91	9,536.82	865.01	15,903.11	7,787.66
Chronic obstructive pulmonary disease, asthma	45,262.78	11,923.53	12,464.81	1,642.40	15,150.31	4,081.72
Hypertension	32,558.58	8,632.91	3,060.29	587.39	16,683.24	3,594.74
Osteoarthritis and other nontraumatic joint disorders	32,235.96	10,710.16	9,975.91	402.97	6,287.39	4,859.53
Diabetes mellitus	27,279.53	6,838.07	5,874.96	181.19	10,636.06	3,749.26
Normal birth, live born	23,406.15	5,982.19	16,673.74	494.35	216.20	39.66
Back problems	22,818.78	12,289.35	5,696.16	748.89	2,638.55	1,445.84
Other circulatory conditions of arteries, veins, and lymphatics	18,955.63	4,353.90	11,384.14	471.48	1,395.69	1,350.43
Kidney disease	18,268.64	11,343.81	4,804.85	1,138.84	520.43	460.72
Disorders of the upper gastrointestinal tract	17,308.46	3,875.07	4,073.91	590.32	8,217.26	551.91
Infectious diseases	17,115.61	3,263.12	7,774.12	528.41	4,192.72	1,357.24
Other central nervous system disorders	16,800.19	8,513.20	3,058.96	545.15	1,272.88	3,410.00
Skin disorders	15,936.09	6,747.82	4,196.56	395.93	2,830.64	1,765.13
Systemic lupus and connective tissue disorders	15,849.36	8,506.13	2,279.43	506.18	2,182.54	2,375.08
Other care and screening	15,258.00	4,656.95	463.45	54.09	9,189.20	894.30
Gall bladder, pancreatic, and liver disease	13,761.19	2,352.45	9,345.36	344.22	362.75	1,356.41
Hyperlipidemia	13,611.51	3,440.19	355.86	35.17	9,491.65	288.66
Residual codes	12,822.77	4,379.37	3,383.42	279.68	2,849.30	1,931.00
Pneumonia	12,669.61	1,237.70	9,851.49	700.22	357.67	522.53
Cerebrovascular disease	12,507.87	1,738.69	7,834.32	321.32	679.60	1,933.93
Female genital disorders and contraception	10,209.11	3,791.66	2,501.38	350.63	3,564.81	0.63
Other eye disorders	9,617.33	5,352.23	648.02	128.06	996.51	2,492.51
Other endocrine, nutritional, and immune disorders	9,504.57	3,241.50	2,841.97	403.63	2,440.16	577.31
Acute bronchitis, upper respiratory infections	9,289.48	4,815.86	1,206.40	501.16	2,587.56	178.50
Other gastrointestinal disorders	8,729.01	2,441.29	3,341.48	643.62	1,517.39	785.24
Symptoms	8,473.37	2,180.23	4,435.79	853.45	455.74	548.16
Other stomach and intestinal disorders	8,014.89	1,350.08	6,178.85	131.54	267.38	87.03
Epilepsy and convulsions	7,192.49	667.06	2,816.43	359.38	1,316.23	2,033.39
Other bone and musculoskeletal diseases	6,622.36	2,815.49	788.44	73.34	1,984.25	960.84
Cataract	6,403.93	5,995.64	65.32	1.61	247.00	94.36
Hereditary, degenerative, and other nervous system disorders	6,038.35	1,122.10	1,509.95	32.03	1,723.91	1,650.36
Perinatal conditions	5,619.32	139.04	5,403.62	2.98	26.12	47.56
Headache	5,037.40	2,192.91	635.75	497.80	1,553.95	156.99

(continued)

	total spent on health events	visits to outpatient and office-based medical providers	hospital inpatient stays	visits to emergency rooms	prescriptions	home health care visits
Congenital anomalies	$4,922.96	$1,694.08	$2,075.00	$19.68	$187.65	$946.55
Urinary tract infections	4,915.78	1,249.25	1,318.70	558.22	437.45	1,352.16
Thyroid disease	4,427.55	1,955.24	662.94	18.25	1,553.94	237.17
Nonmalignant neoplasms	4,321.85	2,621.46	1,528.18	59.91	99.45	12.86
Hernias	4,270.76	2,240.17	1,338.04	58.56	562.67	71.32
Male genital disorders	3,620.94	1,564.46	1,087.19	267.97	660.69	40.63
Other urinary disorders	3,468.76	1,185.14	616.11	192.42	964.97	510.13
Appendicitis	3,388.34	109.02	3,016.07	256.91	6.34	–
Otitis media	3,234.61	2,206.41	154.00	212.61	658.12	3.47
Anemia and other deficiencies	3,097.93	1,737.95	982.54	82.35	159.19	135.90
Paralysis	3,041.79	411.26	49.27	2.19	45.99	2,533.08
Glaucoma	2,740.40	1,383.45	33.39	0.67	1,123.37	199.54
Poisoning by medical, nonmedical substances	2,357.54	476.77	1,375.79	417.68	83.27	4.02
Intestinal infection	2,104.07	785.05	608.27	419.75	251.57	39.43
Hemorrhagic, coagulation, and disorders of white blood cells	2,024.08	668.25	980.70	66.63	294.23	14.27
Nonmalignant breast disease	1,976.07	1,639.10	258.97	5.33	36.60	36.06
Complications of surgery or device	1,765.42	390.55	1,182.64	70.47	80.08	41.68
Allergic reactions	1,714.55	917.28	0.42	192.91	600.84	3.10
Central nervous system infection	1,682.76	78.01	1,486.01	31.32	15.11	72.30
Complications of pregnancy and birth	1,487.73	456.68	819.72	129.58	76.47	5.28
Disorders of teeth and jaw	1,354.38	518.70	460.39	45.38	329.91	–
Influenza	795.40	390.22	130.64	140.10	134.44	–
Tonsillitis	652.40	506.78	35.83	29.99	79.80	–
Coma, brain damage	302.24	34.66	122.12	0.51	0.14	144.81
Disorders of mouth and esophagus	286.87	202.00	–	28.22	56.65	–

Note: (–) means sample is too small to make a reliable estimate.
Source: Center for Financing, Access and Cost Trends, Agency for Healthcare Research and Quality: Medical Expenditure Panel Survey, 2002; Internet site http://www.meps.ahrq.gov/CompendiumTables/TC_TOC.htm

(average expense per health event by condition and type of service, 2002; in dollars; ranked by overall average)

	average expense per event	visit to outpatient and office-based medical providers	hospital inpatient stay	visit to emergency room	prescriptions	home health care visits
Perinatal conditions	$4,074.92	$122.94	$68,400.25	$186.25	$357.81	$594.50
Appendicitis	2,167.84	182.31	9,030.15	865.02	18.98	–
Central nervous system infection	1,380.44	131.55	12,180.41	230.29	68.06	495.21
Coma, brain damage	1,087.19	288.83	6,784.44	170.00	35.00	1,088.80
Gall bladder, pancreatic, and liver disease	1,060.51	286.26	9,180.12	425.49	159.45	2,070.86
Other stomach and intestinal disorders	1,027.29	323.76	13,947.74	382.38	102.60	362.63
Pneumonia	754.50	177.37	7,062.00	472.80	57.52	725.74
Cerebrovascular disease	687.47	174.94	9,141.56	454.48	187.06	632.21
Complications of surgery or device	626.70	268.97	7,211.22	355.91	88.98	408.63
Cancer	620.70	322.55	13,036.66	495.71	193.26	1,050.11
Other circulatory conditions of arteries, veins, and lymphatics	529.43	191.14	11,160.92	649.42	145.63	796.71
Paralysis	525.99	103.96	2,898.24	219.00	177.57	1,643.79
Epilepsy and convulsions	512.29	124.04	8,308.05	509.76	193.99	2,438.12
Heart conditions	511.70	193.54	10,690.18	669.55	122.23	744.41
Hernias	500.38	425.16	5,087.60	476.01	213.70	288.75
Hereditary, degenerative, and other nervous system disorders	489.69	184.22	11,102.57	444.86	419.44	858.22
Congenital anomalies	454.11	194.88	9,696.26	345.26	166.65	1,260.39
Normal birth, live born	451.09	141.28	5,023.72	479.49	42.85	262.65
Symptoms	430.43	187.47	9,222.02	557.81	81.64	1,183.93
Nonmalignant neoplasm	384.27	276.09	6,761.86	450.45	71.86	1,607.50
Complications of pregnancy and birth	379.33	206.36	3,760.18	528.90	63.25	150.86
Other gastrointestinal disorders	377.31	215.60	5,988.32	742.35	152.87	1,703.34
Poisoning by medical and nonmedical substances	374.99	146.83	4,827.33	469.30	48.92	24.81
Hemorrhagic, coagulation, and disorders of white blood cells	349.58	158.32	4,103.35	447.18	267.97	171.93
Infectious diseases	341.59	115.67	10,269.64	376.90	218.95	2,312.16
Cataract	336.61	397.04	2,252.41	84.74	69.09	313.49
Male genital disorders	316.41	241.95	7,395.85	1,927.84	143.66	436.88
Disorders of the upper gastrointestinal tract	308.13	193.17	7,572.32	490.30	244.56	717.70
Kidney disease	302.26	217.02	6,272.65	838.62	99.13	579.52
Trauma-related disorders	297.07	139.23	9,885.06	485.88	73.43	1,199.70
Other central nervous system disorders	275.45	188.09	8,028.77	465.54	105.39	1,624.58
Nonmalignant breast disease	270.88	248.35	4,624.46	133.25	68.03	581.61
Other urinary disorders	269.19	190.84	6,417.81	832.99	161.88	1,314.77
Osteoarthritis, other nontraumatic joint disorders	258.61	141.01	13,952.32	460.54	155.82	719.50
Residual codes	255.95	218.24	5,404.82	494.13	107.64	815.46
Other eye disorders	250.66	202.18	6,056.26	295.07	103.80	1,421.04
Urinary tract infections	248.17	135.88	5,635.47	554.89	50.41	1,939.97

(continued)

	average expense per event	visit to outpatient and office-based medical providers	hospital inpatient stay	visit to emergency room	prescriptions	home health care visits
Anemia and other deficiencies	$247.70	$188.56	$5,064.64	$633.46	$61.06	$377.50
Diabetes mellitus	229.26	129.52	7,199.71	243.86	177.95	770.66
Other endocrine, nutritional, immune disorders	222.94	177.57	5,423.61	553.68	110.47	557.25
Mental disorders	220.43	105.18	6,991.80	506.45	212.35	777.52
Other bone and musculoskeletal disease	204.31	143.57	9,386.19	321.67	180.85	632.55
Female genital disorders and contraception	201.22	201.67	5,310.79	626.13	115.87	4.57
Systemic lupus and connective tissue disorders	199.14	146.46	8,288.84	572.60	120.33	1,073.73
Hyperlipidemia	197.90	117.87	5,833.77	901.79	243.15	628.89
Skin disorders	193.83	149.95	7,728.47	404.01	83.49	985.56
Chronic obstructive pulmonary disease, asthma	190.67	116.36	8,935.35	390.49	120.74	1,064.06
Hypertension	168.01	129.89	6,553.08	701.78	136.64	914.93
Glaucoma	165.80	168.65	5,565.00	223.33	138.57	954.74
Back problems	162.73	107.28	10,028.45	522.97	121.12	765.81
Other care and screening	157.38	123.36	3,484.59	380.92	159.07	774.96
Tonsillitis	156.00	215.47	2,559.29	208.26	47.70	–
Headache	153.27	121.71	6,357.50	443.28	115.29	1,075.27
Intestinal infection	135.17	97.44	4,109.93	394.13	40.08	2,075.26
Disorders of mouth and esophagus	130.28	226.71	–	293.96	46.63	–
Thyroid disease	104.87	118.90	11,630.53	214.71	61.47	671.87
Acute bronchitis and upper respiratory infections	96.03	104.34	6,186.67	290.53	53.44	725.61
Disorders of teeth and jaw	91.18	187.39	6,975.61	158.12	28.12	–
Influenza	90.46	91.43	1,949.85	379.67	32.93	–
Allergic reactions	84.78	86.69	42.00	350.11	66.34	129.17
Otitis media	81.29	103.27	3,276.60	179.27	38.31	247.86

Note: (–) means sample is too small to make a reliable estimate.
Source: Center for Financing, Access and Cost Trends, Agency for Healthcare Research and Quality: Medical Expenditure Panel Survey, 2002; Internet site http://www.meps.ahrq.gov/CompendiumTables/TC_TOC.htm

Table 9.36 Average Expense Per Person Experiencing Health Event, by Condition and Type of Service, 2002

(average expense per person experiencing health event by condition and type of service, 2002; in dollars; ranked by overall average)

	average expense per person with event	visit to outpatient and office-based medical providers	hospital inpatient stay	visit to emergency room	prescriptions	home health care visits
Perinatal conditions	$23,810.68	$747.53	$69,277.18	$186.25	$522.40	$1,398.82
Appendicitis	8,048.31	360.99	9,223.46	991.93	27.45	–
Paralysis	7,604.48	1,432.96	2,898.24	219.00	330.86	17,115.41
Central nervous system infection	7,160.68	614.25	16,329.78	396.46	117.13	2,008.33
Coma, brain damage	6,869.09	1,925.56	8,141.33	170.00	35.00	6,582.27
Kidney disease	5,151.90	3,988.68	7,915.73	1,101.39	247.35	2,387.15
Cerebrovascular disease	5,113.60	1,015.00	11,240.06	537.32	510.59	4,529.11
Gall bladder, pancreatic, and liver diseases	4,803.21	1,026.37	10,500.40	542.08	305.35	16,955.13
Cancer	4,462.34	2,056.03	17,514.39	875.88	438.53	3,037.47
Other stomach and intestinal disorders	4,200.68	941.48	16,007.38	431.28	234.54	1,130.26
Hereditary, degenerative, and other nervous system disorders	3,938.91	984.30	15,894.21	525.08	1,406.13	8,090.00
Normal birth, live born	3,800.93	1,041.65	5,376.89	603.60	67.00	413.13
Heart conditions	3,433.78	864.96	14,235.09	862.43	455.66	3,990.78
Congenital anomalies	3,409.25	1,343.44	11,338.80	410.00	392.57	9,279.90
Epilepsy and consulsions	2,929.73	476.13	9,356.91	697.83	597.47	12,103.51
Pneumonia	2,828.04	388.97	8,611.44	533.70	105.41	2,548.93
Other circulatory conditions of arteries, veins, and lymphatics	2,670.56	816.71	13,849.32	818.54	332.31	4,055.35
Hemorrhagic, coagulation, and disorders of white blood cells	2,214.53	976.97	9,709.90	616.94	573.55	528.52
Diabetes mellitus	1,945.90	619.33	10,008.45	331.85	807.66	4,324.41
Complications of surgery or device	1,825.67	838.09	7,679.48	393.69	140.99	926.22
Hernias	1,759.69	1,308.51	5,267.87	542.22	373.37	1,517.45
Trauma-related disorders	1,561.00	708.79	11,280.60	565.68	124.78	5,401.31
Mental disorders	1,522.43	712.61	9,872.48	714.88	598.31	4,855.15
Cataract	1,505.04	1,445.78	2,252.41	84.74	138.07	1,072.27
Osteoarthritis and other nontraumatic joint disorders	1,372.97	636.37	19,147.62	605.97	364.85	4,167.69
Back problems	1,254.81	789.70	10,627.16	636.27	284.94	3,707.28
Other central nervous system disorders	1,192.26	720.72	9,499.88	544.06	191.61	6,959.18
Complications of pregnancy and birth	1,151.49	640.51	4,291.73	685.61	92.13	586.67
Anemia and other deficiencies	1,131.04	984.12	6,179.50	722.37	100.56	1,493.41
Symptoms	1,091.23	417.27	11,229.85	653.98	122.05	4,983.27
Male genital disorders	1,069.70	684.07	8,985.04	1,999.78	283.68	655.32
Other gastrointestinal disorders	1,062.96	543.96	7,139.91	906.51	278.83	6,384.07
Systemic lupus, connective tissue disorders	1,045.06	699.06	8,800.89	778.74	253.25	7,661.55
Poisoning by medical, nonmedical substances	1,036.74	334.11	5,459.48	480.64	79.84	160.80
Infectious diseases	960.04	252.29	13,543.76	435.26	375.89	6,996.08

(continued)

	average expense per person with event	visit to outpatient and office-based medical providers	hospital inpatient stay	visit to emergency room	prescriptions	home health care visits
Disorders of the upper gastrointestinal tract	$923.07	$463.41	$9,237.89	$578.75	$500.23	$2,844.90
Chronic obstructive pulmonary disease, asthma	901.00	404.39	11,119.37	508.01	339.80	5,708.70
Nonmalignant neoplasm	888.72	550.84	6,761.86	651.20	116.86	1,607.50
Hypertension	877.92	407.62	7,374.19	841.53	467.63	5,438.34
Other bone and musculoskeletal disease	848.26	575.76	10,108.21	520.14	387.02	2,826.00
Residual codes	805.35	728.07	7,153.11	734.07	216.05	4,378.68
Other urinary disorders	801.65	512.16	7,248.35	1,195.16	295.55	8,097.30
Other endocrine, nutritional, immune disorders	785.50	625.17	6,085.59	588.38	252.76	2,229.00
Glaucoma	773.03	455.38	5,565.00	223.33	422.32	2,660.53
Nonmalignant breast disease	766.81	655.90	4,624.46	144.05	82.99	1,163.23
Hyperlipidemia	700.43	310.37	6,714.34	901.79	547.89	2,532.11
Urinary tract infections	695.89	238.00	5,809.25	667.73	73.27	11,268.00
Other eye disorders	652.38	413.33	6,480.20	371.19	158.88	9,265.84
Skin disorders	637.70	361.23	9,162.79	459.32	164.55	5,131.19
Headache	600.98	438.76	6,357.50	641.49	252.55	4,617.35
Female genital disorders and contraception	555.17	532.09	5,461.53	732.00	231.59	22.50
Other care and screening	554.70	374.99	3,707.60	470.35	415.03	3,312.22
Tonsillitis	486.87	440.68	2,559.29	239.92	78.16	–
Thyroid disease	381.13	339.98	14,732.00	253.47	143.67	3,248.90
Allergic reactions	276.14	210.68	42.00	385.82	120.29	516.67
Intestinal infection	272.90	130.28	4,109.93	416.42	56.30	2,464.38
Otitis media	270.54	221.97	3,276.60	203.65	62.12	433.75
Acute bronchitis and upper respiratory infections	266.35	167.80	7,054.97	318.40	92.61	2,176.83
Disorders of mouth and esophagus	250.76	427.06	–	366.49	60.65	–
Influenza	197.76	123.72	2,214.24	383.84	47.98	–
Disorders of teeth and jaw	162.45	386.22	6,975.61	193.11	43.32	–

Note: (–) means sample is too small to make a reliable estimate.
Source: Center for Financing, Access and Cost Trends, Agency for Healthcare Research and Quality: Medical Expenditure Panel Survey, 2002; Internet site http://www.meps.ahrq.gov/CompendiumTables/TC_TOC.htm

10

Health Care Visits

■ **Americans made more than 1 million health care visits in 2002.**

Physician office visits accounted for 82 percent of the total, while 10 percent were visits to ERs and 8 percent to hospital outpatient departments.

■ **Most people think highly of their physician.**

Eighty-nine percent say they trust their doctor's judgments about their medical care.

■ **Only 16 percent of physician office visits were for preventive care.**

Acute health problems, such as colds, the flu, and accidents, bring the largest share of people to the doctor (36 percent). Ranking second are routine visits for chronic health problems (30 percent).

■ **Most doctor visits last less than 15 minutes.**

The median amount of time people spend with the doctor is just 14.7 minutes.

■ **Drugs are prescribed in nearly two-thirds of office visits.**

The drugs most commonly prescribed are Lipitor, Albuterol, Amoxicillin, and Synthroid.

■ **Sixty-nine percent of Americans have had their teeth cleaned in the past year.**

One in four adults has avoided going to the dentist for at least two years.

Four Out of Five Health Care Visits Are to Physicians' Offices

Many substitute a visit to the ER for a visit to the doctor, however.

Americans made over 1 million visits to doctors' offices, hospital outpatient departments, and hospital emergency rooms in 2002. Physician office visits account for 82 percent of total, while 10 percent of visits are to ERs and 8 percent to hospital outpatient departments.

Emergency rooms account for the largest share of health care visits among 15-to-24-year-olds (16 percent). At this age, many people do not need routine health care, but they are more likely to sustain accidental injuries. Lack of access to a regular health care provider also influences the type of health care setting people use. Twenty-four percent of health care visits by American Indians and 19 percent of those by blacks are to emergency rooms. Many may use ERs in lieu of a physician's office because they lack insurance coverage.

Sixty percent of the cost of physician office visits is paid for by private insurance and 21 percent by Medicare. Hospital outpatient and emergency departments, on the other hand, rely more heavily on public funding. Medicare or Medicaid/State Children's Health Insurance Program pays for 42 percent of the expenses for hospital outpatient department visits. Private insurance covers only 37 percent of the cost.

■ Better access to health care clinics could lower health care costs by diverting emergency room visits to a less-expensive setting.

Ten percent of health care visits are to emergency rooms

(percent distribution of health care visits, by place of care, 2002)

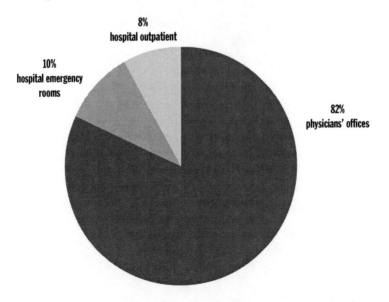

8%
hospital outpatient

10%
hospital emergency
rooms

82%
physicians' offices

Table 10.1 Health Care Visits by Sex, Age, and Race, 2002

(number and percent distribution of visits to physicians' offices, hospital outpatient departments, and emergency rooms, by sex, age, race, and place of care, 2002; numbers in thousands)

	total	physicians' offices	hospital outpatient departments	hospital emergency rooms
Total visits	**1,083,474**	**889,980**	**83,339**	**110,155**
Sex				
Female	639,683	529,075	51,014	59,594
Male	443,791	360,905	32,325	50,561
Age				
Under age 15	202,259	159,235	18,947	24,077
Aged 15 to 24	98,919	71,865	9,839	17,215
Aged 25 to 44	245,928	192,359	21,137	32,432
Aged 45 to 64	283,521	242,142	21,436	19,943
Aged 65 to 74	122,476	109,331	6,386	6,759
Aged 75 or older	130,372	115,049	5,595	9,728
Race				
American Indian	3,429	2,237	383	809
Asian	30,848	26,341	2,334	2,173
Black	132,980	89,455	18,664	24,861
Native Hawaiian	4,301	3,430	436	435
White	909,115	766,096	61,315	81,704
Multiple races	2,801	2,421	207	173
PERCENT DISTRIBUTION BY PLACE OF CARE				
Total visits	**100.0%**	**82.1%**	**7.7%**	**10.2%**
Sex				
Female	100.0	82.7	8.0	9.3
Male	100.0	81.3	7.3	11.4
Age				
Under age 15	100.0	78.7	9.4	11.9
Aged 15 to 24	100.0	72.7	9.9	17.4
Aged 25 to 44	100.0	78.2	8.6	13.2
Aged 45 to 64	100.0	85.4	7.6	7.0
Aged 65 to 74	100.0	89.3	5.2	5.5
Aged 75 or older	100.0	88.2	4.3	7.5
Race				
American Indian	100.0	65.2	11.2	23.6
Asian	100.0	85.4	7.6	7.0
Black	100.0	67.3	14.0	18.7
Native Hawaiian	100.0	79.7	10.1	10.1
White	100.0	84.3	6.7	9.0
Multiple races	100.0	86.4	7.4	6.2

(continued)

PERCENT DISTRIBUTION BY SEX, AGE, AND RACE	total	physicians' offices	hospital outpatient departments	hospital emergency rooms
Total visits	100.0%	100.0%	100.0%	100.0%
Sex				
Female	59.0	59.4	61.2	54.1
Male	41.0	40.6	38.8	45.9
Age				
Under age 15	18.7	17.9	22.7	21.9
Aged 15 to 24	9.1	8.1	11.8	15.6
Aged 25 to 44	22.7	21.6	25.4	29.4
Aged 45 to 64	26.2	27.2	25.7	18.1
Aged 65 to 74	11.3	12.3	7.7	6.1
Aged 75 or older	12.0	12.9	6.7	8.8
Race				
American Indian	0.3	0.3	0.5	0.7
Asian	2.8	3.0	2.8	2.0
Black	12.3	10.1	22.4	22.6
Native Hawaiian	0.4	0.4	0.5	0.4
White	83.9	86.1	73.6	74.2
Multiple races	0.3	0.3	0.2	0.2

Source: National Center for Health Statistics, National Ambulatory Medical Care Survey: 2002 Summary, *Advance Data No. 346, 2004;* National Hospital Ambulatory Medical Care Survey: 2002 Outpatient Department Summary, *Advance Data No. 345, 2004;* National Hospital Ambulatory Medical Care Survey: 2002 Emergency Department Summary, *Advance Data No. 340, 2004; Internet site http://www.cdc.gov/nchs/about/major/ahcd/adata.htm; calculations by New Strategist*

Table 10.2 Health Care Visits by Primary Source of Payment, 2002

(number and percent distribution of visits to physicians' offices, hospital outpatient departments, and emergency rooms, by primary expected source of payment, 2002; numbers in thousands)

	total		physicians' offices		hospital outpatient departments		emergency department	
	number	percent distribution	number	percent distribution	number	percent distribution	number	percent distribution
Total visits	**1,083,474**	**100.0%**	**889,980**	**100.0%**	**83,339**	**100.0%**	**110,155**	**100.0%**
Private insurance	599,385	55.3	525,520	59.0	31,063	37.3	42,802	38.9
Medicare	232,707	21.5	188,207	21.1	22,749	27.3	21,751	19.7
Medicaid/SCHIP	96,066	8.9	67,110	7.5	11,992	14.4	16,964	15.4
Self-pay	61,586	5.7	39,526	4.4	6,125	7.3	15,935	14.5
Worker's Compensation	19,495	1.8	14,658	1.6	2,689	3.2	2,148	1.9
No charge	4,652	0.4	2,485	0.3	1,012	1.2	1,155	1.0
Other/unknown/blank	69,582	6.4	52,474	5.9	7,709	9.3	9,399	8.5

Source: National Center for Health Statistics, National Ambulatory Medical Care Survey: 2002 Summary, Advance Data No. 346, 2004; National Hospital Ambulatory Medical Care Survey: 2002 Outpatient Department Summary, Advance Data No. 345, 2004; National Hospital Ambulatory Medical Care Survey: 2002 Emergency Department Summary, Advance Data No. 340, 2004; Internet site http://www.cdc.gov/nchs/about/major/ahcd/adata.htm; calculations by New Strategist

Women Are More Likely than Men to Visit Health Care Providers

Men are less likely to visit and wait longer between visits.

More than 163 million Americans made at least one visit to the office of a health care provider in 2002. Most visited a doctor or other health care provider at least twice during the year, and 38 percent visited four or more times.

Men are less likely than women to visit a health care provider. Twenty-six percent of men did not visit a health care provider at all in 2002 compared with only 12 percent of women. A substantial 45 percent of women made four or more visits to a health care provider during the year compared with only 30 percent of men. Younger adults are less likely than older ones to visit a health care provider—24 percent of people aged 18 to 44 made no visits in 2002. Hispanics are least likely to visit a health care provider (33 percent made no visits in 2002), while non-Hispanic whites are most likely (only 16 percent made no visits in 2002).

Almost 8 million people have not visited a health care provider in more than five years. Although this figure represents only about 4 percent of adults, it is still a significant number of people. For most adults, their last office visit was within the past six months.

■ With some important health problems, such as high cholesterol, presenting no symptoms, many people would benefit from some type of annual checkup.

More than one in four men has not visited a health care provider in the past year

(percent distribution of people aged 18 or older by number of office visits to a health care professional in the past twelve months, by sex, 2002)

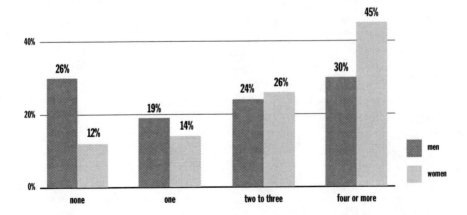

Table 10.3 Number of Office Visits to Health Care Professionals by Selected Characteristics, 2002

(total number of people aged 18 or older and distribution by number of office visits to health care professionals in past twelve months, by selected characteristics, 2002; numbers in thousands)

	total	number of office visits in past twelve months				
		none	one	two to three	four to nine	ten or more
Total adults	**205,825**	**38,413**	**33,616**	**51,514**	**49,630**	**28,585**
Sex						
Men	98,749	25,415	18,614	23,373	19,586	9,923
Women	107,076	12,998	15,002	28,141	30,044	18,662
Age						
Aged 18 to 44	108,114	25,787	20,507	27,657	20,116	12,202
Aged 45 to 64	64,650	9,797	10,034	16,581	17,075	9,801
Aged 65 to 74	17,809	1,628	1,811	4,142	6,595	3,239
Aged 75 or older	15,252	1,201	1,264	3,135	5,843	3,343
Race and Hispanic origin						
Asian	7,270	1,894	1,416	1,829	1,331	603
Black	23,499	4,443	3,777	6,118	5,713	2,807
Hispanic	22,691	7,416	3,998	4,439	4,016	2,456
Non-Hispanic white	149,584	24,102	23,953	38,644	37,858	22,250
Education						
Less than high school	28,248	6,342	3,614	5,616	7,401	4,575
High school graduate	52,556	9,744	8,272	12,678	13,159	7,652
Some college	48,091	8,199	7,941	12,460	11,499	7,226
College graduate	47,197	6,454	8,392	13,201	12,420	6,121
Household income						
Less than $20,000	37,369	8,381	4,809	7,638	9,090	6,776
$20,000 to $34,999	29,671	6,454	4,654	6,558	7,345	4,330
$35,000 to $54,999	31,814	6,266	5,518	7,882	7,492	4,386
$55,000 to $74,999	23,984	4,289	4,223	6,625	5,824	2,852
$75,000 or more	41,572	5,788	7,508	12,428	10,492	4,946
Health insurance coverage among adults under age 65						
Private	124,786	20,206	23,145	35,161	29,235	15,139
Medicaid	11,165	1,333	1,092	2,242	2,832	3,369
Other	4,541	598	468	919	1,300	1,190
Uninsured	31,374	13,229	5,695	5,760	3,696	2,248

Note: Office visits include visits to physicians' offices and clinics but exclude overnight hospitalizations, visits to hospital emergency rooms, home visits, and telephone calls. Numbers by race and Hispanic origin will not sum to total because not all races are shown and Hispanics may be of any race.

Source: National Center for Health Statistics, Summary Health Statistics for U.S. Adults: National Health Interview Survey, 2002, Series 10, No. 222, 2004; Internet site http://www.cdc.gov/nchs/nhis.htm

Table 10.4 Percent Distribution of Office Visits to Health Care Professionals by Selected Characteristics, 2002

(percent distribution of people aged 18 or older by number of office visits to health care professionals in past twelve months, by selected characteristics, 2002)

| | total | number of office visits in past twelve months | | | | |
		none	one	two to three	four to nine	ten or more
Total adults	100.0%	18.7%	16.3%	25.0%	24.1%	13.9%
Sex						
Men	100.0	25.7	18.8	23.7	19.8	10.0
Women	100.0	12.1	14.0	26.3	28.1	17.4
Age						
Aged 18 to 44	100.0	23.9	19.0	25.6	18.6	11.3
Aged 45 to 64	100.0	15.2	15.5	25.6	26.4	15.2
Aged 65 to 74	100.0	9.1	10.2	23.3	37.0	18.2
Aged 75 or older	100.0	7.9	8.3	20.6	38.3	21.9
Race and Hispanic origin						
Asian	100.0	26.1	19.5	25.2	18.3	8.3
Black	100.0	18.9	16.1	26.0	24.3	11.9
Hispanic	100.0	32.7	17.6	19.6	17.7	10.8
Non-Hispanic white	100.0	16.1	16.0	25.8	25.3	14.9
Education						
Less than high school	100.0	22.5	12.8	19.9	26.2	16.2
High school graduate	100.0	18.5	15.7	24.1	25.0	14.6
Some college	100.0	17.0	16.5	25.9	23.9	15.0
College graduate	100.0	13.7	17.8	28.0	26.3	13.0
Household income						
Less than $20,000	100.0	22.4	12.9	20.4	24.3	18.1
$20,000 to $34,999	100.0	21.8	15.7	22.1	24.8	14.6
$35,000 to $54,999	100.0	19.7	17.3	24.8	23.5	13.8
$55,000 to $74,999	100.0	17.9	17.6	27.6	24.3	11.9
$75,000 or more	100.0	13.9	18.1	29.9	25.2	11.9
Health insurance coverage among adults under age 65						
Private	100.0	16.2	18.5	28.2	23.4	12.1
Medicaid	100.0	11.9	9.8	20.1	25.4	30.2
Other	100.0	13.2	10.3	20.2	28.6	26.2
Uninsured	100.0	42.2	18.2	18.4	11.8	7.2

Note: Office visits include visits to physicians' offices and clinics but exclude overnight hospitalizations, visits to hospital emergency rooms, home visits, and telephone calls. Numbers by race and Hispanic origin will not sum to total because not all races are shown and Hispanics may be of any race.
Source: National Center for Health Statistics, Summary Health Statistics for U.S. Adults: National Health Interview Survey, 2002, Series 10, No. 222, 2004; Internet site http://www.cdc.gov/nchs/nhis.htm

Table 10.5 Length of Time Since Last Office Visit to a Health Care Professional by Selected Characteristics, 2002

(total number of people aged 18 or older and distribution by length of time since last office visit to a health care professional, by selected characteristics, 2002; numbers in thousands)

| | total | time since last office visit | | | | | |
		six months or less	six months but less than one year	more than one year but less than two years	more than two years but less than five years	more than five years	never
Total adults	205,825	140,382	28,198	16,381	10,396	5,286	2,632
Sex							
Men	98,749	59,212	14,539	10,522	7,504	3,913	1,613
Women	107,076	81,169	13,660	5,858	2,892	1,373	1,019
Age							
Aged 18 to 44	108,114	65,721	17,504	11,236	7,295	3,200	1,784
Aged 45 to 64	64,650	46,683	8,229	4,267	2,526	1,558	620
Aged 65 to 74	17,809	14,904	1,441	495	336	341	108
Aged 75 or older	15,252	13,074	1,024	382	239	188	121
Race and Hispanic origin							
Asian	7,270	4,296	1,026	868	506	267	148
Black	23,499	15,703	3,464	1,700	1,117	613	374
Hispanic	22,691	12,183	3,461	2,394	1,875	1,344	1,138
Non-Hispanic white	149,584	106,407	19,751	11,183	6,758	2,975	957
Education							
Less than high school	28,248	19,031	3,070	2,122	1,617	1,360	734
High school graduate	52,556	35,986	7,310	3,949	2,581	1,565	530
Some college	48,091	33,574	6,640	3,697	2,366	1,065	396
College graduate	47,197	34,043	6,597	3,278	1,831	565	360
Household income							
Less than $20,000	37,369	25,616	4,040	2,891	2,195	1,500	731
$20,000 to $34,999	29,671	19,704	3,889	2,581	1,829	965	542
$35,000 to $54,999	31,814	21,477	4,617	2,472	1,926	789	333
$55,000 to $74,999	23,984	16,366	3,622	1,946	1,125	509	305
$75,000 or more	41,572	29,658	6,048	3,440	1,252	538	301
Health insurance coverage among adults under age 65							
Private	124,786	86,176	19,073	9,974	5,206	1,953	1,147
Medicaid	11,165	8,771	1,150	594	211	104	172
Other	4,541	3,621	388	303	123	57	22
Uninsured	31,374	13,408	5,004	4,531	4,231	2,600	1,061

Note: Office visits include visits to physicians' offices and clinics but exclude overnight hospitalizations, visits to hospital emergency rooms, home visits, and telephone calls. Numbers by race and Hispanic origin will not sum to total because not all races are shown and Hispanics may be of any race.
Source: National Center for Health Statistics, Summary Health Statistics for U.S. Adults: National Health Interview Survey, 2002, *Series 10, No. 222, 2004; Internet site http://www.cdc.gov/nchs/nhis.htm*

Table 10.6 Percent Distribution by Length of Time Since Last Office Visit to a Health Care Professional, 2002

(percent distribution of people aged 18 or older by length of time since last office visit to a health care professional, by selected characteristics, 2002)

		time since last office visit					
	total	six months or less	more than six months but less than one year	more than one year but less than two years	more than two years but less than five years	more than five years	never
Total adults	100.0%	68.2%	13.7%	8.0%	5.1%	2.6%	1.3%
Sex							
Men	100.0	60.0	14.7	10.7	7.6	4.0	1.6
Women	100.0	75.8	12.8	5.5	2.7	1.3	1.0
Age							
Aged 18 to 44	100.0	60.8	16.2	10.4	6.7	3.0	1.7
Aged 45 to 64	100.0	72.2	12.7	6.6	3.9	2.4	1.0
Aged 65 to 74	100.0	83.7	8.1	2.8	1.9	1.9	0.6
Aged 75 or older	100.0	85.7	6.7	2.5	1.6	1.2	0.8
Race and Hispanic origin							
Asian	100.0	59.1	14.1	11.9	7.0	3.7	2.0
Black	100.0	66.8	14.7	7.2	4.8	2.6	1.6
Hispanic	100.0	53.7	15.3	10.6	8.3	5.9	5.0
Non-Hispanic white	100.0	71.1	13.2	7.5	4.5	2.0	0.6
Education							
Less than high school	100.0	67.4	10.9	7.5	5.7	4.8	2.6
High school graduate	100.0	68.5	13.9	7.5	4.9	3.0	1.0
Some college	100.0	69.8	13.8	7.7	4.9	2.2	0.8
College graduate	100.0	72.1	14.0	6.9	3.9	1.2	0.8
Household income							
Less than $20,000	100.0	68.5	10.8	7.7	5.9	4.0	2.0
$20,000 to $34,999	100.0	66.4	13.1	8.7	6.2	3.3	1.8
$35,000 to $54,999	100.0	67.5	14.5	7.8	6.1	2.5	1.0
$55,000 to $74,999	100.0	68.2	15.1	8.1	4.7	2.1	1.3
$75,000 or more	100.0	71.3	14.5	8.3	3.0	1.3	0.7
Health insurance coverage among adults under age 65							
Private	100.0	69.1	15.3	8.0	4.2	1.6	0.9
Medicaid	100.0	78.6	10.3	5.3	1.9	0.9	1.5
Other	100.0	79.7	8.5	6.7	2.7	1.3	0.5
Uninsured	100.0	42.7	15.9	14.4	13.5	8.3	3.4

Note: Office visits include visits to physicians' offices and clinics but exclude overnight hospitalizations, visits to hospital emergency rooms, home visits, and telephone calls. Numbers by race and Hispanic origin will not sum to total because not all races are shown and Hispanics may be of any race.
Source: National Center for Health Statistics, Summary Health Statistics for U.S. Adults: National Health Interview Survey, 2002, Series 10, No. 222, 2004; Internet site http://www.cdc.gov/nchs/nhis.htm

Teenagers Are Least Likely to Visit a Doctor Frequently

Younger children make more well visits—and have more colds and other illnesses.

Of the 73 million children under age 18 in the United States in 2002, more than 7 million had no health insurance. The lack of health insurance reduces the likelihood that children will get the health care they need, particularly "well visits," which are important for diagnosing conditions with no obvious symptoms. Hispanic children are twice as likely as the average child to have no health insurance (21 versus 10 percent).

Children aged 12 to 17 are more likely than those under age 12 to have no usual place for health care, perhaps because parents are more relaxed about the health of teenagers. Teens are also less likely to get the ear infections and respiratory illnesses that drive younger children to the doctor.

Most children see a doctor regularly. Seventy-four percent last visited a health care provider within the past six months. As children age, their office visits become less frequent. Among children under age 5, fully 87 percent had been to a health care provider within the past six months. Only 68 percent of children aged 12 to 17 had made an office visit that recently.

■ Teenagers may not need to see a physician as often as toddlers, but many would benefit from getting a checkup at least once a year.

One in ten children does not have health insurance

(percent of children with selected problems in accessing health care, 2002)

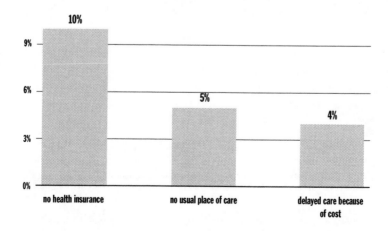

Table 10.7 Health Care Access for Children under Age 18 by Selected Characteristics, 2002

(total number of people under age 18, and number with health care access problems, by selected characteristics, 2002; numbers in thousands)

	total	no health insurance	unmet medical need	delayed care because of cost	no usual place of care	two or more visits to emergency room in past 12 months
Total children	**72,970**	**7,378**	**1,595**	**2,525**	**3,888**	**5,395**
Sex						
Female	35,659	3,597	819	1,258	1,891	2,578
Male	37,311	3,781	776	1,267	1,997	2,817
Age						
Aged 0 to 4	19,827	1,880	344	679	726	2,132
Aged 5 to 11	28,780	2,825	646	964	1,507	1,834
Aged 12 to 17	24,363	2,673	605	881	1,656	1,429
Race and Hispanic origin						
Asian	2,554	322	60	63	309	91
Black	10,578	1,021	289	400	564	1,159
Hispanic	12,563	2,659	353	545	1,446	1,003
Non-Hispanic white	45,253	3,078	824	1,386	1,467	2,858
Family structure						
Mother and father	52,588	4,860	795	1,491	2,344	3,233
Mother, no father	16,175	1,899	731	934	1,079	1,838
Father, no mother	2,124	274	39	60	208	121
Neither mother nor father	2,081	345	29	39	258	202
Parent's education						
Less than high school diploma	9,438	2,006	366	399	1,108	991
High school diploma	16,411	1,944	419	679	940	1,433
More than high school	44,560	2,930	773	1,395	1,542	2,750
Household income						
Less than $20,000	12,299	1,763	519	626	1,015	1,677
$20,000 to $34,999	10,174	1,678	462	687	805	944
$35,000 to $54,999	11,667	1,317	239	467	563	721
$55,000 to $74,999	9,565	531	94	172	385	546
$75,000 or more	16,223	444	86	200	288	813
Health insurance status						
Private	46,640	–	461	919	1,114	2,583
Medicaid/other public	17,243	–	405	592	763	2,176
Other	1,464	–	9	18	48	82
Uninsured	7,378	7,378	692	982	1,937	521

Note: Mother and father includes biological, adoptive, step, in-law, and foster relationships. Legal guardians are classified as neither mother nor father. Parent's education is the education level of the parent with the higher level of education. Unmet medical need is defined as being unable to afford necessary medical care in the past twelve months. Delayed care is defined as delaying medical care because of cost. (–) means not applicable.
Source: National Center for Health Statistics, Summary Health Statistics for U.S. Children: National Health Interview Survey, *2002, Series 10, No. 221, 2004; Internet site http://www.cdc.gov/nchs/nhis.htm*

Table 10.8 Percent of Children under Age 18 with Problems Accessing Health Care, 2002

(percent of people under age 18 with problems accessing health care, by selected characteristics, 2002)

	total	no health insurance	unmet medical need	delayed care because of cost	no usual place of care	two or more visits to emergency room in past 12 months
Total children	**100.0%**	**10.1%**	**2.2%**	**3.5%**	**5.3%**	**7.4%**
Sex						
Female	100.0	10.1	2.3	3.5	5.3	7.2
Male	100.0	10.1	2.1	3.4	5.4	7.6
Age						
Aged 0 to 4	100.0	9.5	1.7	3.4	3.7	10.8
Aged 5 to 11	100.0	9.8	2.2	3.3	5.2	6.4
Aged 12 to 17	100.0	11.0	2.5	3.6	6.8	5.9
Race and Hispanic origin						
Asian	100.0	12.6	2.3	2.5	12.1	3.6
Black	100.0	9.7	2.7	3.8	5.3	11.0
Hispanic	100.0	21.2	2.8	4.3	11.5	8.0
Non-Hispanic white	100.0	6.8	1.8	3.1	3.2	6.3
Family structure						
Mother and father	100.0	9.2	1.5	2.8	4.5	6.1
Mother, no father	100.0	11.7	4.5	5.8	6.7	11.4
Father, no mother	100.0	12.9	1.8	2.8	9.8	5.7
Neither mother nor father	100.0	16.6	1.4	1.9	12.4	9.7
Parent's education						
Less than high school diploma	100.0	21.3	3.9	4.2	11.7	10.5
High school diploma	100.0	11.8	2.6	4.1	5.7	8.7
More than high school	100.0	6.6	1.7	3.1	3.5	6.2
Household income						
Less than $20,000	100.0	14.3	4.2	5.1	8.3	13.6
$20,000 to $34,999	100.0	16.5	4.5	6.8	7.9	9.3
$35,000 to $54,999	100.0	11.3	2.0	4.0	4.8	6.2
$55,000 to $74,999	100.0	5.6	1.0	1.8	4.0	5.7
$75,000 or more	100.0	2.7	0.5	1.2	1.8	5.0
Health insurance status						
Private	100.0	–	1.0	2.0	2.4	5.5
Medicaid/other public	100.0	–	2.3	3.4	4.4	12.6
Other	100.0	–	0.6	1.2	3.3	5.6
Uninsured	100.0	100.0	9.4	13.3	26.3	7.1

Note: Mother and father includes biological, adoptive, step, in-law, and foster relationships. Legal guardians are classified as neither mother nor father. Parent's education is the education level of the parent with the higher level of education. Unmet medical need is defined as being unable to afford necessary medical care in the past twelve months. Delayed care is defined as delaying medical care because of cost. (–) means not applicable.
Source: National Center for Health Statistics, Summary Health Statistics for U.S. Children: National Health Interview Survey, 2002, *Series 10, No. 221, 2004; Internet site http://www.cdc.gov/nchs/nhis.htm*

Table 10.9 Length of Time Since Child's Last Office Visit to a Health Care Professional By Selected Characteristics, 2002

(total number of people under age 18 and distribution by length of time since last office visit to a health care professional, by selected characteristics, 2002; numbers in thousands)

	total	six months or less	more than six months but less than one year	more than one year but less than two years	more than two years but less than five years	more than five years
Total children	72,970	54,345	10,611	4,408	1,144	1,681
Sex						
Female	35,659	26,494	5,257	2,150	596	770
Male	37,311	27,851	5,354	2,257	548	911
Age						
Aged 0 to 4	19,827	17,182	1,646	411	35	403
Aged 5 to 11	28,780	20,658	4,673	2,044	478	625
Aged 12 to 17	24,363	16,505	4,292	1,952	632	652
Race and Hispanic origin						
Asian	2,554	1,689	432	213	52	82
Black	10,578	7,696	1,734	612	187	185
Hispanic	12,563	8,440	1,857	940	305	851
Non-Hispanic white	45,253	34,920	6,317	2,562	580	535
Family structure						
Mother and father	52,588	39,455	7,549	3,127	808	1,189
Mother, no father	16,175	11,970	2,440	868	259	392
Father, no mother	2,124	1,443	321	241	52	32
Neither mother nor father	2,081	1,475	301	173	26	68
Parent's education						
Less than high school diploma	9,438	6,390	1,241	719	284	646
High school diploma	16,411	11,720	2,570	1,177	291	437
More than high school	44,560	34,473	6,464	2,305	531	515
Household income						
Less than $20,000	12,299	9,120	1,590	789	216	421
$20,000 to $34,999	10,174	7,211	1,625	656	202	375
$35,000 to $54,999	11,667	8,601	1,771	776	208	256
$55,000 to $74,999	9,565	7,043	1,602	532	124	216
$75,000 or more	16,223	12,844	2,268	786	87	140
Health insurance status						
Private	46,640	35,709	6,955	2,457	493	681
Medicaid/other public	17,243	13,556	2,039	820	181	374
Other	1,464	1,123	161	122	24	15
Uninsured	7,378	3,805	1,398	997	439	601

Note: Mother and father can include biological, adoptive, step, in-law, or foster relationships. Legal guardians are classified as neither mother nor father. Parent's education is the education level of the parent with the higher level of education.
Source: National Center for Health Statistics, Summary Health Statistics for U.S. Children: National Health Interview Survey, 2002, Series 10, No. 221, 2004; Internet site http://www.cdc.gov/nchs/nhis.htm

Table 10.10 Percent Distribution of Children by Length of Time Since Child's Last Office Visit to a Health Care Professional, 2002

(percent distribution of people under age 18 by length of time since last office visit to a health care professional, by selected characteristics, 2002)

		time since last office visit				
	total	six months or less	more than six months but less than one year	more than one year but less than two years	more than two years but less than five years	more than five years
Total children	100.0%	74.5%	14.5%	6.0%	1.6%	2.3%
Sex						
Female	100.0	74.3	14.7	6.0	1.7	2.2
Male	100.0	74.6	14.3	6.0	1.5	2.4
Age						
Aged 0 to 4	100.0	86.7	8.3	2.1	0.2	2.0
Aged 5 to 11	100.0	71.8	16.2	7.1	1.7	2.2
Aged 12 to 17	100.0	67.7	17.6	8.0	2.6	2.7
Race and Hispanic origin						
Asian	100.0	66.1	16.9	8.3	2.0	3.2
Black	100.0	72.8	16.4	5.8	1.8	1.7
Hispanic	100.0	67.2	14.8	7.5	2.4	6.8
Non-Hispanic white	100.0	77.2	14.0	5.7	1.3	1.2
Family structure						
Mother and father	100.0	75.0	14.4	5.9	1.5	2.3
Mother, no father	100.0	74.0	15.1	5.4	1.6	2.4
Father, no mother	100.0	67.9	15.1	11.3	2.4	1.5
Neither mother nor father	100.0	70.9	14.5	8.3	1.2	3.3
Parent's education						
Less than high school diploma	100.0	67.7	13.1	7.6	3.0	6.8
High school diploma	100.0	71.4	15.7	7.2	1.8	2.7
More than high school	100.0	77.4	14.5	5.2	1.2	1.2
Household income						
Less than $20,000	100.0	74.2	12.9	6.4	1.8	3.4
$20,000 to $34,999	100.0	70.9	16.0	6.4	2.0	3.7
$35,000 to $54,999	100.0	73.7	15.2	6.7	1.8	2.2
$55,000 to $74,999	100.0	73.6	16.7	5.6	1.3	2.3
$75,000 or more	100.0	79.2	14.0	4.8	0.5	0.9
Health insurance status						
Private	100.0	76.6	14.9	5.3	1.1	1.5
Medicaid/other public	100.0	78.6	11.8	4.8	1.0	2.2
Other	100.0	76.7	11.0	8.3	1.6	1.0
Uninsured	100.0	51.6	18.9	13.5	6.0	8.1

Note: Mother and father can include biological, adoptive, step, in-law, or foster relationships. Legal guardians are classified as neither mother nor father. Parent's education is the education level of the parent with the higher level of education.
Source: National Center for Health Statistics, Summary Health Statistics for U.S. Children: National Health Interview Survey, 2002, Series 10, No. 221, 2004; Internet site http://www.cdc.gov/nchs/nhis.htm

Most People Think Highly of Their Physician

The majority trusts their doctor's judgment about medical care.

Americans have lofty opinions of physicians, in spite of the public's discontent with the overall health care system. Asked to agree or disagree with the statement, "I trust my doctor's judgments about my medical care," 89 percent agree. The share agreeing "strongly" was a sizable 42 percent. Relatively few worry that their doctor will put profits before patients, with 84 percent saying they agree that their doctor puts their medical needs above other considerations.

A slightly smaller share (78 percent) feel their physician is a "real expert" when it comes to medical problems like theirs. Seventy-one percent trust their doctor to tell them if a mistake is made, and 68 percent disagree with the statement, "I doubt my doctor really cares about me as a person."

■ While most people have confidence in their physician, some have doubts.

Trust is high on a number of issues

(percent of people aged 18 or older who agree with selected statements, 2002)

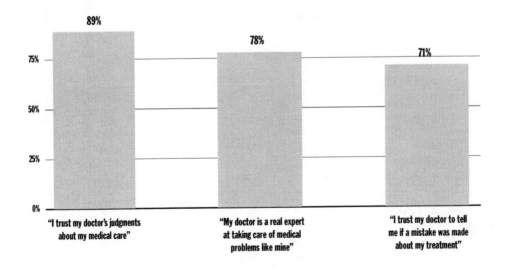

Table 10.11 Attitudes toward Doctors, 2002

"As you read each of the following statements, please think about the medical care you are now receiving. If you have not received any medical care recently, circle the answer based on what you would expect if you had to seek care today."

(number of respondents aged 18 or older and percent distribution by response, 2002)

	number of respondents	percent distribution
"I doubt my doctor really cares about me as a person."		
TOTAL RESPONDENTS	1,393	100.0%
Strongly agree	91	6.5
Agree somewhat	190	13.6
Neither agree nor disagree	132	9.5
Disagree somewhat	378	27.1
Strongly disagree	571	41.0
Don't know	22	1.6
No answer	9	0.6
"I trust my doctor's judgments about my medical care."		
TOTAL RESPONDENTS	1,393	100.0
Strongly agree	589	42.3
Agree somewhat	645	46.3
Neither agree nor disagree	51	3.7
Disagree somewhat	61	4.4
Strongly disagree	19	1.4
Don't know	20	1.4
No answer	8	0.6
"I trust my doctor to put my medical needs above all other considerations when treating my medical problems."		
TOTAL RESPONDENTS	1,393	100.0
Strongly agree	597	42.9
Agree somewhat	571	41.0
Neither agree nor disagree	76	5.5
Disagree somewhat	95	6.8
Strongly disagree	25	1.8
Don't know	21	1.5
No answer	8	0.6

(continued)

	number of respondents	percent distribution
"My doctor is a real expert in taking care of medical problems like mine."		
TOTAL RESPONDENTS	**1,393**	**100.0%**
Strongly agree	503	36.1
Agree somewhat	585	42.0
Neither agree nor disagree	149	10.7
Disagree somewhat	93	6.7
Strongly disagree	17	1.2
Don't know	35	2.5
No answer	11	0.8
"I trust my doctor to tell me if a mistake was made about my treatment."		
TOTAL RESPONDENTS	**1,393**	**100.0**
Strongly agree	516	37.0
Agree somewhat	476	34.2
Neither agree nor disagree	108	7.8
Disagree somewhat	148	10.6
Strongly disagree	111	8.0
Don't know	26	1.9
No answer	8	0.6

Source: General Social Survey, National Opinion Research Center, University of Chicago

Women Seek Health Care More Often than Men

Men average one fewer physician visit per year.

On average, Americans made 3.1 visits to a doctor's office in 2002. Visits are least frequent among people aged 15 to 24 (who are generally in good health), rising with age to a peak of 7.2 visits per year among people aged 75 or older.

Women average 3.6 doctor visits a year compared with an average of 2.6 visits for men. Health care visits are about the same for boys and girls under age 15, but in all other age groups women go to the doctor more often than men. Behind this difference is the fact that women are more willing than men to seek health care treatment.

Whites visit doctors more often than blacks, regardless of age. The lower visit rate of blacks is a reflection of the fact that they are less likely to be covered by private health insurance, which reduces access to health care.

■ The growing number of Americans without health insurance could lower the average number of office visits people make since the uninsured tend to forego medical care until it becomes absolutely necessary.

Older women visit doctors the most

(average number of physician office visits per person per year, by sex and age, 2002)

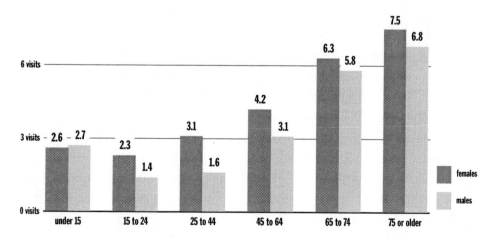

Table 10.12 Physician Office Visits by Sex and Age, 2002

(total number, percent distribution, and number of physician office visits per person per year, by sex and age, 2002; numbers in thousands)

	total	percent distribution	average number of visits per year
Total visits	**889,980**	**100.0%**	**3.1**
Under age 15	159,235	17.9	2.6
Aged 15 to 24	71,865	8.1	1.8
Aged 25 to 44	192,359	21.6	2.3
Aged 45 to 64	242,142	27.2	3.7
Aged 65 to 74	109,331	12.3	6.1
Aged 75 or older	115,049	12.9	7.2
Visits by females	**529,075**	**59.4**	**3.6**
Under age 15	76,382	8.6	2.6
Aged 15 to 24	44,909	5.0	2.3
Aged 25 to 44	128,743	14.5	3.1
Aged 45 to 64	144,205	16.2	4.2
Aged 65 to 74	61,819	6.9	6.3
Aged 75 or older	73,017	8.2	7.5
Visits by males	**360,905**	**40.6**	**2.6**
Under age 15	82,853	9.3	2.7
Aged 15 to 24	26,958	3.0	1.4
Aged 25 to 44	63,616	7.1	1.6
Aged 45 to 64	97,937	11.0	3.1
Aged 65 to 74	47,512	5.3	5.8
Aged 75 or older	42,032	4.7	6.8

Source: National Center for Health Statistics, National Ambulatory Medical Care Survey: 2002 Summary, *Advance Data No. 346, 2004; Internet site http://www.cdc.gov/nchs/about/major/ahcd/adata.htm*

Table 10.13 Physician Office Visits by Race and Age, 2002

(total number, percent distribution, and number of physician office visits per person per year, by race and age, 2002; numbers in thousands)

	total	percent distribution	average number of visits per year
Total visits	**889,980**	**100.0%**	**3.1**
Under age 15	159,235	17.9	2.6
Aged 15 to 24	71,865	8.1	1.8
Aged 25 to 44	192,359	21.6	2.3
Aged 45 to 64	242,142	27.2	3.7
Aged 65 to 74	109,331	12.3	6.1
Aged 75 or older	115,049	12.9	7.2
Visits by blacks	**89,455**	**10.1**	**2.5**
Under age 15	19,867	2.2	2.1
Aged 15 to 24	8,071	0.9	1.4
Aged 25 to 44	18,750	2.1	1.8
Aged 45 to 64	22,496	2.5	3.2
Aged 65 to 74	10,733	1.2	6.6
Aged 75 or older	9,538	1.1	8.1
Visits by whites	**766,096**	**86.1**	**3.3**
Under age 15	131,023	14.7	2.8
Aged 15 to 24	61,012	6.9	2.0
Aged 25 to 44	164,890	18.5	2.5
Aged 45 to 64	211,162	23.7	3.8
Aged 65 to 74	95,465	10.7	6.1
Aged 75 or older	102,544	11.5	7.2
American Indians	**2,237**	**0.3**	**0.8**
Asians	**26,341**	**3.0**	**2.3**
Native Hawaiians	**3,430**	**0.4**	**7.2**
Multiple races	**2,421**	**0.3**	**0.6**

Source: National Center for Health Statistics, National Ambulatory Medical Care Survey: 2002 Summary, *Advance Data No. 346, 2004; Internet site http://www.cdc.gov/nchs/about/major/ahcd/adata.htm*

Preventive Care Visits Are Most Common among the Young

Only 16 percent of the population made a preventive care visit in the past year.

Preventive care office visits may seem like a waste of time and money to many people, but checkups are important in identifying illnesses that present few, if any symptoms. Well visits are the norm for children, which explains why people under age 15 accounted for 30 percent of preventive care visits in 2002.

Acute health problems, such as colds, flu, and injuries sustained in accidents, bring the largest share of people to the doctor (36 percent). Ranking second are routine visits for chronic health problems (30 percent). Preventive care visits rank third, at 16 percent. Nine percent of visits are due to flare-ups of chronic conditions, while 5 percent are pre- or postsurgery visits.

An examination of the specific diagnoses made by doctors reveals the many different reasons patients come in the door. Hypertension accounts for the largest single primary diagnosis group, but only 5 percent of all office visits in 2002 were for hypertension.

■ Annual physical exams for all could improve the health of the nation as a whole.

Illnesses and injuries account for the largest share of doctor visits

(percent distribution of physician office visits by major reason for visit, 2002)

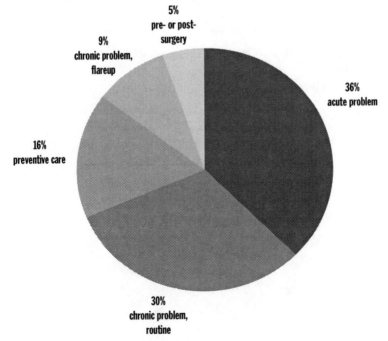

5%
pre- or post-
surgery

9%
chronic problem,
flareup

36%
acute problem

16%
preventive care

30%
chronic problem,
routine

Table 10.14 Physician Office Visits for Preventive Care by Sex, Age, and Race, 2002

(total number and percent distribution of physician office visits for preventive care, and number per person per year, by sex, age, race, and primary expected source of payment, 2002; numbers in thousands)

	total	percent distribution	average number of visits per year
Total preventive care visits	**144,851**	**100.0%**	**0.5**
Under age 15	43,557	30.1	0.7
Aged 15 to 24	15,872	11.0	0.4
Aged 25 to 44	39,865	27.5	0.5
Aged 45 to 64	27,316	18.9	0.4
Aged 65 to 74	10,642	7.3	0.6
Aged 75 or older	7,598	5.2	0.5
Total females	**97,008**	**67.0**	**0.7**
Under age 15	21,106	14.6	0.7
Aged 15 to 24	12,606	8.7	0.6
Aged 25 to 44	34,003	23.5	0.8
Aged 45 to 64	18,471	12.8	0.5
Aged 65 to 74	5,853	4.0	0.6
Aged 75 or older	4,968	3.4	0.5
Total males	**47,843**	**33.0**	**0.3**
Under age 15	22,451	15.5	0.7
Aged 15 to 24	3,266	2.3	0.2
Aged 25 to 44	5,862	4.0	0.1
Aged 45 to 64	8,844	6.1	0.3
Aged 65 to 74	4,789	3.3	0.6
Aged 75 or older	2,630	1.8	0.4
Race			
Black	17,502	12.1	0.5
White	120,074	82.9	0.5
Other	7,275	5.0	0.4
Primary expected source of payment			
Private insurance	97,348	67.2	0.5
Medicaid/SCHIP	17,872	12.3	0.5
Medicare	14,712	10.2	0.4
Self pay/charity/no charge	5,834	4.0	0.1

Source: National Center for Health Statistics, National Ambulatory Medical Care Survey: 2002 Summary, *Advance Data No. 346, 2004; Internet site http://www.cdc.gov/nchs/about/major/ahcd/adata.htm*

Table 10.15 Physician Office Visits by Major Reason for Visit, 2002

(number and percent distribution of physician office visits by sex, age, race, and major reason for visit, 2002; numbers in thousands)

	total	acute problem	chronic problem, routine	chronic problem, flare-up	pre- or post-surgery	preventive care
Total visits	**889,980**	**323,541**	**264,452**	**76,383**	**46,153**	**144,851**
Sex						
Female	529,075	185,407	153,009	46,087	27,177	97,008
Male	360,905	138,134	111,443	30,296	18,976	47,843
Age						
Under age 15	159,235	82,771	17,133	7,758	2,552	43,557
Aged 15 to 24	71,865	32,191	13,004	4,906	2,957	15,872
Aged 25 to 44	192,359	71,598	46,366	16,383	10,606	39,865
Aged 45 to 64	242,142	77,842	88,022	25,908	13,211	27,316
Aged 65 to 74	109,331	27,665	47,987	10,702	7,636	10,642
Aged 75 or older	115,049	31,474	51,841	10,726	9,191	7,598
Race						
Black	89,455	31,165	27,961	5,358	3,763	17,502
White	766,096	280,834	226,296	68,513	41,432	120,074
Other	34,429	11,542	10,194	2,512	958	7,275
Percent distribution by reason						
Total visits	**100.0%**	**36.4%**	**29.7%**	**8.6%**	**5.2%**	**16.3%**
Sex						
Female	100.0	35.0	28.9	8.7	5.1	18.3
Male	100.0	38.3	30.9	8.4	5.3	13.3
Age						
Under age 15	100.0	52.0	10.8	4.9	1.6	27.4
Aged 15 to 24	100.0	44.8	18.1	6.8	4.1	22.1
Aged 25 to 44	100.0	37.2	24.1	8.5	5.5	20.7
Aged 45 to 64	100.0	32.1	36.4	10.7	5.5	11.3
Aged 65 to 74	100.0	25.3	43.9	9.8	7.0	9.7
Aged 75 or older	100.0	27.4	45.1	9.3	8.0	6.6
Race						
Black	100.0	34.8	31.3	6.0	4.2	19.6
White	100.0	36.7	29.5	8.9	5.4	15.7
Other	100.0	33.5	29.6	7.3	2.8	21.1

Note: Numbers will not add to total because blank and unknown are not shown.
Source: National Center for Health Statistics, National Ambulatory Medical Care Survey: 2002 Summary, Advance Data No. 346, 2004; Internet site http://www.cdc.gov/nchs/about/major/ahcd/adata.htm

Table 10.16 Physician Office Visits by Detailed Reason for Visit, 2002

(number and percent distribution of physician office visits by the twenty principal reasons for visit most frequently mentioned by patients, 2002; numbers in thousands)

	number	percent distribution
Total visits	**889,980**	**100.0%**
General medical exam	64,726	7.3
Progress visit, not otherwise specified	40,983	4.6
Cough	28,469	3.2
Postoperative visit	22,083	2.5
Routine prenatal exam	19,582	2.2
Symptoms referable to throat	18,515	2.1
Hypertension	17,195	1.9
Knee symptoms	14,803	1.7
Well baby exam	14,293	1.6
Medication	14,076	1.6
Stomach pain, cramps, and spasms	13,547	1.5
Earache or ear infection	13,160	1.5
Back symptoms	12,902	1.4
Vision dysfunctions	12,897	1.4
Blood pressure test	12,630	1.4
Fever	12,258	1.4
Nasal congestion	12,149	1.4
Skin rash	11,887	1.3
Chest pain and related symptoms	11,189	1.3
Diabetes mellitus	11,189	1.3
All other reasons	511,446	57.5

Source: National Center for Health Statistics, National Ambulatory Medical Care Survey: 2002 Summary, *Advance Data No. 346, 2004; Internet site http://www.cdc.gov/nchs/about/major/ahcd/adata.htm*

Table 10.17 Physician Office Visits by Major Disease Category and Primary Diagnosis Group, 2002

(number and percent distribution of physician office visits by major disease category and primary diagnosis group, 2002; numbers in thousands)

	number	percent distribution
MAJOR DISEASE CATEGORY		
Total visits	**889,980**	**100.0%**
Infectious and parasitic diseases	24,431	2.7
Neoplasms	25,321	2.8
Endocrine, nutritional, metabolic diseases, and immunity disorders	52,672	5.9
Mental disorders	40,016	4.5
Diseases of the nervous system and sense organs	79,417	8.9
Diseases of the circulatory system	80,092	9.0
Diseases of the respiratory system	112,107	12.6
Diseases of the digestive system	30,132	3.4
Diseases of the genitourinary system	42,706	4.8
Diseases of the skin and subcutaneous tissue	42,743	4.8
Diseases of the musculoskeletal system and connective tissue	66,575	7.5
Symptoms, signs, and ill-defined conditions	55,674	6.3
Injuries and poisonings	53,143	6.0
Supplementary classification	146,162	16.4
All other diagnoses	15,787	1.8
Unknown	23,002	2.6
PRIMARY DIAGNOSIS GROUP		
Total visits	**889,980**	**100.0**
Essential hypertension	48,180	5.4
Routine infant or child health check	35,935	4.0
Acute upper respiratory infections, excl. pharyngitis	30,141	3.4
Diabetes mellitus	24,877	2.8
Arthropathies and related disorders	23,725	2.7
General medical examination	22,362	2.5
Spinal disorders	20,444	2.3
Rheumatism, excluding back	17,766	2.0
Normal pregnancy	17,585	2.0
Otitis media and eustachian tube disorders	16,702	1.9
Malignant neoplasms	15,651	1.8
Chronic sinusitis	14,197	1.6
Allergic rhinitis	14,101	1.6
Asthma	12,692	1.4
Gynecological examination	11,883	1.3
Disorder of lipoid metabolism	11,767	1.3
Heart disease, excluding ischemic	11,670	1.3
Ischemic heart disease	10,970	1.2
Acute pharyngitis	10,090	1.1
Follow-up exam	9,995	1.1
All other diagnoses	509,248	57.2

Source: National Center for Health Statistics, National Ambulatory Medical Care Survey: 2002 Summary, *Advance Data No. 346, 2004; Internet site http://www.cdc.gov/nchs/about/major/ahcd/adata.htm*

Nearly Half of Office Visits include a Blood Pressure Reading

Other tests and procedures are much less common.

The most common diagnostic test performed during a doctor visit is a blood pressure reading, taken during 48 percent of all visits. Laboratory tests and cultures of any kind are far less common. The most common laboratory test is a urinalysis, performed in 10 percent of office visits. The most common culture is a throat culture or rapid strep test, but fewer than 2 percent of office visits require this service. Only 11 percent of office visits require imaging of some type, primarily X-rays.

Overall, half of office visits are to a primary care provider, with the remainder at some type of specialist. Many of those seeing specialists were referred by another physician, but most were not.

Three-quarters of office visits are to self-employed physicians, while the remainder is to physicians employed by or contracting with a health care business. Fully 86 percent of visits are to practices owned by physicians either alone or in a group.

■ Basic procedures, such as blood pressure readings and blood tests, could be beneficial if performed more often on more patients.

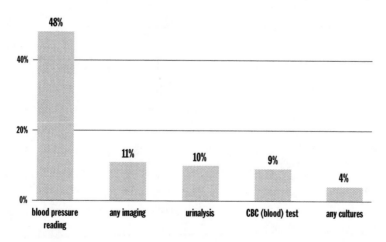

Fewer than 10 percent of office visits involve blood tests

(percent of physician office visits by selected services ordered or provided, 2002)

Table 10.18 Physician Office Visits by Services Provided, 2002

(number and percent of physician office visits by services ordered or provided, 2002; numbers in thousands)

	number	percent
Total visits	**889,980**	**100.0%**
None	126,218	14.2
Examinations		
General medical	442,299	49.7
Other	206,336	23.2
Diagnostic tests		
Blood pressure	428,011	48.1
EKG	31,790	3.6
Any scope procedure	18,882	2.1
Sigmoidoscopy/colonoscopy	9,772	1.1
Endoscopy	6,387	0.7
Cystoscopy	1,874	0.2
Tuberculin skin test	3,740	0.4
Audiometry	3,706	0.4
Fetal monitoring	2,839	0.3
Cardiac stress test	825	0.1
EEG	1,526	0.2
Laboratory tests		
CBC	78,118	8.8
Urinalysis	85,723	9.6
Pap test	46,260	5.2
Cholesterol	14,870	1.7
Hematocrit/hemoglobin	28,321	3.2
PSA	36,341	4.1
Cultures		
Any cultures	31,331	3.5
Throat/rapid strep test	15,036	1.7
Urine	6,066	0.7
Cervical/urethral	1,886	0.2
Stool	3,933	0.4
Imaging		
Any imaging	96,781	10.9
X-ray	53,458	6.0
Mammography	8,578	1.0
Ultrasound	17,560	2.0
Other imaging	32,298	3.6

Source: National Center for Health Statistics, National Ambulatory Medical Care Survey: 2002 Summary, Advance Data No. 346, 2004; Internet site http://www.cdc.gov/nchs/about/major/ahcd/adata.htm

Table 10.19 Physician Office Visits by Specialty and Referral Status, 2002

(number and percent distribution of physician office visits by specialty and referral status, 2002; numbers in thousands)

| | total | | visit to primary care provider | visit to nonprimary care provider | |
	number	percent		referred by another physician	not referred by another physician
Total visits	**889,980**	**100.0%**	**50.4%**	**13.7%**	**23.9%**
General and family practice	215,466	100.0	84.1	2.8	6.5
Internal medicine	156,692	100.0	82.3	2.9	6.0
Pediatrics	120,018	100.0	88.2	2.0	5.5
Obstetrics and gynecology	70,324	100.0	15.3	10.0	54.0
Ophthalmology	49,937	100.0	2.0	20.7	61.7
Orthopedic surgery	38,028	100.0	5.3	45.5	36.9
Dermatology	32,227	100.0	–	18.9	58.7
Cardiovascular diseases	21,659	100.0	–	15.9	64.6
Psychiatry	20,822	100.0	13.4	40.2	40.6
General surgery	17,133	100.0	8.1	41.0	40.2
Otolaryngology	17,080	100.0	–	39.8	42.4
Urology	17,000	100.0	3.8	50.9	33.9
Neurology	9,622	100.0	2.6	55.2	29.6
All other specialties	103,974	100.0	13.1	27.7	34.2

Note: Percentages will not sum to 100 because unknown is not shown; (–) means sample is too small to make a reliable estimate.

Source: National Center for Health Statistics, National Ambulatory Medical Care Survey: 2002 Summary, Advance Data No. 346, 2004; Internet site http://www.cdc.gov/nchs/about/major/ahcd/adata.htm

Table 10.20 Physician Office Visits by Practice Characteristics, 2002

(number and percent distribution of physician office visits by physician practice characteristics, 2002; numbers in thousands)

	number	percent distribution
Total visits	**889,980**	**100.0%**
Physician employment status		
Owner	664,121	74.6
Employee	189,987	21.3
Contractor	35,873	4.0
Ownership		
Physician/group	767,468	86.2
Other health care corporation	42,497	4.8
Other hospital	33,188	3.7
Medical/academic health center	19,794	2.2
HMO	14,885	1.7
Other	12,149	1.4
Practice size		
Solo	313,795	35.3
2 to 4	290,632	32.7
5 to 9	180,825	20.3
10 to 39	80,796	9.1
40 or more	19,505	2.2
Type of practice		
Single-specialty group	366,676	41.2
Multispecialty group	209,510	23.5
Solo	313,795	35.3
Office type		
Private practice	817,154	91.8
Clinic/urgicenter	46,380	5.2
Other	26,447	3.0

Note: Numbers may not add to total because blank is not shown.
Source: National Center for Health Statistics, National Ambulatory Medical Care Survey: 2002 Summary, *Advance Data No. 346, 2004; Internet site http://www.cdc.gov/nchs/about/major/ahcd/adata.htm*

Most Doctor Visits Last Less than Fifteen Minutes

Some specialists spend more time with patients, however.

On average, patients spend only 18.4 minutes with the doctor during an office visit. The median is just 14.7 minutes, meaning half the patients saw a physician for less than 14.7 minutes. In 26 percent of office visits, in fact, the physician spent 10 or fewer minutes with the patient.

Psychiatrists spend the most time with their patients. But the average length of a visit to a psychiatrist—35.2 minutes—suggests that the "50-minute hour" has gotten even shorter. Neurologists also spend more time than average with patients, as do cardiovascular specialists. Often these physicians treat patients with serious, ongoing illnesses that require careful examinations and a wider range of services.

Of the nearly 890 million physician office visits in 2002, 87 percent were by established patients, most of whom had been to the doctor's office three or more times before. Primary care physicians are more likely than surgical or medical specialists to see established patients. In the 64 percent majority of office visits, patients see the same doctor they saw in the past.

■ Although some office visits require little time, hurried examinations can lead to missed problems and a sense on the patient's part that he or she is not getting the best care.

Few patients spend more than half an hour with the doctor

(percent distribution of physician office visits by time spent with physician, 2002)

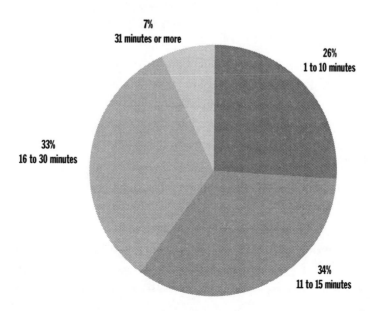

7%
31 minutes or more

26%
1 to 10 minutes

33%
16 to 30 minutes

34%
11 to 15 minutes

Table 10.21 Physician Office Visits by Continuity of Care, 2002

(number and percent distribution of physician office visits by continuity of care and specialty type, 2002; numbers in thousands)

	total	specialty type		
		primary care	surgical	medical
Total visits	**889,980**	**558,402**	**177,397**	**154,181**
Established patient	771,679	508,721	139,308	123,651
No prior visits	56,080	33,204	13,640	9,236
1 to 2 visits	245,048	151,762	57,049	36,237
3 to 5 visits	225,822	155,650	37,519	32,654
6 or more visits	201,998	136,529	24,844	40,625
Unknown	42,731	31,576	6,255	4,898
New patient	108,049	42,481	36,507	29,061
Unknown if patient previously seen	10,252	7,200	1,582	1,470
Do other physicians share care of patient?				
Yes	202,393	102,662	55,996	43,736
No	570,326	384,892	104,432	81,002
Unknown	117,261	70,848	16,969	29,444
Episode of care				
Initial visit for problem	273,910	189,092	47,167	37,651
Follow-up visit for problem	401,767	196,012	103,529	102,227
Unknown/blank	69,452	43,046	17,384	9,022
Not applicable (preventive care visit)	144,851	130,253	9,316	5,282
PERCENT DISTRIBUTION				
Total visits	**100.0%**	**100.0%**	**100.0%**	**100.0%**
Established patient	86.7	91.1	78.5	80.2
No prior visits	6.3	5.9	7.7	6.0
1 to 2 visits	27.5	27.2	32.2	23.5
3 to 5 visits	25.4	27.9	21.1	21.2
6 or more visits	22.7	24.4	14.0	26.3
Unknown	4.8	5.7	3.5	3.2
New patient	12.1	7.6	20.6	18.8
Unknown if patient previously seen	1.2	1.3	0.9	1.0
Do other physicians share care of patient?				
Yes	22.7	18.4	31.6	28.4
No	64.1	68.9	58.9	52.5
Unknown	13.2	12.7	9.6	19.1
Episode of care				
Initial visit for problem	30.8	33.9	26.6	24.4
Follow-up visit for problem	45.1	35.1	58.4	66.3
Unknown/blank	7.8	7.7	9.8	5.9
Not applicable (preventive care visit)	16.3	23.3	5.3	3.4

Source: National Center for Health Statistics, National Ambulatory Medical Care Survey: 2002 Summary, *Advance Data No. 346, 2004; Internet site http://www.cdc.gov/nchs/about/major/ahcd/adata.htm*

Table 10.22 Physician Office Visits by Time Spent with Physician, 2002

(number and percent distribution of physician office visits by time spent with physician; mean and median amount of time spent with physician by specialty, 2002; numbers in thousands)

	number	percent distribution
PHYSICIAN SEEN		
Total visits	**889,980**	**100.0%**
No physician seen	43,813	4.9
Physician seen	846,167	95.1
TIME SPENT WITH PHYSICIAN		
Total visits with physician	**846,167**	**100.0**
1 to 5 minutes	38,393	4.5
6 to 10 minutes	181,078	21.4
11 to 15 minutes	290,573	34.3
16 to 30 minutes	275,653	32.6
31 to 60 minutes	57,693	6.8
61 minutes or more	2,777	0.3

	minutes	
	mean	median
Total visits with physician	**18.4**	**14.7**
Psychiatry	35.2	29.6
Neurology	27.9	24.1
Cardiovascular diseases	21.4	18.0
Internal medicine	20.0	17.1
General surgery	19.6	14.5
Urology	18.2	14.8
Obstetrics and gynecology	18.1	14.7
Ophthalmology	17.3	14.4
Orthopedic surgery	17.1	14.3
General and family practice	16.1	14.5
Pediatrics	16.1	14.5
Dermatology	15.2	14.1
Otolaryngology	15.1	14.3
All other specialties	21.3	15.0

Source: National Center for Health Statistics, National Ambulatory Medical Care Survey: 2002 Summary, Advance Data No. 346, 2004; Internet site http://www.cdc.gov/nchs/about/major/ahcd/adata.htm

Most Patients Prefer to See a Doctor

But highly trained nurses could handle more health problems.

Although there has been increased reliance on nurse practitioners and other health care professionals to supplement physicians' services, fully 95 percent of visits to physicians' offices involve a doctor. Often, patients see other types of health care providers as well—most commonly a medical or nursing assistant (27 percent of visits), followed by a registered nurse (17 percent).

Over the past few years, the nursing field has developed into a multi-tiered profession, with those at the top able to perform many services previously limited to physicians. Many patients are not convinced, however, and continue to prefer to see a physician. This accounts, in part, for the small number of office visits in which patients see a registered nurse. Resistance by doctors to professional nursing is another factor behind the small showing for nurses.

Most health insurance plans include relatively generous benefits for physician office visits. Private insurance covers the majority of payments for these visits (59 percent), with an additional 33 percent covered by government (Medicare and Medicaid/SCHIP) and worker's compensation. Less than 5 percent of payments for physician office visits are "self-pay."

■ The need to control health care costs may eventually require more visits to health care professionals other than physicians.

Registered nurses are seen on only 17 percent of doctor visits

(percent of physician office visits in which patients see provider, by type of provider, 2002)

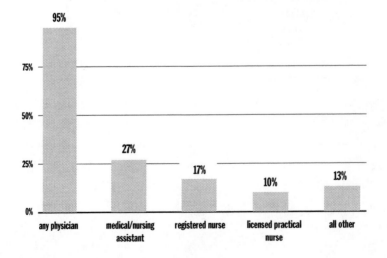

Table 10.23 Physician Office Visits by Providers Seen and Primary Source of Payment, 2002

(number and percent distribution of physician office visits by providers seen and primary expected source of payment, 2002; numbers in thousands)

	number	percent distribution
PROVIDER SEEN		
Total visits	**889,980**	**100.0%**
Any physician	846,167	95.1
Medical/nursing assistant	243,082	27.3
Registered nurse	146,513	16.5
Licensed practical nurse	88,902	10.0
Medical technician/technologist	54,983	6.2
Other provider	31,784	3.6
Physician assistant	16,264	1.8
Nurse practitioner/midwife	11,176	1.3
PRIMARY EXPECTED SOURCE OF PAYMENT		
Total visits	**889,980**	**100.0**
Private insurance	525,520	59.0
Medicare	188,207	21.1
Medicaid/SCHIP	67,110	7.5
Self-pay	39,526	4.4
Worker's Compensation	14,658	1.6
No charge	2,485	0.3
Other	21,456	2.4
Unknown/blank	31,018	3.5

Source: National Center for Health Statistics, National Ambulatory Medical Care Survey: 2002 Summary, *Advance Data No. 346, 2004; Internet site http://www.cdc.gov/nchs/about/major/ahcd/adata.htm*

Drugs Are Prescribed More Often than Lifestyle Change

Drugs are prescribed or provided in nearly two-thirds of office visits.

Although some physicians still do not discuss lifestyle issues with patients, more are beginning to do so. In 2002, 14 percent of physician office visits involved counseling about diet and nutrition. Exercise was prescribed in 10 percent of visits. Only 2 percent of visits include counseling about weight reduction, however, a relatively small share considering that most Americans are overweight.

While lifestyle changes may not be a routine part of physicians' recommendations, drug therapy has become standard. During 65 percent of physician office visits, one or more drugs were prescribed. The share is even higher during visits to general/family practice physicians (77 percent), internists (74 percent), cardiovascular disease specialists (76 percent), and psychiatrists (83 percent).

Given the enormous number of prescription drugs on the market, it is not surprising that no specific class of drugs accounts for more than 5 percent of the total. Among the most common are NSAIDs (nonsteroidal anti-inflammatory drugs), antidepressants, and antihistamines. The most common drugs prescribed are Lipitor, Albuterol, Amoxicillin, and Synthroid.

■ Many patients do not want to hear about lifestyle changes, which is why few doctors counsel them on the topic.

Psychiatrists are most likely to prescribe drugs

(percent of physician office visits during which one or more drugs are provided or prescribed, by physician specialty, 2002)

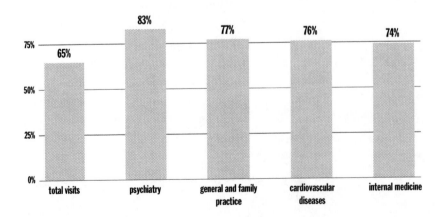

Table 10.24 Physician Office Visits by Therapeutic Services Ordered or Provided, 2002

(number and percent distribution of physician office visits by therapeutic services ordered or provided, 2002; numbers in thousands)

	number	percent
Total visits	**889,980**	**100.0%**
None	473,435	53.2
Diet/nutrition	127,699	14.3
Exercise	89,087	10.0
Growth/development	40,764	4.6
Psychotherapy	32,050	3.6
Mental health/stress management	29,100	3.3
Tobacco use/exposure	23,674	2.7
Asthma education	22,531	2.5
Weight reduction	18,339	2.1
Physiotherapy	18,231	2.0
Other	190,849	21.4

Source: National Center for Health Statistics, National Ambulatory Medical Care Survey: 2002 Summary, *Advance Data No. 346, 2004; Internet site http://www.cdc.gov/nchs/about/major/ahcd/adata.htm*

Table 10.25 Physician Office Visits by Drug Therapy and Physician Specialty, 2002

(total number of physician office visits, and number and percent distribution of physician office visits at which one or more drugs were provided or prescribed by the physician, by physician specialty, 2002; numbers in thousands)

	total	drug visits		drugs provided or prescribed		drug visits as percent of total	number of drugs provided or prescribed per visit
		number	percent distribution	number	percent distribution		
Total visits	**889,980**	**577,075**	**100.0%**	**1,347,312**	**100.0%**	**64.8%**	**1.5**
General and family practice	215,466	165,371	28.7	402,067	29.8	76.8	1.9
Internal medicine	156,692	115,219	20.0	310,006	23.0	73.5	2.0
Pediatrics	120,018	80,814	14.0	149,572	11.1	67.3	1.2
Obstetrics and gynecology	70,324	34,355	6.0	57,937	4.3	48.9	0.8
Ophthalmology	49,937	25,066	4.3	54,150	4.0	50.2	1.1
Dermatology	32,227	21,292	3.7	39,180	2.9	66.1	1.2
Psychiatry	20,822	17,901	3.1	39,735	2.9	82.6	1.8
Cardiovascular diseases	21,659	15,889	2.8	64,088	4.8	76.3	3.1
Orthopedic surgery	38,028	14,293	2.5	23,214	1.7	37.6	0.6
Urology	17,000	8,352	1.4	11,760	0.9	48.8	0.7
Otolaryngology	17,080	8,033	1.4	14,329	1.1	47.0	0.8
Neurology	9,622	5,799	1.0	12,368	0.9	60.3	1.3
General surgery	17,133	4,733	0.8	10,314	0.8	28.1	0.6
All other specialties	103,974	59,919	10.4	158,593	11.8	57.6	1.5

Source: National Center for Health Statistics, National Ambulatory Medical Care Survey: 2002 Summary, *Advance Data No. 346, 2004; Internet site http://www.cdc.gov/nchs/about/major/ahcd/adata.htm*

Table 10.26 Medications Prescribed during Physician Office Visits by Therapeutic Class, 2002

(number and percent distribution of drugs provided or prescribed during physician office visits, for the twenty most frequently occurring therapeutic classes, 2002; numbers in thousands)

	number	percent distribution of drugs provided or prescribed
Total drugs provided or prescribed	**1,347,312**	**100.0%**
NSAIDs	66,328	4.9
Antidepressants	60,367	4.5
Antihistamines	58,060	4.3
Antiasthmatics/bronchodilators	54,562	4.0
Vaccines/antisera	53,785	4.0
Antihypertensive agents	49,298	3.7
Hyperlipidemia	44,065	3.3
Blood glucose regulators	41,865	3.1
ACE inhibitors	40,927	3.0
Disorders, acid/peptic	40,812	3.0
Analgesics, nonnarcotic	39,753	3.0
Penicillins	38,075	2.8
Diuretics	35,942	2.7
Antipyretics	34,784	2.6
Analgesics, narcotic	34,739	2.6
Beta blockers	33,090	2.5
Calcium channel blockers	31,998	2.4
Vitamins/minerals	30,154	2.2
Antiarthritics	28,955	2.1
Estrogens/progestins	28,359	2.1
All other drugs	501,394	37.2

Source: National Center for Health Statistics, National Ambulatory Medical Care Survey: 2002 Summary, Advance Data No. 346, 2004; Internet site http://www.cdc.gov/nchs/about/major/ahcd/adata.htm

Table 10.27 Medications Prescribed during Physician Office Visits by Drug Name, 2002

(number and percent distribution of drugs provided or prescribed during physician office visits, for the twenty most frequently prescribed drugs, 2002; numbers in thousands)

	number	percent distribution of drugs provided or prescribed
Total drugs provided or prescribed	**1,347,312**	**100.0%**
Lipitor	18,842	1.4
Albuterol	15,442	1.1
Amoxicillin	14,690	1.1
Synthroid	14,525	1.1
Lasix	14,004	1.0
Celebrex	13,763	1.0
Tylenol	12,919	1.0
Vioxx	12,650	0.9
Augmentin	11,995	0.9
Norvasc	11,853	0.9
Zyrtec	11,573	0.9
Zocor	11,429	0.8
Acetylsalicylic acid	10,670	0.8
Prednisone	10,422	0.8
Allegra	10,420	0.8
Coumadin	10,090	0.7
Atenolol	9,694	0.7
Claritin	9,208	0.7
Paxil	9,118	0.7
Prevacid	8,981	0.7
All other drugs	1,105,025	82.0

Source: National Center for Health Statistics, National Ambulatory Medical Care Survey: 2002 Summary, *Advance Data No. 346, 2004; Internet site http://www.cdc.gov/nchs/about/major/ahcd/adata.htm*

More than One Million Americans Receive Home Health Care

Most home health care patients are older women.

Home health care is increasingly recognized as a cost-effective alternative to hospitalization. It is also much preferred by many patients and families. In 2000, there were almost 1.4 million home health care patients. Seven out of ten home health care patients are aged 65 or older. Almost two-thirds are women, as would be expected given that there are more women than men in the older age groups.

The most common diagnosis among people receiving home health care is some type of circulatory system disease (24 percent of the total), primarily heart disease (11 percent). Ten percent have some type of disease of the musculoskeletal system and connective tissue, such as osteoarthritis.

■ The need for home health care will increase substantially as the number of older adults rises with the aging of the baby-boom generation.

People aged 65 or older account for 70 percent of patients

(percent distribution of home health care patients, by age, 2000)

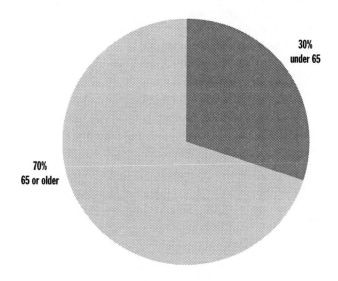

30%
under 65

70%
65 or older

Table 10.28 Home Health Care Patients, 2000

(number and percent distribution of home health care patients by sex, age, and primary admission diagnosis, 2000)

	number	percent
Total home health care patients	**1,355,290**	**100.0%**
Sex		
Females	878,228	64.8
Males	477,062	35.2
Age		
Under age 65	399,811	29.5
Aged 65 or older	955,479	70.5
Aged 65 to 74	234,465	17.3
Aged 75 to 84	424,206	31.3
Aged 85 or older	296,809	21.9
Primary admission diagnosis		
Malignant neoplasms	66,409	4.9
Diabetes	105,713	7.8
Diseases of the nervous system and sense organs	82,673	6.1
Diseases of the circulatory system	319,848	23.6
Diseases of the heart	147,727	10.9
Cerebrovascular diseases	98,936	7.3
Diseases of the respiratory system	92,160	6.8
Decubitus ulcers	25,751	1.9
Diseases of the musculoskeletal system and connective tissue	132,818	9.8
Osteoarthritis	47,435	3.5
Fractures, all sites	55,567	4.1
Fracture of neck of femur (hip)	20,329	1.5
Other	472,996	34.9

Source: National Center for Health Statistics, Health, United States, 2004, *Internet site http://www.cdc.gov/nchs/hus.htm; calculations by New Strategist*

Most People See a Dentist Regularly

Many uninsured children are not getting needed care, however.

Regular dental cleanings are a standard part of dental care for most Americans, with 69 percent saying they had their teeth cleaned in the past year. The percentage varies by race and Hispanic origin, however, with non-Hispanic whites more likely than others to have had an annual dental cleaning.

People aged 65 or older are most likely to have skipped a dental visit for two or more years. Overall, 25 percent of people aged 18 or older have avoided the dentist for that long, but among people aged 75 or older the share is 38 percent. Some older adults may no longer have their natural teeth and think they no longer need to see a dentist.

The majority of children aged 2 to 17 have seen a dentist within the past six months, and nearly three-quarters had a dental visit within the past year. Children aged 12 to 17, however, are less likely to have had a recent dental visit and are more likely than younger children to have an unmet dental need. Children without health insurance are most likely to have an unmet dental need.

■ Traditionally, dental care is not covered under standard health insurance policies although dental problems can affect overall health.

Fifteen percent of children without health insurance have an unmet dental need

(percent of people aged 2 to 17 with an unmet dental need, by insurance status, 2002)

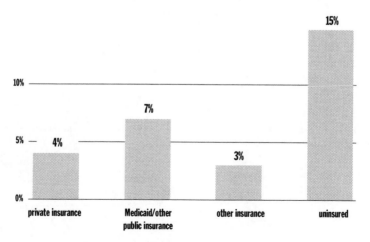

Table 10.29 Dental Cleaning in Past Year by Selected Characteristics, 2002

(percent distribution of people aged 18 or older by whether they had their teeth cleaned by a dentist or dental hygienist in the past year, by selected characteristics, 2002)

	yes	no
Total people	**69.2%**	**30.7%**
Sex		
Men	66.8	33.1
Women	71.9	28.1
Age		
Aged 18 to 24	69.9	30.1
Aged 25 to 34	65.9	34.1
Aged 35 to 44	68.9	31.0
Aged 45 to 54	71.1	28.8
Aged 55 to 64	72.5	27.5
Aged 65 or older	71.9	28.1
Race and Hispanic origin		
Black	62.3	37.6
Hispanic	65.4	34.6
White	72.1	27.9
Multiracial	56.2	41.7
Other	64.1	35.8
Household income		
Under $15,000	48.6	51.4
$15,000 to $24,999	56.1	43.9
$25,000 to $34,999	64.6	35.4
$35,000 to $49,999	72.3	27.6
$50,000 or more	80.6	19.3
Education		
Not a high school graduate	47.2	52.7
High school graduate	64.7	35.2
Some college	72.4	27.6
College graduate	79.2	20.8

Source: Centers for Disease Control and Prevention, Behavorial Risk Factor Surveillance System, Prevalence Data, Internet site http://apps.nccd.cdc.gov/brfss/; calculations by New Strategist

Table 10.30 Length of Time Since Last Dental Visit by Selected Characteristics, 2002

(total number of people aged 18 or older and distribution by length of time since last dental visit, by selected characteristics, 2002; numbers in thousands)

	total	six months or less	more than six months but less than one year	more than one year but less than two years	more than two years but less than five years	more than five years	never
Total adults	**205,825**	**89,244**	**35,466**	**25,652**	**24,717**	**25,357**	**1,908**
Sex							
Men	98,749	39,979	16,478	12,642	13,169	13,514	1,251
Women	107,076	49,265	18,988	13,010	11,548	11,843	657
Age							
Aged 18 to 44	108,114	44,635	20,454	15,452	14,146	10,175	1,577
Aged 45 to 64	64,650	31,222	10,540	7,314	6,893	7,474	210
Aged 65 to 74	17,809	7,784	2,324	1,684	2,018	3,640	30
Aged 75 or older	15,252	5,603	2,147	1,202	1,661	4,068	91
Race and Hispanic origin							
Asian	7,270	2,865	1,403	1,021	811	578	304
Black	23,499	7,287	4,396	3,833	3,642	3,375	248
Hispanic	22,691	6,920	4,118	3,189	3,372	3,653	1,021
Non-Hispanic white	149,584	71,299	24,948	17,109	16,542	17,373	301
Education							
Less than high school	28,248	6,434	3,712	3,561	4,902	8,376	730
High school graduate	52,556	20,260	8,882	7,058	6,994	8,164	254
Some college	48,091	22,952	8,561	6,159	5,264	4,484	179
College graduate	47,197	28,623	8,095	4,493	3,472	1,980	130
Household income							
Less than $20,000	37,369	10,205	5,975	5,274	5,932	8,705	607
$20,000 to $34,999	29,671	10,309	4,850	4,096	4,701	5,115	381
$35,000 to $54,999	31,814	13,310	6,001	4,452	3,975	3,572	218
$55,000 to $74,999	23,984	12,063	4,334	2,743	2,539	2,048	111
$75,000 or more	41,572	25,118	7,204	4,337	2,721	1,785	144
Health insurance coverage among adults under age 65							
Private	124,786	64,596	23,579	14,953	11,408	8,394	483
Medicaid	11,165	3,203	1,912	1,758	1,879	1,956	162
Other	4,541	1,546	832	661	729	702	4
Uninsured	31,374	6,313	4,559	5,312	6,801	6,506	1,135

Note: Numbers by race and Hispanic origin will not sum to total because not all races are shown and Hispanics may be of any race.
Source: National Center for Health Statistics, Summary Health Statistics for U.S. Adults: National Health Interview Survey, 2002, Series 10, No. 222, 2004; Internet site http://www.cdc.gov/nchs/nhis.htm

Table 10.31 **Percent Distribution by Length of Time since Last Dental Visit By Selected Characteristics, 2002**

(percent distribution of people aged 18 or older by length of time since last dental visit, by selected characteristics, 2002)

	total	six months or less	more than six months but less than one year	more than one year but less than two years	more than two years but less than five years	more than five years	never
				time since last dental visit			
Total adults	100.0%	43.4%	17.2%	12.5%	12.0%	12.3%	0.9%
Sex							
Men	100.0	40.5	16.7	12.8	13.3	13.7	1.3
Women	100.0	46.0	17.7	12.2	10.8	11.1	0.6
Age							
Aged 18 to 44	100.0	41.3	18.9	14.3	13.1	9.4	1.5
Aged 45 to 64	100.0	48.3	16.3	11.3	10.7	11.6	0.3
Aged 65 to 74	100.0	43.7	13.0	9.5	11.3	20.4	0.2
Aged 75 or older	100.0	36.7	14.1	7.9	10.9	26.7	0.6
Race and Hispanic origin							
Asian	100.0	39.4	19.3	14.0	11.2	8.0	4.2
Black	100.0	31.0	18.7	16.3	15.5	14.4	1.1
Hispanic	100.0	30.5	18.1	14.1	14.9	16.1	4.5
Non-Hispanic white	100.0	47.7	16.7	11.4	11.1	11.6	0.2
Education							
Less than high school	100.0	22.8	13.1	12.6	17.4	29.7	2.6
High school graduate	100.0	38.5	16.9	13.4	13.3	15.5	0.5
Some college	100.0	47.7	17.8	12.8	10.9	9.3	0.4
College graduate	100.0	60.6	17.2	9.5	7.4	4.2	0.3
Household income							
Less than $20,000	100.0	27.3	16.0	14.1	15.9	23.3	1.6
$20,000 to $34,999	100.0	34.7	16.3	13.8	15.8	17.2	1.3
$35,000 to $54,999	100.0	41.8	18.9	14.0	12.5	11.2	0.7
$55,000 to $74,999	100.0	50.3	18.1	11.4	10.6	8.5	0.5
$75,000 or more	100.0	60.4	17.3	10.4	6.5	4.3	0.3
Health insurance coverage among adults under age 65							
Private	100.0	51.8	18.9	12.0	9.1	6.7	0.4
Medicaid	100.0	28.7	17.1	15.7	16.8	17.5	1.5
Other	100.0	34.0	18.3	14.6	16.1	15.5	0.1
Uninsured	100.0	20.1	14.5	16.9	21.7	20.7	3.6

Source: National Center for Health Statistics, Summary Health Statistics for U.S. Adults: National Health Interview Survey, 2002, *Series 10, No. 222, 2004; Internet site http://www.cdc.gov/nchs/nhis.htm*

Table 10.32 Dental Care Access and Length of Time Since Last Dental Visit For Children under Age 18, 2002

(total number of people aged 2 to 17 and distribution by access to dental care and length of time since last dental visit, by selected characteristics, 2002; numbers in thousands)

				time since last dental visit				
	total	unmet dental need	met dental need	six months or less	more than six months but less than one year	more than one year but less than two years	more than two years but less than five years	more than five years
Total children	**65,153**	**3,819**	**61,031**	**36,232**	**11,558**	**5,051**	**2,086**	**9,379**
Sex								
Female	31,826	2,062	29,646	18,011	5,534	2,380	951	4,572
Male	33,327	1,757	31,385	18,221	6,023	2,671	1,135	4,808
Age								
Aged 2 to 4	12,010	302	11,630	3,824	991	384	101	6,557
Aged 5 to 11	28,780	1,824	26,827	17,959	5,649	2,201	800	1,889
Aged 12 to 17	24,363	1,694	22,574	14,449	4,918	2,467	1,185	933
Race and Hispanic origin								
Asian	2,254	56	2,194	1,123	337	206	88	432
Black	9,447	553	8,837	4,088	2,242	1,053	460	1,361
Hispanic	10,957	796	10,110	4,645	2,076	1,256	543	2,248
Non-Hispanic white	40,748	2,228	38,327	25,458	6,608	2,378	925	5,061
Family structure								
Mother and father	46,429	2,260	43,965	27,283	7,756	2,945	1,226	6,757
Mother, no father	14,741	1,311	13,350	7,023	3,078	1,660	651	2,065
Father, no mother	2,064	127	1,925	1,113	319	173	66	342
Neither mother nor father	1,920	122	1,791	813	404	273	142	216
Parent's education								
Less than high school diploma	8,067	724	7,296	3,064	1,737	1,008	431	1,664
High school diploma	14,721	1,107	13,517	7,081	3,027	1,343	608	2,461
More than high school	40,009	1,854	38,040	25,166	6,314	2,374	880	4,983
Household income								
Less than $20,000	10,498	1,030	9,429	4,586	2,139	1,213	513	1,835
$20,000 to $34,999	9,012	892	8,071	4,116	1,809	860	432	1,740
$35,000 to $54,999	10,386	796	9,569	5,220	1,898	925	389	1,852
$55,000 to $74,999	8,628	255	8,360	5,409	1,453	504	197	1,030
$75,000 or more	14,822	373	14,417	10,677	1,861	633	181	1,390
Health insurance status								
Private	42,301	1,673	40,490	26,745	6,821	2,467	931	5,011
Medicaid/other public	14,652	1,063	13,478	6,599	3,219	1,561	550	2,403
Other	1,236	34	1,195	713	232	106	23	145
Uninsured	6,756	1,021	5,693	2,078	1,239	908	556	1,811

Note: Mother and father includes biological, adoptive, step, in-law, and foster relationships. Legal guardians are classified as neither mother nor father. Parents' education is the education level of the parent with the higher level of education. Unmet dental need is defined as being unable to afford necessary dental care including check-ups in the past twelve months. (–) means not applicable.
Source: National Center for Health Statistics, Summary Health Statistics for U.S. Children: National Health Interview Survey, 2002, Series 10, No. 221, 2004; Internet site http://www.cdc.gov/nchs/nhis.htm

Table 10.33 Percent Distribution of Children under Age 18 by Dental Care Access and Length of Time Since Last Dental Visit, 2002

(percent distribution of people aged 2 to 17 by access to dental care and length of time since last dental visit, by selected characteristics, 2002)

	total	unmet dental need	met dental need	six months or less	more than six months but less than one year	more than one year but less than two years	more than two years but less than five years	more than five years
Total children	100.0%	5.9%	93.7%	55.6%	17.7%	7.8%	3.2%	14.4%
Sex								
Female	100.0	6.5	93.2	56.6	17.4	7.5	3.0	14.4
Male	100.0	5.3	94.2	54.7	18.1	8.0	3.4	14.4
Age								
Aged 2 to 4	100.0	2.5	96.8	31.8	8.3	3.2	0.8	54.6
Aged 5 to 11	100.0	6.3	93.2	62.4	19.6	7.6	2.8	6.6
Aged 12 to 17	100.0	7.0	92.7	59.3	20.2	10.1	4.9	3.8
Race and Hispanic origin								
Asian	100.0	2.5	97.3	49.8	15.0	9.1	3.9	19.2
Black	100.0	5.9	93.5	43.3	23.7	11.1	4.9	14.4
Hispanic	100.0	7.3	92.3	42.4	18.9	11.5	5.0	20.5
Non-Hispanic white	100.0	5.5	94.1	62.5	16.2	5.8	2.3	12.4
Family structure								
Mother and father	100.0	4.9	94.7	58.8	16.7	6.3	2.6	14.6
Mother, no father	100.0	8.9	90.6	47.6	20.9	11.3	4.4	14.0
Father, no mother	100.0	6.2	93.3	53.9	15.5	8.4	3.2	16.6
Neither mother nor father	100.0	6.4	93.3	42.3	21.0	14.2	7.4	11.3
Parent's education								
Less than high school diploma	100.0	9.0	90.4	38.0	21.5	12.5	5.3	20.6
High school diploma	100.0	7.5	91.8	48.1	20.6	9.1	4.1	16.7
More than high school	100.0	4.6	95.1	62.9	15.8	5.9	2.2	12.5
Household income								
Less than $20,000	100.0	9.8	89.8	43.7	20.4	11.6	4.9	17.5
$20,000 to $34,999	100.0	9.9	89.6	45.7	20.1	9.5	4.8	19.3
$35,000 to $54,999	100.0	7.7	92.1	50.3	18.3	8.9	3.7	17.8
$55,000 to $74,999	100.0	3.0	96.9	62.7	16.8	5.8	2.3	11.9
$75,000 or more	100.0	2.5	97.3	72.0	12.6	4.3	1.2	9.4
Health insurance status								
Private	100.0	4.0	95.7	63.2	16.1	5.8	2.2	11.8
Medicaid/other public	100.0	7.3	92.0	45.0	22.0	10.7	3.8	16.4
Other	100.0	2.8	96.7	57.7	18.8	8.6	1.9	11.7
Uninsured	100.0	15.1	84.3	30.8	18.3	13.4	8.2	26.8

Note: Mother and father includes biological, adoptive, step, in-law, and foster relationships. Legal guardians are classified as neither mother nor father. Parents' education is the education level of the parent with the higher level of education. Unmet dental need is defined as being unable to afford necessary dental care including check-ups in the past twelve months. (–) means not applicable.

Source: National Center for Health Statistics, Summary Health Statistics for U.S. Children: National Health Interview Survey, 2002, Series 10, No. 221, 2004; Internet site http://www.cdc.gov/nchs/nhis.htm

11

Hospital Care

■ **Thirty-six percent of visits to hospital outpatient departments are due to acute health problems.**

Respiratory illness is the most common diagnosis for people visiting hospital outpatient facilities, accounting for 11 percent of the total.

■ **The oldest Americans are most likely to use emergency rooms.**

People aged 15-to-24 have the second-highest rate of visits to emergency rooms.

■ **People aged 45 or older account for most hospital discharges.**

In 2002, hospitals discharged more than 33 million people. People aged 45 or older accounted for fully 61 percent of discharges.

■ **Heart disease is one of the most common reasons for hospitalization.**

Diseases related to the circulatory system account for 19 percent of hospitalizations, while respiratory illness accounts for 11 percent.

■ **The average length of a hospital stay has declined.**

In 1980, the average hospital stay was 7.3 days. By 2002, it had fallen to 4.9 days.

■ **In 2002, the nation's hospitals performed more than 42 million procedures.**

The largest share of procedures (16 percent) is performed on the cardiovascular system, while another 16 percent are obstetrical.

Big Differences in the Use of Hospital Outpatient Services

Older blacks are particularly likely to use hospital outpatient departments.

Americans use hospital outpatient facilities for a variety of reasons—to see physicians, undergo tests, or for care related to chronic conditions. In 2002, there were 29.4 visits to hospital outpatient departments for every 100 people. This figure does not mean that 29 percent of Americans visited an outpatient department during the year, however, since some people visited outpatient departments more than once.

The use of outpatient departments is highest among people aged 65 or older, which is predictable since older adults tend to have more health problems. Women are more likely than men to visit hospital outpatient departments. There are also differences by age in the pattern of visits to these facilities. Women aged 25 to 64 account for one-third of visits to outpatient departments, while men in that age group account for a much smaller 18 percent of visits to these facilities.

The use of hospital outpatient facilities is much higher among blacks than whites. One reason for the difference is that blacks have less access to private physicians because of their lower incomes. Many blacks use public hospitals for much of their medical care. Blacks aged 65 or older are especially likely to use hospital outpatient departments, with a rate in 2002 of more than 85 visits per 100 people—much higher than the rate of 30 to 31 among whites aged 65 or older.

■ Private clinics are increasingly offering services that were once the purview of hospital outpatient facilities, such as mammograms. As competition increases, the rate of hospital outpatient department visits could decline.

The black rate is more than double the white rate

(number of visits to hospital outpatient departments per 100 people aged 65 or older, by race, 2002)

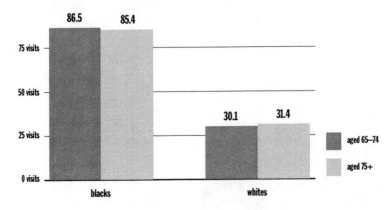

Table 11.1 Visits to Hospital Outpatient Departments by Sex and Age, 2002

(number, percent distribution, and rate of hospital outpatient department visits by sex and age, 2002; numbers in thousands)

	number	percent distribution	number of visits per 100 people per year
Total visits	**83,339**	**100.0%**	**29.4**
Under age 15	18,947	22.7	31.3
Aged 15 to 24	9,839	11.8	24.9
Aged 25 to 44	21,137	25.4	25.5
Aged 45 to 64	21,436	25.7	32.4
Aged 65 to 74	6,386	7.7	35.4
Aged 75 or older	5,595	6.7	35.1
Total females	**51,014**	**61.2**	**35.2**
Under age 15	9,452	11.3	31.9
Aged 15 to 24	6,874	8.2	35.0
Aged 25 to 44	14,317	17.2	34.1
Aged 45 to 64	13,100	15.7	38.4
Aged 65 to 74	3,585	4.3	36.4
Aged 75 or older	3,687	4.4	37.7
Total males	**32,325**	**38.8**	**23.4**
Under age 15	9,495	11.4	30.6
Aged 15 to 24	2,965	3.6	14.9
Aged 25 to 44	6,820	8.2	16.7
Aged 45 to 64	8,336	10.0	26.0
Aged 65 to 74	2,801	3.4	34.2
Aged 75 or older	1,908	2.3	31.1

Source: National Center for Health Statistics, National Hospital Ambulatory Medical Care Survey: 2002 Outpatient Department Summary, *Advance Data, No. 345, 2004; Internet site http://www.cdc.gov/nchs/about/major/ahcd/adata.htm*

Table 11.2 Visits to Hospital Outpatient Departments by Race and Age, 2002

(number, percent distribution, and rate of hospital outpatient department visits by race and age, 2002; numbers in thousands)

	number	percent distribution	number of visits per 100 people per year
Total visits	**83,339**	**100.0%**	**29.4**
Under age 15	18,947	22.7	31.3
Aged 15 to 24	9,839	11.8	24.9
Aged 25 to 44	21,137	25.4	25.5
Aged 45 to 64	21,436	25.7	32.4
Aged 65 to 74	6,386	7.7	35.4
Aged 75 or older	5,595	6.7	35.1
Total blacks	**18,664**	**22.4**	**52.8**
Under age 15	4,602	5.5	48.5
Aged 15 to 24	2,332	2.8	41.0
Aged 25 to 44	4,764	5.7	46.0
Aged 45 to 64	4,552	5.5	64.6
Aged 65 to 74	1,409	1.7	86.5
Aged 75 or older	1,004	1.2	85.4
Total whites	**61,315**	**73.6**	**26.8**
Under age 15	13,471	16.2	29.1
Aged 15 to 24	7,161	8.6	23.2
Aged 25 to 44	15,474	18.6	23.3
Aged 45 to 64	16,032	19.2	28.9
Aged 65 to 74	4,702	5.6	30.1
Aged 75 or older	4,475	5.4	31.4
American Indians	**383**	**0.5**	**14.2**
Asians	**2,334**	**2.8**	**20.3**
Native Hawaiians	**436**	**0.5**	**91.8**
Multiple races	**207**	**0.2**	**5.0**

Source: National Center for Health Statistics, National Hospital Ambulatory Medical Care Survey: 2002 Outpatient Department Summary, Advance Data, No. 345, 2004; Internet site http://www.cdc.gov/nchs/about/major/ahcd/adata.htm

Acute Health Problems Are the Most Common Reason for Visiting a Hospital Outpatient Department

But people receive many types of services from these facilities.

Acute health problems account for the largest share (36 percent) of visits to hospital outpatient departments. This broad general category includes injuries and illnesses of relatively short duration, such as respiratory infections. Among children under age 15, acute illnesses account for nearly half of visits to outpatient facilities. The most commonly cited detailed reason for an outpatient department visit is a general medical exam or progress visit.

Respiratory illness is the most common diagnosis (11 percent) among people visiting hospital outpatient facilities. The majority of patients see a staff physician during their visit, although 69 percent see a registered nurse, medical or nursing assistant, or licensed practical nurse in addition to or in lieu of a doctor. Most patients receive a general medical exam and a blood pressure test. The wide variety of services provided, however, means that no other single type of service is performed on most patients. Among the therapeutic services provided, the most common is related to diet and nutrition, given to 12 percent of patients.

■ Medicare and Medicaid cover a larger share of hospital outpatient visits (42 percent) than private insurance (37 percent) does.

Acute problems account for fewer than one-third of visits by people aged 45 or older

(percent of hospital outpatient department visits because of acute health problems, by age, 2002)

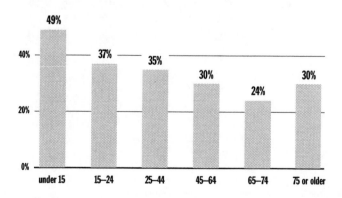

Table 11.3 Hospital Outpatient Department Visits by Major Reason for Visit, 2002

(number and percent distribution of hospital outpatient department visits by age, sex, race, and major reason for visit, 2002; numbers in thousands)

	total	acute problem	chronic problem, routine	chronic problem, flare-up	pre- or post-surgery/injury follow-up	nonillness care
Total visits	**83,339**	**29,903**	**25,339**	**4,968**	**3,376**	**15,025**
Age						
Under age 15	18,947	9,270	3,535	670	278	4,449
Aged 15 to 24	9,839	3,656	1,879	409	347	3,091
Aged 25 to 44	21,137	7,423	5,848	1,430	894	4,304
Aged 45 to 64	21,436	6,364	8,752	1,603	1,154	2,111
Aged 65 to 74	6,386	1,527	2,920	483	427	544
Aged 75 or older	5,595	1,664	2,405	373	276	525
Sex						
Female	51,014	17,414	15,127	3,015	1,803	10,745
Male	32,325	12,489	10,212	1,953	1,573	4,280
Race						
Black	18,664	5,384	6,086	1,183	798	4,376
White	61,315	23,434	18,367	3,646	2,409	9,888
Other	3,361	1,086	886	138	168	761
PERCENT DISTRIBUTION						
Total visits	**100.0%**	**35.9%**	**30.4%**	**6.0%**	**4.1%**	**18.0%**
Age						
Under age 15	100.0	48.9	18.7	3.5	1.5	23.5
Aged 15 to 24	100.0	37.2	19.1	4.2	3.5	31.4
Aged 25 to 44	100.0	35.1	27.7	6.8	4.2	20.4
Aged 45 to 64	100.0	29.7	40.8	7.5	5.4	9.8
Aged 65 to 74	100.0	23.9	45.7	7.6	6.7	8.5
Aged 75 or older	100.0	29.7	43.0	6.7	4.9	9.4
Sex						
Female	100.0	34.1	29.7	5.9	3.5	21.1
Male	100.0	38.6	31.6	6.0	4.9	13.2
Race						
Black	100.0	28.8	32.6	6.3	4.3	23.4
White	100.0	38.2	30.0	5.9	3.9	16.1
Other	100.0	32.3	26.4	4.1	5.0	22.6

Note: Numbers will not add to total because blank and unknown are not shown.
Source: National Center for Health Statistics, National Hospital Ambulatory Medical Care Survey: 2002 Outpatient Department Summary, Advance Data, No. 345, 2004; Internet site http://www.cdc.gov/nchs/about/major/ahcd/adata.htm

Table 11.4 Visits to Hospital Outpatient Departments by Detailed Reason for Visit, 2002

(number and percent distribution of hospital outpatient department visits by the twenty principal reasons for visit most frequently mentioned by patients, 2002; numbers in thousands)

	number	percent distribution
Total visits	**83,339**	**100.0%**
General medical examination	5,926	7.1
Progress visit	5,842	7.0
Prenatal examination, routine	2,772	3.3
Cough	2,241	2.7
Throat symptoms	2,119	2.5
Diabetes mellitus	1,476	1.8
Well-baby examination	1,367	1.6
Stomach and abdominal pain	1,320	1.6
Medication, other and unspecified	1,298	1.6
Postoperative visit	1,216	1.5
Hypertension	1,166	1.4
Fever	1,149	1.4
Back symptoms	1,100	1.3
Headache, pain in head	1,080	1.3
Earache or ear infection	1,039	1.2
Counseling, not otherwise stated	1,020	1.2
Skin rash	969	1.2
Low back symptoms	939	1.1
Depression	884	1.1
Knee symptoms	765	0.9
All other reasons	47,652	57.2

Source: National Center for Health Statistics, National Hospital Ambulatory Medical Care Survey: 2002 Outpatient Department Summary, *Advance Data, No. 345, 2004; Internet site http://www.cdc.gov/nchs/about/major/ahcd/adata.htm*

Table 11.5 Visits to Hospital Outpatient Departments by Primary Diagnosis, 2002

(number and percent distribution of hospital outpatient department visits by primary diagnosis, 2002; numbers in thousands)

	number	percent distribution
Total visits	**83,339**	**100.0%**
Infectious and parasitic diseases	2,996	3.6
Neoplasms	2,644	3.2
Endocrine, nutritional, metabolic diseases, and immunity disorders	5,034	6.0
Mental disorders	4,966	6.0
Diseases of the nervous system and sense organs	5,651	6.8
Diseases of the circulatory system	6,024	7.2
Diseases of the respiratory system	9,193	11.0
Diseases of the digestive system	2,293	2.8
Diseases of the genitourinary system	3,348	4.0
Diseases of the skin and subcutaneous tissue	2,941	3.5
Diseases of the musculoskeletal system and connective tissue	6,093	7.3
Symptoms, signs, and ill-defined conditions	5,960	7.2
Injury and poisoning	5,341	6.4
Supplementary classification	15,884	19.1
All other diagnoses	3,399	4.1
Unknown	1,572	1.9

Source: National Center for Health Statistics, National Hospital Ambulatory Medical Care Survey: 2002 Outpatient Department Summary, *Advance Data, No. 345, 2004; Internet site http://www.cdc.gov/nchs/about/major/ahcd/adata.htm*

Table 11.6   Visits to Hospital Outpatient Departments by Providers Seen And Primary Source of Payment, 2002

(number and percent distribution of hospital outpatient department visits by providers seen and primary expected source of payment, 2002; numbers in thousands)

	number	percent distribution
PROVIDER SEEN		
Total visits	**83,339**	**100.0%**
Any physician	66,976	80.4
Staff physician	60,159	72.2
Resident/intern	13,490	16.2
Other physician	2,991	3.6
Registered nurse	32,580	39.1
Medical/nursing assistant	15,360	18.4
Licensed practical nurse	9,761	11.7
Nurse practitioner/midwife	6,553	7.9
Medical technician/technologist	4,602	5.5
Physician assistant	3,664	4.4
Other provider	6,144	7.4
PRIMARY EXPECTED SOURCE OF PAYMENT		
Total visits	**83,339**	**100.0**
Private insurance	31,063	37.3
Medicare	22,749	27.3
Medicaid/SCHIP	11,992	14.4
Self-pay	6,125	7.3
Worker's Compensation	2,689	3.2
No charge	1,012	1.2
Other	3,037	3.6
Unknown/blank	4,672	5.6

Source: National Center for Health Statistics, National Hospital Ambulatory Medical Care Survey: 2002 Outpatient Department Summary, *Advance Data, No. 345, 2004; Internet site http://www.cdc.gov/nchs/about/major/ahcd/adata.htm*

Table 11.7 Visits to Hospital Outpatient Departments by Services Ordered or Provided, 2002

(number and percent of hospital outpatient department visits by services ordered or provided, 2002; numbers in thousands)

	number	percent
Total visits	**83,339**	**100.0%**
None	8,926	10.7
Examinations		
General medical	48,684	58.4
Other	15,612	18.7
Diagnostic tests		
Blood pressure	43,021	51.6
EKG	3,012	3.6
Any scope procedure	1,388	1.7
Sigmoidoscopy/colonoscopy	754	0.9
Endoscopy	581	0.7
Cystoscopy	126	0.2
Tuberculin skin test	588	0.7
Audiometry	307	0.4
Fetal monitoring	297	0.4
Cardiac stress test	293	0.4
EEG	144	0.2
Laboratory tests		
CBC	8,288	9.9
Urinalysis	7,277	8.7
Pap test	2,948	3.5
Cholesterol	2,446	2.9
Hematocrit/hemoglobin	2,170	2.6
PSA	470	0.6
Cultures		
Any cultures	3,667	4.4
Throat/rapid strep test	1,619	1.9
Urine	773	0.9
Cervical/urethral	751	0.9
Stool	200	0.2
Imaging		
Any imaging	10,384	12.5
X-ray	5,886	7.1
Mammography	1,490	1.8
Ultrasound	1,243	1.5
Other imaging	3,771	4.5

Source: National Center for Health Statistics, National Hospital Ambulatory Medical Care Survey: 2002 Outpatient Department Summary, *Advance Data, No. 345, 2004; Internet site http://www.cdc.gov/nchs/about/major/ahcd/adata.htm*

Table 11.8   Visits to Hospital Outpatient Departments by Therapeutic Services Ordered or Provided, 2002

(number and percent distribution of hospital outpatient department visits by therapeutic services ordered or provided, 2002; numbers in thousands)

	number	percent distribution
Total visits	**83,339**	**100.0%**
No therapeutic services	45,823	55.0
Diet/nutrition	10,290	12.3
Exercise	4,958	5.9
Growth/development	2,944	3.5
Psychotherapy	2,545	3.1
Mental health/stress management	2,473	3.0
Tobacco use/exposure	2,413	2.9
Asthma education	1,221	1.5
Weight reduction	1,124	1.3
Physiotherapy	1,119	1.3
Other	21,414	25.7

Source: National Center for Health Statistics, National Hospital Ambulatory Medical Care Survey: 2002 Outpatient Department Summary, *Advance Data, No. 345, 2004; Internet site http://www.cdc.gov/nchs/about/major/ahcd/adata.htm*

Emergency Room Visits Rise Sharply after Age 74

The oldest age group has the highest rate of emergency room visits.

People aged 75 or older have the highest rate of visits to hospital emergency rooms, with 61.1 visits per 100 people in the age group per year. This figure compares with a rate of 38.9 visits per 100 people among the total population. The second-highest emergency room visit rate (43.6 per 100) is found among people aged 15 to 24. At this age, many are prone to behavior that can lead to accidents and injuries, necessitating a trip to the local ER. People aged 75 or older accounted for only 9 percent of total ER visits in 2002 because they make up a relatively small share of the total population.

Blacks are far more likely than the general population to visit a hospital emergency room, with 70.3 visits per 100 blacks in the population versus a rate of 35.7 per 100 among whites. The rate is especially high for blacks aged 75 or older, at 91.7 per 100. The low incomes of blacks, which limit their access to private physicians, are one reason for their higher rate of emergency room use.

■ As the population ages, the need for emergency care will increase.

The rate of emergency room visits is lowest among 45-to-64-year-olds

(number of hospital emergency room visits per 100 people, by age, 2002)

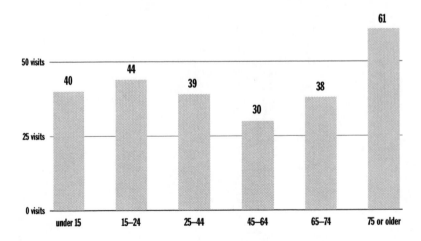

Table 11.9 Visits to Hospital Emergency Departments by Sex and Age, 2002

(number, percent distribution, and rate of hospital emergency department visits by sex and age, 2002; numbers in thousands)

	number	percent distribution	number of visits per 100 people per year
Total visits	**110,155**	**100.0%**	**38.9**
Under age 15	24,077	21.9	39.7
Aged 15 to 24	17,215	15.6	43.6
Aged 25 to 44	32,432	29.4	39.2
Aged 45 to 64	19,943	18.1	30.1
Aged 65 to 74	6,759	6.1	37.5
Aged 75 or older	9,728	8.8	61.1
Total females	**59,594**	**54.1**	**41.1**
Under age 15	11,262	10.2	38.1
Aged 15 to 24	9,756	8.9	49.7
Aged 25 to 44	17,852	16.2	42.5
Aged 45 to 64	10,877	9.9	31.9
Aged 65 to 74	3,653	3.3	37.1
Aged 75 or older	6,194	5.6	63.3
Total males	**50,561**	**45.9**	**36.6**
Under age 15	12,815	11.6	41.3
Aged 15 to 24	7,459	6.8	37.5
Aged 25 to 44	14,580	13.2	35.7
Aged 45 to 64	9,065	8.2	28.3
Aged 65 to 74	3,106	2.8	37.9
Aged 75 or older	3,534	3.2	57.6

Source: National Center for Health Statistics, National Hospital Ambulatory Medical Care Survey: 2002 Emergency Department Summary, *Advance Data, No. 340, 2004; Internet site http://www.cdc.gov/nchs/about/major/ahcd/adata.htm*

Table 11.10 Visits to Hospital Emergency Departments by Race and Age, 2002

(number, percent distribution, and rate of hospital emergency department visits by race and age, 2002; numbers in thousands)

	number	percent distribution	number of visits per 100 people per year
Total visits	**110,155**	**100.0%**	**38.9**
Under age 15	24,077	21.9	39.7
Aged 15 to 24	17,215	15.6	43.6
Aged 25 to 44	32,432	29.4	39.2
Aged 45 to 64	19,943	18.1	30.1
Aged 65 to 74	6,759	6.1	37.5
Aged 75 or older	9,728	8.8	61.1
Total blacks	**24,861**	**22.6**	**70.3**
Under age 15	6,201	5.6	65.4
Aged 15 to 24	4,362	4.0	76.8
Aged 25 to 44	7,811	7.1	75.5
Aged 45 to 64	4,301	3.9	61.0
Aged 65 to 74	1,109	1.0	68.1
Aged 75 or older	1,077	1.0	91.7
Total whites	**81,704**	**74.2**	**35.7**
Under age 15	16,952	15.4	36.6
Aged 15 to 24	12,323	11.2	39.9
Aged 25 to 44	23,612	21.4	35.6
Aged 45 to 64	14,980	13.6	27.0
Aged 65 to 74	5,427	4.9	34.8
Aged 75 or older	8,410	7.6	59.1
American Indians	**809**	**0.7**	**30.0**
Asians	**2,173**	**2.0**	**18.9**
Native Hawaiians	**435**	**0.4**	**91.6**
Multiple races	**173**	**0.2**	**4.2**

Source: National Center for Health Statistics, National Hospital Ambulatory Medical Care Survey: 2002 Emergency Department Summary, *Advance Data, No. 340, 2004; Internet site http://www.cdc.gov/nchs/about/major/ahcd/adata.htm*

ER Visits by Older Adults Are Most Likely to Be Extremely Urgent

The youngest patients are most likely to have nonemergency conditions.

Most visits (57 percent) to hospital emergency rooms are for medical problems that are truly dire ("emergent" conditions) or require urgent care. Another 19 percent are for "semiurgent" conditions, while 10 percent are for conditions that do not require emergency treatment. Visits by people aged 65 or older are most likely to fall into the emergent category, while the highest share of nonurgent visits is found among people under age 15.

The principal reasons people visit an ER vary widely. The most commonly given reason is stomach pain, cramps, and spasms, although these symptoms accounted for only 6.5 percent of ER visits in 2002. Among the specific diagnoses given to ER patients, injuries and poisonings account for the largest share (26 percent).

Nearly all patients visiting an ER are seen by a physician, with most (88 percent) seen by a staff physician and/or a registered nurse (89 percent). Most (63 percent) are given basic medical screening and one-third has some type of blood test. X-rays and other imaging techniques are also commonly used, with 41 percent of visits including these services.

■ The burden on hospital emergency rooms is growing because people without easy access to private physicians use them for basic medical care.

Many visits to emergency rooms are not for emergencies

(percent distribution of visits to emergency rooms by urgency of problem, 2002)

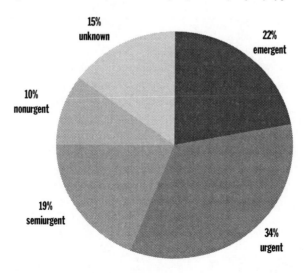

15%
unknown

22%
emergent

10%
nonurgent

19%
semiurgent

34%
urgent

Table 11.11 Emergency Department Visits by Selected Characteristics and Urgency of Problem, 2002

(number of visits to emergency rooms and percent distribution by urgency of problem, by age, sex, and race, 2002; numbers in thousands)

| | number | percent distribution by urgency of problem | | | | | |
		total	emergent	urgent	semiurgent	nonurgent	unknown
Total visits	**110,155**	**100.0%**	**22.3%**	**34.2%**	**18.5%**	**10.2%**	**14.8%**
Age							
Under age 15	24,077	100.0	16.3	33.5	19.7	15.6	14.9
Aged 15 to 24	17,215	100.0	18.6	33.9	20.8	11.6	15.1
Aged 25 to 44	32,432	100.0	20.7	34.3	20.1	10.1	14.9
Aged 45 to 64	19,943	100.0	24.8	34.4	17.5	8.1	15.2
Aged 65 to 74	6,759	100.0	32.4	35.1	13.6	4.1	14.8
Aged 75 or older	9,728	100.0	36.9	34.6	12.1	3.1	13.3
Sex							
Female	59,594	100.0	22.0	34.9	18.7	9.6	14.7
Male	50,561	100.0	22.6	33.3	18.4	10.8	15.0
Race							
Black	24,861	100.0	17.8	34.5	19.7	14.4	13.6
White	81,704	100.0	23.6	34.0	18.3	9.1	15.1
Other	3,590	100.0	23.2	36.6	16.5	6.1	17.6

Note: Emergent is a visit in which the patient should be seen in less than 15 minutes; urgent is a visit in which the patient should be seen within 15 to 60 minutes; semiurgent is a visit in which the patient should be seen within 61 to 120 minutes; nonurgent is a visit in which the patient should be seen within 121 minutes to 24 hours; unknown is a visit with no mention of immediacy or triage, or the patient was dead on arrival.
Source: National Center for Health Statistics, National Hospital Ambulatory Medical Care Survey: 2002 Emergency Department Summary, Advance Data, *No. 340, 2004; Internet site http://www.cdc.gov/nchs/about/major/ahcd/adata.htm*

Table 11.12 Visits to Hospital Emergency Departments by Reason for Visit, 2002

(number and percent distribution of hospital emergency department visits by the twenty principal reasons most frequently mentioned by patients for visit, 2002; numbers in thousands)

	number	percent distribution
Total visits	**110,155**	**100.0%**
Stomach pain, cramps, and spasms	7,152	6.5
Chest pain and related symptoms	5,637	5.1
Fever	5,310	4.8
Cough	3,016	2.7
Shortness of breath	2,943	2.7
Headache, pain in head	2,844	2.6
Back symptoms	2,713	2.5
Symptoms referable to throat	2,483	2.3
Vomiting	2,422	2.2
Pain, site not referable to specific body system	2,176	2.0
Laceration and cuts—upper extremity	2,161	2.0
Motor vehicle accident, type of injury not specified	1,758	1.6
Earache or ear infection	1,748	1.6
Accident, not otherwise specified	1,729	1.6
Vertigo, dizziness	1,578	1.4
Injury to head, neck, and face	1,468	1.3
Low back symptoms	1,438	1.3
Labored or difficult breathing (dyspnea)	1,387	1.3
Skin rash	1,376	1.2
Nausea	1,355	1.2
All other reasons	57,462	52.2

Source: National Center for Health Statistics, National Hospital Ambulatory Medical Care Survey: 2002 Emergency Department Summary, *Advance Data, No. 340, 2004; Internet site http://www.cdc.gov/nchs/about/major/ahcd/adata.htm*

Table 11.13 Visits to Hospital Emergency Departments by Primary Diagnosis, 2002

(number and percent distribution of hospital emergency department visits by primary diagnosis, 2002; numbers in thousands)

	number	percent distribution
Total visits	**110,155**	**100.0%**
Infectious and parasitic diseases	3,422	3.1
Neoplasms	257	0.2
Endocrine, nutritional and metabolic diseases and immunity disorders	1,637	1.5
Mental disorders	3,487	3.2
Diseases of the nervous system and sense organs	6,244	5.7
Diseases of the circulatory system	4,648	4.2
Diseases of the respiratory system	12,978	11.8
Diseases of the digestive system	6,657	6.0
Diseases of the genitourinary system	4,949	4.5
Diseases of the skin and subcutaneous tissue	3,166	2.9
Diseases of the musculoskeletal system and connective tissue	5,939	5.4
Symptoms, signs, and ill-defined conditions	19,574	17.8
Injury and poisoning	28,749	26.1
Fractures	3,705	3.4
Sprains	6,164	5.6
Intracranial	293	0.3
Open wounds	6,507	5.9
Superficial	1,750	1.6
Contusions	4,692	4.3
Foreign bodies	538	0.5
Burns	164	0.1
Trauma complications and unspecified injuries	1,607	1.5
Poisoning and toxic effects	889	0.8
Surgical and medical complications	454	0.4
Other injuries	1,986	1.8
Supplementary classification	2,973	2.7
All other diagnoses	3,744	3.4
Unknown	1,729	1.6

Source: National Center for Health Statistics, National Hospital Ambulatory Medical Care Survey: 2002 Emergency Department Summary, *Advance Data, No. 340, 2004; Internet site http://www.cdc.gov/nchs/about/major/ahcd/adata.htm*

Table 11.14 Visits to Hospital Emergency Departments by Providers Seen And Primary Source of Payment, 2002

(number and percent distribution of hospital emergency department visits by providers seen and primary expected source of payment, 2002; numbers in thousands)

	number	percent distribution
PROVIDER SEEN		
Total visits	**110,155**	**100.0%**
Any physician	103,020	93.5
Staff physician	96,644	87.7
Resident/intern	9,955	9.0
Other physician	9,778	8.9
Registered nurse	97,504	88.5
Other technician	26,421	24.0
Licensed practical nurse	8,491	7.7
E.M.T.	7,874	7.1
Physician assistant	5,367	4.9
Nurse practitioner	1,803	1.6
Other provider	6,253	5.7
PRIMARY EXPECTED SOURCE OF PAYMENT		
Total visits	**110,155**	**100.0**
Private insurance	42,802	38.9
Medicaid/SCHIP	21,751	19.7
Medicare	16,964	15.4
Self-pay	15,935	14.5
Worker's Compensation	2,148	1.9
No charge	1,155	1.0
Other	2,551	2.3
Unknown	6,848	6.2

Source: National Center for Health Statistics, National Hospital Ambulatory Medical Care Survey: 2002 Outpatient Department Summary, *Advance Data, No. 345, 2004; Internet site http://www.cdc.gov/nchs/about/major/ahcd/adata.htm*

Table 11.15 Visits to Hospital Emergency Departments by Diagnostic and Screening Services Ordered or Provided, 2002

(number and percent of hospital emergency department visits by diagnostic and screening services ordered or provided, 2002; numbers in thousands)

	number	percent
Total visits	**110,155**	**100.0%**
None	12,788	11.6
Examinations and tests		
Medical screening	69,269	62.9
Pulse oximetry	21,043	19.1
Urinalysis	17,704	16.1
EKG/ECG	16,533	15.0
Mental status exam	11,359	10.3
Cardiac monitor	7,377	6.7
Pregnancy test	3,551	3.2
EEG	281	0.3
Imaging		
Chest X-ray	20,412	18.5
Extremity X-ray	11,057	10.0
Other X-ray	10,290	9.3
MRI/CAT scan	7,857	7.1
Ultrasound	2,257	2.0
Other imaging	1,771	1.6
Any imaging	44,828	40.7
Blood tests		
CBC	33,503	30.4
Other blood chemistry	19,336	17.6
BUN	16,596	15.1
Glucose	15,366	13.9
Creatinine	15,348	13.9
Cholesterol	3,947	3.6
HgbA1C	2,113	1.9
BAC	1,517	1.4
HIV serology	163	0.1
Any blood test listed	36,632	33.3
Cultures		
Urine	4,638	4.2
Blood	2,768	2.5
Throat/rapid strep test	2,138	1.9
Cervical urethral	825	0.7
Stool	670	0.6
Any culture listed	9,529	8.7

Source: National Center for Health Statistics, National Hospital Ambulatory Medical Care Survey: 2002 Emergency Department Summary, *Advance Data, No. 340, 2004; Internet site http://www.cdc.gov/nchs/about/major/ahcd/adata.htm*

Older Adults Are Far More Likely to Need Hospitalization

The rate is lowest among children.

The rate of hospitalization increases with age as health problems become more serious. Among people under age 15, the discharge rate from nonfederal short-stay hospitals in 2002 was 418.7 per 10,000 population. This figure compares with a much higher rate of 3,574.9 per 10,000 among people aged 65 or older.

The hospitalization rate varies by sex as well as age. Among children under age 15, the rate is higher for males than females. Among people aged 45 or older, the rate for men and women is almost the same. Among those aged 15 to 44, women are far more likely to have a hospital stay. The primary reason is childbearing and conditions related to the reproductive system necessitating procedures such as hysterectomies.

Among people aged 15 to 64, men have longer hospital stays, on average, than women. The difference in average length of stay by sex is particularly large in the 15-to-44 age group. Men in the age group who were hospitalized in 2002 had an average hospital stay of 4.9 days; women had a stay of just 3.3 days. Behind women's shorter length of stay is the brief time most women spend in the hospital following childbirth.

■ Hospital birthing centers, which provide a homelike environment, effectively halted the trend toward home births that had been gaining momentum a few decades ago.

Among older men and women, hospital stays are the same length

(average length of hospital stay for inpatients discharged from nonfederal short-stay hospitals, by sex and age, 2002)

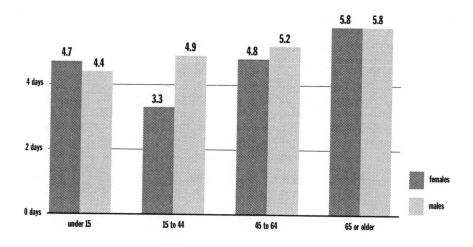

Table 11.16 People with Overnight Hospital Stays by Selected Characteristics, 2002

(total number of people, and percent distribution by number of overnight hospital stays in past twelve months, by selected characteristics, 2002; numbers in thousands)

	total			one or more			
	number	percent	none	total	one	two	three or more
Total people	**278,789**	**100.0%**	**90.7%**	**8.4%**	**6.5%**	**1.2%**	**0.7%**
Sex							
Female	142,731	100.0	89.1	9.9	7.8	1.4	0.8
Male	136,058	100.0	92.3	6.8	5.2	1.0	0.6
Age							
Under age 12	48,356	100.0	91.4	7.9	6.9	0.7	0.3
Aged 12 to 17	24,612	100.0	96.8	2.6	2.1	0.3	0.1
Aged 18 to 44	108,111	100.0	92.2	7.1	5.8	0.8	0.5
Aged 45 to 64	64,650	100.0	90.8	8.1	5.9	1.3	0.8
Aged 65 or older	33,060	100.0	79.9	18.5	12.7	3.6	2.2
Race and Hispanic origin							
Asian	10,740	100.0	94.0	4.4	4.0	0.3	0.1
Black	34,037	100.0	90.3	8.7	6.4	1.4	0.9
Hispanic	35,254	100.0	92.3	7.3	5.8	1.0	0.5
Non-Hispanic white	193,860	100.0	90.3	8.8	6.8	1.3	0.7
Household income							
Under $20,000	46,934	100.0	87.4	12.1	8.7	2.0	1.4
$20,000 to $34,999	36,568	100.0	90.2	9.8	7.3	1.5	1.0
$35,000 to $54,999	40,451	100.0	91.3	8.5	6.8	1.2	0.5
$55,000 to $74,999	31,344	100.0	93.2	6.8	5.5	0.9	0.4
$75,000 or more	55,653	100.0	93.7	6.3	5.2	0.7	0.3
Education							
Not a high school graduate	27,467	100.0	86.0	13.6	9.3	2.6	1.7
High school graduate	52,064	100.0	90.0	9.8	7.2	1.6	1.0
Some college	46,703	100.0	89.8	10.0	7.6	1.4	0.9
College graduate	45,541	100.0	92.4	7.4	5.9	0.9	0.5
Health insurance coverage among people under age 65							
Private	169,418	100.0	93.2	6.5	5.3	0.8	0.3
Medicaid	27,538	100.0	86.9	12.6	9.3	1.9	1.4
Other	5,883	100.0	86.1	13.0	9.0	2.3	1.8
Uninsured	40,127	100.0	93.0	5.3	4.3	0.6	0.3

Note: Numbers by race and Hispanic origin will not sum to total because not all races are shown and Hispanics may be of any race.
Source: National Center for Health Statistics, Summary Health Statistics for the U.S. Population: National Health Interview Survey, 2002, Vital and Health Statistics, Series 10, No. 220, 2004; Internet site http://www.cdc.gov/nchs/nhis.htm; calculations by New Strategist

Table 11.17 Hospital Discharges and Length of Stay, 2002

(number of hospital discharges, discharge rate per 10,000 population, and average length of stay in days, for inpatients from nonfederal short-stay hospitals by age and sex, 2002; excludes newborn infants)

	total	female	male
Total discharges			
(in 000s)	**33,727**	**20,338**	**13,389**
Under age 15	2,540	1,128	1,412
Aged 15 to 44	10,736	7,830	2,906
Aged 45 to 64	7,723	3,968	3,755
Aged 65 or older	12,727	7,412	5,315
DISCHARGE RATE (PER 10,000 POPULATION)			
Total	**1,174.6**	**1,388.0**	**952.3**
Under age 15	418.7	380.8	454.9
Aged 15 to 44	864.2	1,265.7	466.0
Aged 45 to 64	1,158.9	1,159.7	1,158.1
Aged 65 or older	3,574.9	3,558.3	3,598.4
AVERAGE LENGTH OF STAY (DAYS)			
Total	**4.9**	**4.6**	**5.3**
Under age 15	4.5	4.7	4.4
Aged 15 to 44	3.7	3.3	4.9
Aged 45 to 64	5.0	4.8	5.2
Aged 65 or older	5.8	5.8	5.8

Source: National Center for Health Statistics, 2002 National Hospital Discharge Survey, Advance Data, No. 342, 2004; Internet site http://www.cdc.gov/nchs/about/major/hdasd/listpubs.htm; calculations by New Strategist

The Oldest Account for the Largest Share of Hospitalizations

Younger adults are most likely to be hospitalized for certain conditions, however.

In 2002, hospitals discharged more than 33 million people, more than one-third of them aged 65 or older. Older adults account for more than half of discharged patients with certain health conditions. People aged 65 or older account for 53 percent of patients discharged with a diagnosis of malignant neoplasm (cancer) and 64 percent of patients with any type of heart disease. Among all hospitalizations for pneumonia, 59 percent were among people aged 65 or older.

People aged 15 to 44 account for the largest share of hospitalizations for some conditions, however. As would be expected, nearly everyone who gave birth in a hospital was in this age group. But the age group also made up more than half of those hospitalized for poisoning, appendicitis, and mental health conditions—including pyschoses and alcohol dependence.

■ Hospice care, which allows the terminally ill to spend their final days in the comfort of their home or a homelike setting, is one of the few substitutes for hospital care.

People aged 45 or older account for most hospital discharges

(percent distribution of hospital discharges from nonfederal short-stay hospitals by age, 2002)

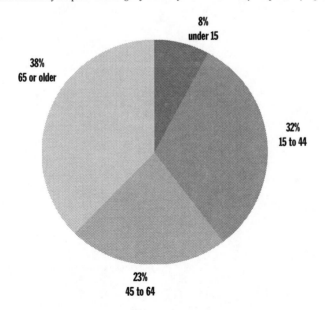

8%
under 15

38%
65 or older

32%
15 to 44

23%
45 to 64

Table 11.18 Number of Hospital Discharges by Diagnosis and Age, 2002

(number of hospital discharges from nonfederal short-stay hospitals by first-listed diagnosis and age, 2002; numbers in thousands)

	total	under 15	15 to 44	45 to 64	65 or older
All conditions	**33,727**	**2,540**	**10,736**	**7,723**	**12,727**
Infectious and parasitic diseases	877	156	204	185	332
Septicemia	341	12	34	76	219
Neoplasms	1,682	33	313	611	725
Malignant neoplasms	1,208	25	121	419	643
Malignant neoplasm of large intestine and rectum	159	–	5	46	107
Malignant neoplasm of trachea, bronchus, lung	160	–	5	55	100
Malignant neoplasm of breast	85	–	11	36	38
Benign neoplasms	427	–	183	178	61
Endocrine, nutritional, and metabolic diseases and immunity disorders	1,619	187	328	454	649
Diabetes mellitus	577	33	147	205	193
Volume depletion	508	129	53	77	249
Diseases of the blood and blood-forming organs	446	71	106	81	188
Mental disorders	2,464	149	1,422	620	273
Psychoses	1,704	–	957	431	224
Alcohol dependence syndrome	145	–	87	53	–
Diseases of the nervous system and sense organs	518	81	134	114	189
Diseases of the circulatory system	6,373	31	434	1,871	4,037
Heart disease	4,446	17	273	1,313	2,843
Acute myocardial infarction	818	–	57	259	501
Coronary atherosclerosis	1,096	–	48	432	615
Other ischemic heart disease	211	–	18	86	107
Cardiac dysrhythmias	788	–	45	174	562
Congestive heart failure	970	–	32	219	717
Cerebrovascular disease	942	–	40	229	669
Diseases of the respiratory system	3,542	730	382	697	1,732
Acute bronchitis and bronchiolitis	279	209	8	22	40
Pneumonia	1,312	204	116	216	776
Chronic bronchitis	520	–	16	161	343
Asthma	484	187	109	109	80
Diseases of the digestive system	3,320	216	839	955	1,310
Appendicitis	295	70	155	50	21
Noninfectious enteritis and colitis	310	54	89	66	100
Diverticula of intestine	262	–	36	77	149
Cholelithiasis	359	–	116	109	133
Diseases of the genitourinary system	1,817	88	580	458	690
Calculus of kidney and ureter	176	–	81	62	29
Complications of pregnancy, childbirth, and the puerperium	528	–	524	–	–
Diseases of the skin and subcutaneous tissue	601	–	158	151	199
Cellulitis and abscess	422	41	109	126	147

(continued)

	total	under 15	15 to 44	45 to 64	65 or older
Diseases of the musculoskeletal system and connective tissue	1,736	41	326	598	770
Osteoarthrosis and allied disorders	568	–	20	193	356
Intervertebral disc disorders	353	–	133	153	67
Congenital anomalies	178	124	31	15	7
Certain conditions originating in the perinatal period	166	165	–	–	–
Symptoms, signs, and ill-defined conditions	283	63	99	68	54
Injury and poisoning	2,697	233	780	621	1,063
Fractures, all sites	995	68	239	165	524
Fracture of neck of femur	315	–	6	24	282
Poisonings	214	18	120	48	28
Supplementary classifications	4,880	75	4,073	224	508
Females with deliveries	3,951	12	3,934	5	–

Note: (–) means category not applicable or sample is too small to make a reliable estimate.
Source: National Center for Health Statistics, 2002 National Hospital Discharge Survey, *Advance Data, No. 342, 2004; Internet site http://www.cdc.gov/nchs/about/major/hdasd/listpubs.htm; calculations by New Strategist*

Table 11.19 Percent Distribution of Hospital Discharges by Diagnosis and Age, 2002

(percent distribution of hospital discharges from nonfederal short-stay hospitals by first-listed diagnosis and age, 2002)

	total	under 15	15 to 44	45 to 64	65 or older
All conditions	100.0%	7.5%	31.8%	22.9%	37.7%
Infectious and parasitic diseases	100.0	17.8	23.3	21.1	37.9
Septicemia	100.0	3.5	10.0	22.3	64.2
Neoplasms	100.0	2.0	18.6	36.3	43.1
Malignant neoplasms	100.0	2.1	10.0	34.7	53.2
Malignant neoplasm of large intestine and rectum	100.0	–	3.1	28.9	67.3
Malignant neoplasm of trachea, bronchus, lung	100.0	–	3.1	34.4	62.5
Malignant neoplasm of breast	100.0	–	12.9	42.4	44.7
Benign neoplasms	100.0	–	42.9	41.7	14.3
Endocrine, nutritional, and metabolic diseases and immunity disorders	100.0	11.6	20.3	28.0	40.1
Diabetes mellitus	100.0	5.7	25.5	35.5	33.4
Volume depletion	100.0	25.4	10.4	15.2	49.0
Diseases of the blood and blood-forming organs	100.0	15.9	23.8	18.2	42.2
Mental disorders	100.0	6.0	57.7	25.2	11.1
Psychoses	100.0	–	56.2	25.3	13.1
Alcohol dependence syndrome	100.0	–	60.0	36.6	–
Diseases of the nervous system and sense organs	100.0	15.6	25.9	22.0	36.5
Diseases of the circulatory system	100.0	0.5	6.8	29.4	63.3
Heart disease	100.0	0.4	6.1	29.5	63.9
Acute myocardial infarction	100.0	–	7.0	31.7	61.2
Coronary atherosclerosis	100.0	–	4.4	39.4	56.1
Other ischemic heart disease	100.0	–	8.5	40.8	50.7
Cardiac dysrhythmias	100.0	–	5.7	22.1	71.3
Congestive heart failure	100.0	–	3.3	22.6	73.9
Cerebrovascular disease	100.0	–	4.2	24.3	71.0
Diseases of the respiratory system	100.0	20.6	10.8	19.7	48.9
Acute bronchitis and bronchiolitis	100.0	74.9	2.9	7.9	14.3
Pneumonia	100.0	15.5	8.8	16.5	59.1
Chronic bronchitis	100.0	–	3.1	31.0	66.0
Asthma	100.0	38.6	22.5	22.5	16.5
Diseases of the digestive system	100.0	6.5	25.3	28.8	39.5
Appendicitis	100.0	23.7	52.5	16.9	7.1
Noninfectious enteritis and colitis	100.0	17.4	28.7	21.3	32.3
Diverticula of intestine	100.0	–	13.7	29.4	56.9
Cholelithiasis	100.0	–	32.3	30.4	37.0
Diseases of the genitourinary system	100.0	4.8	31.9	25.2	38.0
Calculus of kidney and ureter	100.0	–	46.0	35.2	16.5
Complications of pregnancy, childbirth, and the puerperium	100.0	–	99.2	–	–
Diseases of the skin and subcutaneous tissue	100.0	–	26.3	25.1	33.1
Cellulitis and abscess	100.0	9.7	25.8	29.9	34.8

(continued)

	total	under 15	15 to 44	45 to 64	65 or older
Diseases of the musculoskeletal system and connective tissue	100.0%	2.4%	18.8%	34.4%	44.4%
Osteoarthrosis and allied disorders	100.0	–	3.5	34.0	62.7
Intervertebral disc disorders	100.0	–	37.7	43.3	19.0
Congenital anomalies	100.0	69.7	17.4	8.4	3.9
Certain conditions originating in the perinatal period	100.0	99.4	–	–	–
Symptoms, signs, and ill-defined conditions	100.0	22.3	35.0	24.0	19.1
Injury and poisoning	100.0	8.6	28.9	23.0	39.4
Fractures, all sites	100.0	6.8	24.0	16.6	52.7
Fracture of neck of femur	100.0	–	1.9	7.6	89.5
Poisonings	100.0	8.4	56.1	22.4	13.1
Supplementary classifications	100.0	1.5	83.5	4.6	10.4
Females with deliveries	100.0	0.3	99.6	0.1	–

Note: (–) means category not applicable or sample is too small to make a reliable estimate.
Source: National Center for Health Statistics, 2002 National Hospital Discharge Survey, Advance Data, No. 342, 2004; Internet site http://www.cdc.gov/nchs/about/major/hdasd/listpubs.htm; calculations by New Strategist

Heart Disease Is Most Likely to Lead to Hospitalization

But heart patients do not stay in the hospital any longer than average.

There are many different health conditions that can lead to a hospital stay. A few conditions account for a sizable share of hospitalizations. Based on the first-listed (primary) diagnosis on discharge, the most common health problems among the hospitalized are related to the circulatory system, accounting for 19 percent. Most of these are heart disease cases (13 percent). Respiratory illnesses are also a major cause of hospitalization, accounting for 11 percent of the total. The only other condition that accounts for a relatively large share of hospital stays is childbirth. Among all discharges in 2002, 12 percent were women who had given birth.

Although heart disease is a leading reason for hospitalization, it does not require as long a hospital stay as some other conditions. The average length of stay for all those with heart disease was 4.6 days, although those with myocardial infarction (heart attack) stayed a longer 5.6 days, on average.

Regardless of diagnosis, the average hospital stay in 2002 was shorter than in 1980. There are two reasons for the decline—insurance limits and treatment protocols. Insurance companies have generally reduced the number of days of hospitalization for which they will pay, which effectively requires patients to be discharged more quickly. But the treatment of many diseases has also changed, often reducing the need for long hospital stays.

■ At first, insurance curbs on hospital stays encouraged a "treat 'em and street 'em" approach. But protests from patients as well as health care providers resulted in more flexibility from insurers.

Hospital stays are getting shorter

(average length of hospital stay in days for discharges from short-stay hospitals, 1980 and 2002)

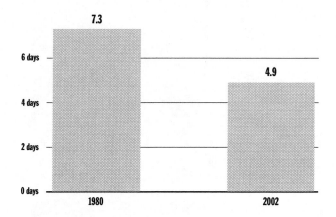

Table 11.20 Number and Rate of Discharges from Hospitals by Diagnosis, 2002

(number and percent distribution of hospital discharges and discharge rate per 10,000 population by first-listed diagnosis, 2002; excludes newborn infants; numbers in thousands)

	number	percent distribution	rate per 10,000 population
Total conditions	**33,727**	**100.0%**	**1,174.6**
Infectious and parasitic diseases	877	2.6	30.5
Septicemia	341	1.0	11.9
Neoplasms	1,682	5.0	58.6
Malignant neoplasms	1,208	3.6	42.1
Malignant neoplasm of large intestine and rectum	159	0.5	5.5
Malignant neoplasm of trachea, bronchus, and lung	160	0.5	5.6
Malignant neoplasm of breast	85	0.3	3.0
Benign neoplasms	427	1.3	14.9
Endocrine, nutritional, and metabolic diseases and immunity disorders	1,619	4.8	56.4
Diabetes mellitus	577	1.7	20.1
Volume depletion	508	1.5	17.7
Diseases of the blood and blood forming organs	446	1.3	15.5
Mental disorders	2,464	7.3	85.8
Psychoses	1,704	5.1	59.4
Alcohol dependence syndrome	145	0.4	5.1
Diseases of the nervous system and sense organs	518	1.5	18.0
Diseases of the circulatory system	6,373	18.9	222.0
Heart disease	4,446	13.2	154.8
Acute myocardial infarction	818	2.4	28.5
Coronary atherosclerosis	1,096	3.2	38.2
Other ischemic heart disease	211	0.6	7.3
Cardiac dysrhythmias	788	2.3	27.5
Congestive heart failure	970	2.9	33.8
Cerebrovascular disease	942	2.8	32.8
Diseases of the respiratory system	3,542	10.5	123.4
Acute bronchitis and bronchiolitis	279	0.8	9.7
Pneumonia	1,312	3.9	45.7
Chronic bronchitis	520	1.5	18.1
Asthma	484	1.4	16.8
Diseases of the digestive system	3,320	9.8	115.6
Appendicitis	295	0.9	10.3
Noninfectious enteritis and colitis	310	0.9	10.8
Diverticula of intestine	262	0.8	9.1
Cholelithiasis	359	1.1	12.5
Diseases of the genitourinary system	1,817	5.4	63.3
Calculus of kidney and ureter	176	0.5	6.1
Complications of pregnancy, childbirth, and the puerperium	528	1.6	18.4

(continued)

	number	percent distribution	rate per 10,000 population
Diseases of the skin and subcutaneous tissue	601	1.8%	20.9
Cellulitis and abscess	422	1.3	14.7
Diseases of the musculoskeletal system and connective tissue	1,736	5.1	60.5
Osteoarthrosis and allied disorders	568	1.7	19.8
Intervertebral disc disorders	353	1.0	12.3
Congenital anomalies	178	0.5	6.2
Certain conditions originating in the perinatal period	166	0.5	5.8
Symptoms, signs, and ill-defined conditions	283	0.8	9.9
Injury and poisoning	2,697	8.0	93.9
Fractures, all sites	995	3.0	34.7
Fracture of neck of femur	315	0.9	11.0
Poisonings	214	0.6	7.4
Supplementary classifications	4,880	14.5	170.0
Females with deliveries	3,951	11.7	137.6

Source: National Center for Health Statistics, 2002 National Hospital Discharge Survey, Advance Data, No. 342, 2004; Internet site http://www.cdc.gov/nchs/about/major/hdasd/listpubs.htm; calculations by New Strategist

Table 11.21 Length of Hospital Stay by Diagnosis, 1980 and 2002

(average length of stay in days for discharges from short-stay hospitals by first-listed diagnosis, 1980 and 2002, and change in days, 1980–2002; excludes newborn infants)

	2002	1980	change, 1980–2002
Total conditions	**4.9**	**7.3**	**–2.4**
Infectious and parasitic diseases	6.4	6.9	–0.5
Septicemia	8.3	14.3	–6.0
Neoplasms	6.1	10.5	–4.4
Malignant neoplasms	7.1	11.9	–4.8
Malignant neoplasm of large intestine and rectum	8.7	15.7	–7.0
Malignant neoplasm of trachea, bronchus, and lung	7.5	12.8	–5.3
Malignant neoplasm of breast	2.9	10.9	–8.0
Benign neoplasms	3.3	6.2	–2.9
Endocrine, nutritional, and metabolic diseases and immunity disorders	4.3	9.6	–5.3
Diabetes mellitus	5.0	10.5	–5.5
Volume depletion	3.8	8.9	–5.1
Diseases of the blood and blood forming organs	4.4	7.2	–2.8
Mental disorders	7.1	11.6	–4.5
Psychoses	8.0	14.8	–6.8
Alcohol dependence syndrome	5.8	10.1	–4.3
Diseases of the nervous system and sense organs	5.1	5.4	–0.3
Diseases of the circulatory system	4.7	10.0	–5.3
Heart disease	4.6	9.5	–4.9
Acute myocardial infarction	5.6	12.6	–7.0
Coronary atherosclerosis	3.5	10.0	–6.5
Other ischemic heart disease	2.6	7.7	–5.1
Cardiac dysrhythmias	3.6	7.6	–4.0
Congestive heart failure	5.4	10.4	–5.0
Cerebrovascular disease	5.3	12.4	–7.1
Diseases of the respiratory system	5.3	6.3	–1.0
Acute bronchitis and bronchiolitis	3.4	4.7	–1.3
Pneumonia	5.7	8.3	–2.6
Chronic bronchitis	5.3	–	–
Asthma	3.2	6.0	–2.8
Diseases of the digestive system	4.9	7.0	–2.1
Appendicitis	3.2	5.5	–2.3
Noninfectious enteritis and colitis	4.7	5.6	–0.9
Diverticula of intestine	5.8	–	–
Cholelithiasis	4.0	9.3	–5.3
Diseases of the genitourinary system	3.7	5.6	–1.9
Calculus of kidney and ureter	2.2	5.0	–2.8
Complications of pregnancy, childbirth, the puerperium	2.7	2.5	0.2

(continued)

	2002	1980	change, 1980–2002
Diseases of the skin and subcutaneous tissue	5.3	8.0	–2.7
Cellulitis and abscess	5.2	8.0	–2.8
Diseases of the musculoskeletal system and connective tissue	3.9	8.3	–4.4
Osteoarthrosis and allied disorders	4.2	–	–
Intervertebral disc disorders	2.8	9.9	–7.1
Congenital anomalies	5.8	6.6	–0.8
Certain conditions originating in the perinatal period	11.1	8.7	2.4
Symptoms, signs, and ill-defined conditions	2.7	4.5	–1.8
Injury and poisoning	5.3	7.7	–2.4
Fractures, all sites	5.4	10.8	–5.4
Fracture of neck of femur	6.6	20.6	–14.0
Poisonings	2.7	–	–
Supplementary classifications	3.8	3.7	0.1
Females with deliveries	2.6	3.8	–1.2

Note: (–) means data not available.
Source: National Center for Health Statistics, Trends in Hospital Utilization: United States, 1988–92, *Vital and Health Statistics, Series 13, No. 124, 1996; and 2002* National Hospital Discharge Survey, *Advance Data, No. 342, 2004; Internet site http://www. cdc.gov/nchs/about/major/hdasd/listpubs.htm; calculations by New Strategist*

Hospitals Provide a Wide Variety of Services

Surgeries account for a sizable share.

Hospitals provide a wide variety of services, from basic support care to diagnostics to surgery and maternity services. In 2002, hospitals performed more than 42 million procedures. The largest share (29 percent) is accounted for by the general category, "miscellaneous diagnostic and therapeutic procedures." Operations on the cardiovascular system make up another 16 percent. Obstetrical procedures also account for about 16 percent of the total. Thirteen percent are operations on the digestive system.

People aged 65 or older account for the largest share of procedures. This group also makes up the largest share of hospital patients, so it is not surprising that they account for more procedures than younger age groups do.

■ Some procedures that were once performed only in a hospital setting have migrated to less expensive venues, including doctor's offices.

Most hospital procedures are performed on people aged 45 or older

(percent distribution of procedures performed in nonfederal short-stay hospitals, by age of patient, 2002)

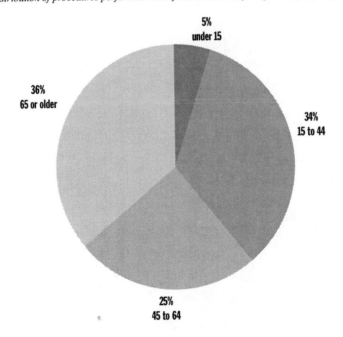

5%
under 15

36%
65 or older

34%
15 to 44

25%
45 to 64

Table 11.22 Number of Hospital Discharges by Procedure and Age, 2002

(number of hospital discharges from nonfederal short-stay hospitals by procedure category and age, 2002; numbers in thousands)

	total	under 15	15 to 44	45 to 64	65 or older
Total procedures	**42,533**	**2,084**	**14,419**	**10,743**	**15,286**
Operations on the nervous system	1,101	215	337	256	293
Spinal tap	316	142	93	42	39
Operations on the endocrine system	102	–	30	40	31
Operations on the eye	86	12	27	21	25
Operations on the ear	46	19	–	7	–
Operations on the nose, mouth, and pharynx	269	66	93	59	52
Operations on the respiratory system	1,022	57	179	304	482
Bronchoscopy with or without biopsy	251	15	39	69	127
Operations on the cardiovascular system	6,813	210	681	2384	3538
Removal of coronary artery obstruction and insertion of stent(s)	1,204	–	76	517	608
Coronary artery bypass graft	515	–	19	217	279
Cardiac catheterization	1,328	–	107	555	659
Insertion, replacement, removal, and revision of pacemaker	420	–	–	47	358
Hemodialysis	552	–	85	210	251
Operations on the hemic and lymphatic system	354	22	55	130	147
Operations on the digestive system	5,597	222	1307	1607	2461
Endoscopy of small intestine with or without biopsy	1,032	16	160	279	577
Endoscopy of large intestine with or without biopsy	578	–	76	137	358
Partial excision of large intestine	263	–	35	79	145
Appendectomy, excluding incidental	329	70	176	57	25
Cholecystectomy	436	–	142	140	151
Lysis of peritoneal adhesions	342	3	143	103	93
Operations on the urinary system	955	38	232	299	386
Cystoscopy with or without biopsy	173	–	40	52	77
Operations on the male genital organs	262	18	12	79	152
Prostatectomy	195	–	–	66	128
Operations on the female genital organs	2,161	5	1256	668	231
Oophorectomy and salpingo-oophorectomy	533	–	224	249	60
Bilateral destruction or occlusion of fallopian tubes	329	–	329	–	–
Hysterectomy	669	–	344	262	63
Obstetrical procedures	6,646	21	6617	8	–
Episiotomy with or without forceps or vacuum extraction	780	–	776	–	–
Artificial rupture of membranes	901	–	899	–	–
Caesarean section	1,059	–	1055	–	–
Repair of current obstetric laceration	1,234	–	1228	–	–
Operations on the musculoskeletal system	3,442	173	811	1087	1371
Partial excision of bone	218	13	67	89	49
Reduction of fracture	606	50	186	122	247
Open reduction of fracture with internal fixation	414	15	129	86	185
Excision or destruction of intervertebral disc	323	–	120	147	55
Total hip replacement	193	–	11	67	114
Total knee replacement	381	–	10	131	241

(continued)

	total	under 15	15 to 44	45 to 64	65 or older
Operations on the integumentary system	1,348	–	388	415	429
Debridement of wound, infection, or burn	361	–	88	114	140
Miscellaneous diagnostic and therapeutic procedures	12,332	890	2382	3381	5679
Computerized axial tomography	703	42	157	169	336
Arteriography and angiocardiography using contrast material	2,058	–	194	823	1028
Diagnostic ultrasound	773	–	133	192	404
Respiratory therapy	1,070	207	144	243	476
Insertion of endotracheal tube	477	48	62	126	241
Injection or infusion of cancer chemotherapeutic substance	217	34	51	72	61

Note: (–) means category not applicable or sample is too small to make a reliable estimate.
Source: National Center for Health Statistics, 2002 National Hospital Discharge Survey, Advance Data, No. 342, 2004; Internet site http://www.cdc.gov/nchs/about/major/hdasd/listpubs.htm; calculations by New Strategist

Table 11.23 Percent Distribution of Hospital Discharges by Procedure and Age, 2002

(percent distribution of hospital discharges from nonfederal short-stay hospitals by procedure category and age, 2002)

	total	under 15	15 to 44	45 to 64	65 or older
Total procedures	**100.0%**	**4.9%**	**33.9%**	**25.3%**	**35.9%**
Operations on the nervous system	100.0	19.5	30.6	23.3	26.6
Spinal tap	100.0	44.9	29.4	13.3	12.3
Operations on the endocrine system	100.0	–	29.4	39.2	30.4
Operations on the eye	100.0	14.0	31.4	24.4	29.1
Operations on the ear	100.0	41.3	–	15.2	–
Operations on the nose, mouth, and pharynx	100.0	24.5	34.6	21.9	19.3
Operations on the respiratory system	100.0	5.6	17.5	29.7	47.2
Bronchoscopy with or without biopsy	100.0	6.0	15.5	27.5	50.6
Operations on the cardiovascular system	100.0	3.1	10.0	35.0	51.9
Removal of coronary artery obstruction and insertion of stent(s)	100.0	–	6.3	42.9	50.5
Coronary artery bypass graft	100.0	–	3.7	42.1	54.2
Cardiac catheterization	100.0	–	8.1	41.8	49.6
Insertion, replacement, removal, and revision of pacemaker	100.0	–	–	11.2	85.2
Hemodialysis	100.0	–	15.4	38.0	45.5
Operations on the hemic and lymphatic system	100.0	6.2	15.5	36.7	41.5
Operations on the digestive system	100.0	4.0	23.4	28.7	44.0
Endoscopy of small intestine with or without biopsy	100.0	1.6	15.5	27.0	55.9
Endoscopy of large intestine with or without biopsy	100.0	–	13.1	23.7	61.9
Partial excision of large intestine	100.0	–	13.3	30.0	55.1
Appendectomy, excluding incidental	100.0	21.3	53.5	17.3	7.6
Cholecystectomy	100.0	–	32.6	32.1	34.6
Lysis of peritoneal adhesions	100.0	0.9	41.8	30.1	27.2
Operations on the urinary system	100.0	4.0	24.3	31.3	40.4
Cystoscopy with or without biopsy	100.0	–	23.1	30.1	44.5
Operations on the male genital organs	100.0	6.9	4.6	30.2	58.0
Prostatectomy	100.0	–	–	33.8	65.6
Operations on the female genital organs	100.0	0.2	58.1	30.9	10.7
Oophorectomy and salpingo-oophorectomy	100.0	–	42.0	46.7	11.3
Bilateral destruction or occlusion of fallopian tubes	100.0	–	100.0	–	–
Hysterectomy	100.0	–	51.4	39.2	9.4
Obstetrical procedures	100.0	0.3	99.6	0.1	–
Episiotomy with or without forceps or vacuum extraction	100.0	–	99.5	–	–
Artificial rupture of membranes	100.0	–	99.8	–	–
Caesarean section	100.0	–	99.6	–	–
Repair of current obstetric laceration	100.0	–	99.5	–	–
Operations on the musculoskeletal system	100.0	5.0	23.6	31.6	39.8
Partial excision of bone	100.0	6.0	30.7	40.8	22.5
Reduction of fracture	100.0	8.3	30.7	20.1	40.8
Open reduction of fracture with internal fixation	100.0	3.6	31.2	20.8	44.7
Excision or destruction of intervertebral disc	100.0	–	37.2	45.5	17.0
Total hip replacement	100.0	–	5.7	34.7	59.1
Total knee replacement	100.0	–	2.6	34.4	63.3

(continued)

	total	under 15	15 to 44	45 to 64	65 or older
Operations on the integumentary system	100.0%	–	28.8%	30.8%	31.8%
Debridement of wound, infection, or burn	100.0	–	24.4	31.6	38.8
Miscellaneous diagnostic and therapeutic procedures	100.0	7.2%	19.3	27.4	46.1
Computerized axial tomography	100.0	6.0	22.3	24.0	47.8
Arteriography and angiocardiography using contrast material	100.0	–	9.4	40.0	50.0
Diagnostic ultrasound	100.0	–	17.2	24.8	52.3
Respiratory therapy	100.0	19.3	13.5	22.7	44.5
Insertion of endotracheal tube	100.0	10.1	13.0	26.4	50.5
Injection or infusion of cancer chemotherapeutic substance	100.0	15.7	23.5	33.2	28.1

Note: (–) means category not applicable or sample is too small to make a reliable estimate.
Source: National Center for Health Statistics, 2002 National Hospital Discharge Survey, Advance Data, No. 342, 2004; Internet site http://www.cdc.gov/nchs/about/major/hdasd/listpubs.htm; calculations by New Strategist

Table 11.24   Discharges from Hospitals by Procedure, 2002

(number and percent distribution of hospital discharges and discharge rate per 10,000 population for all listed procedures, 2002; excludes newborn infants; numbers in thousands)

	number	percent distribution	rate per 10,000 population
Total procedures	**42,533**	**100.0%**	**1,481.4**
Operations on the nervous system	1,101	2.6	38.3
Spinal tap	316	0.7	11.0
Operations on the endocrine system	102	0.2	3.6
Operations on the eye	86	0.2	3.0
Operations on the ear	46	0.1	1.6
Operations on the nose, mouth, and pharynx	269	0.6	9.4
Operations on the respiratory system	1,022	2.4	35.6
Bronchoscopy with or without biopsy	251	0.6	8.7
Operations on the cardiovascular system	6,813	16.0	237.3
Removal of coronary artery obstruction and insertion of stent(s)	1,204	2.8	41.9
Coronary artery bypass graft	515	1.2	17.9
Cardiac catheterization	1,328	3.1	46.2
Insertion, replacement, removal, and revision of pacemaker	420	1.0	14.6
Hemodialysis	552	1.3	19.2
Operations on the hemic and lymphatic system	354	0.8	12.3
Operations on the digestive system	5,597	13.2	194.9
Endoscopy of small intestine with or without biopsy	1,032	2.4	35.9
Endoscopy of large intestine with or without biopsy	578	1.4	20.1
Partial excision of large intestine	263	0.6	9.2
Appendectomy, excluding incidental	329	0.8	11.5
Cholecystectomy	436	1.0	15.2
Lysis of peritoneal adhesions	342	0.8	11.9
Operations on the urinary system	955	2.2	33.2
Cystoscopy with or without biopsy	173	0.4	6.0
Operations on the male genital organs	262	0.6	9.1
Prostatectomy	195	0.5	6.8
Operations on the female genital organs	2,161	5.1	75.3
Oophorectomy and salpingo-oophorectomy	533	1.3	18.6
Bilateral destruction or occlusion of fallopian tubes	329	0.8	11.5
Hysterectomy	669	1.6	23.3
Obstetrical procedures	6,646	15.6	231.5
Episiotomy with or without forceps or vacuum extraction	780	1.8	27.2
Artificial rupture of membranes	901	2.1	31.4
Caesarean section	1,059	2.5	36.9
Repair of current obstetric laceration	1,234	2.9	43.0
Operations on the musculoskeletal system	3,442	8.1	119.9
Partial excision of bone	218	0.5	7.6
Reduction of fracture	606	1.4	21.1
Open reduction of fracture with internal fixation	414	1.0	14.4
Excision or destruction of intervertebral disc	323	0.8	11.3
Total hip replacement	193	0.5	6.7
Total knee replacement	381	0.9	13.3

(continued)

	number	percent distribution	rate per 10,000 population
Operations on the integumentary system	1,348	3.2%	46.9
Debridement of wound, infection, or burn	361	0.8	12.6
Miscellaneous diagnostic and therapeutic procedures	12,332	29.0	429.5
Computerized axial tomography	703	1.7	24.5
Arteriography and angiocardiography using contrast material	2,058	4.8	71.7
Diagnostic ultrasound	773	1.8	26.9
Respiratory therapy	1,070	2.5	37.3
Insertion of endotracheal tube	477	1.1	16.6
Injection or infusion of cancer chemotherapeutic substance	217	0.5	7.6

Source: National Center for Health Statistics, 2002 National Hospital Discharge Survey, *Advance Data, No. 342, 2004; Internet site http://www.cdc.gov/nchs/about/major/hdasd/listpubs.htm; calculations by New Strategist*

12

Mental Health

■ **Twenty-two percent of adults have a diagnosable mental disorder in a given year.**

Among the most common are depressive disorders, which affect nearly 10 percent of adults, and anxiety disorders, which affect 13 percent.

■ **Most Americans would seek help if they had a mental health problem.**

The percentage of Americans who sought help in the past year is highest among people aged 18 to 29, at 20 percent.

■ **Women are more likely than men to report mental health problems.**

Some of the differences between the sexes may be due to women's greater willingness to admit having problems.

■ **Mental health problems are greatest among those with low incomes.**

People living in households with incomes below $20,000 are much more likely than those with higher incomes to feel like "everything is an effort."

■ **Many teenagers have suicidal thoughts.**

Twenty-one percent of girls in grades nine through twelve say they have considered suicide in the past year.

■ **Nine percent of adults had a serious mental illness in 2003.**

Among people with serious mental health problems, only 47 percent received mental health treatment.

More than One in Five Adults Have a Mental Disorder

These can range from phobias to serious mental illness.

Twenty-two percent of adults have a diagnosable mental disorder in a given year, according to the National Institute of Mental Health. Among the most common are depressive disorders, which affect nearly 10 percent of adults, and anxiety disorders, which affect 13 percent. The prevalence of mental disorders in the population means that many Americans know someone who has experienced a mental health problem, even if they have not had a problem themselves.

Most adults believe the medications prescribed for emotional, nervous, or other mental disorders help those with mental problems control their symptoms. But they also have concerns about the drugs, with three out of four agreeing at least somewhat that the medications are addictive and often have unacceptable side effects. Only 15 percent think taking them is a sign of weakness, however.

The public may worry about medications, but most (52 percent) are willing to seek advice when they have a problem. The percentage of people who have sought help from a mental health professional in the past year is highest among those aged 18 to 29 (20 percent), but falls to only 5 percent among people aged 65 or older.

■ Older Americans are less likely to consult a mental health professional, but they are also less likely than younger adults to say their mental health status is only fair or poor.

Young adults are most likely to seek help for mental problems

(percent of people aged 18 or older who sought help from mental health professionals in the past year, 2004)

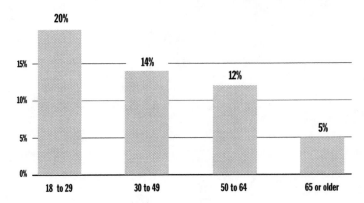

Table 12.1 Prevalence of Mental Disorders, 2001

(percentage or number of people with selected mental disorders, 2001)

	prevalence
Adults aged 18 or older with any diagnosable mental disorder	**22.1% in a given year**
Adults aged 18 or older with any depressive disorder	9.5 % in a given year
Percent with major depressive disorder	5.0 % in a given year
Percent with dysthymic disorder	5.4 % during lifetime
Percent with bipolar disorder	1.2 % in a given year
Adults aged 18 or older with schizophrenia	1.1 % in a given year
Adults aged 18 to 54 with anxiety disorder	13.3 % in a given year
Percent with panic disorder	1.7 % in a given year
Percent with obsessive-compulsive disorder	2.3 % in a given year
Percent with post-traumatic stress disorder	3.6 % in a given year
Percent with generalized anxiety disorder	2.8 % in a given year
Percent with social phobia	3.7 % in a given year
Percent with agoraphobia	2.2 % in a given year
Percent with specific phobia	4.4 % in a given year
Eating disorders	
Anorexia nervosa	0.5 to 3.7% of females during lifetime
Bulimia	1.1 to 4.2% of females during lifetime
Binge eating disorders	2 to 5% of population in 6-month period
Attention deficit hyperactivity disorder	**4.1% of children aged 9 to 17 in 6-month period**
Autism	**1 to 2 people per 1,000 population**
Alzheimer's disease	**4 million**

Source: National Institute of Mental Health, The Numbers Count: Mental Disorders in America, *2001, Internet Site, http://www.nimh.nih.gov/publicat/numbers.cfm*

Table 12.2 **Medications for People with Mental Health Problems, 2002**

"Please tell me how much you agree or disagree with the following statements about medicines prescribed by doctors that are intended to help people who are having problems with their emotions, nerves, or their mental health."

(number of respondents aged 18 or older and percent distribution by response, 2002)

	number of respondents	percent distribution
"These medications help people control their symptoms. Do you strongly agree, agree somewhat, disagree somewhat, or strongly disagree?"		
Total respondents	**1,393**	**100.0%**
Strongly agree	369	26.5
Agree somewhat	809	58.1
Disagree somewhat	103	7.4
Strongly disagree	43	3.1
Don't know	57	4.1
No answer	15	1.1
"These medications are addictive."		
Total respondents	**1,393**	**100.0**
Strongly agree	472	33.9
Agree somewhat	564	40.5
Disagree somewhat	181	13.0
Strongly disagree	53	3.8
Don't know	108	7.8
No answer	15	1.1
"Taking medications is a sign of weakness."		
Total respondents	**1,393**	**100.0**
Strongly agree	59	4.2
Agree somewhat	145	10.4
Disagree somewhat	437	31.4
Strongly disagree	710	51.0
Don't know	31	2.2
No answer	11	0.8
"These medications often have unacceptable side effects."		
Total respondents	**1,393**	**100.0**
Strongly agree	413	29.6
Agree somewhat	646	46.4
Disagree somewhat	186	13.4
Strongly disagree	44	3.2
Don't know	92	6.6
No answer	12	0.9

Source: General Social Survey, National Opinion Research Center, University of Chicago

Table 12.3 Solve Problems on Your Own or Get Advice, 2002

"When you have a problem, do you prefer to solve it on your own or do you like to talk to other people to get advice, help, or information?"

(number of respondents aged 18 or older and percent distribution by response, 2002)

	number of respondents	percent distribution
Total respondents	**1,393**	**100.0%**
On own	593	42.6
Get advice	729	52.3
Something else	50	3.6
Don't know	14	1.0
No answer	7	0.5

Source: General Social Survey, National Opinion Research Center, University of Chicago

Table 12.4 **Self-Reported Mental Health and Help-Seeking Behavior by Selected Characteristics, 2004**

(percent distribution of people aged 18 or older by self-reported mental health status, and percent who sought help from mental health professionals in past year, by selected characteristics, 2004)

SELF-REPORTED MENTAL HEALTH STATUS

	excellent	good	fair/poor
Total people	**51%**	**37%**	**12%**
Age			
Aged 18 to 29	55	29	16
Aged 30 to 49	55	34	11
Aged 50 to 64	43	43	14
Aged 65 or older	43	46	11
Household income			
Under $20,000	31	39	30
$20,000 to $29,999	42	43	15
$30,000 to $49,999	44	41	15
$50,000 to $74,999	62	32	6
$75,000 or more	63	34	3
Education			
High school or less	41	40	19
Some college	52	38	10
College graduate	64	30	6
Postgraduate	61	35	4

PERCENT SEEKING HELP FROM A MENTAL HEALTH PROFESSIONAL IN THE PAST 12 MONTHS

Total people	**12%**
Aged 18 to 29	20
Aged 30 to 49	14
Aged 50 to 64	12
Aged 65 or older	5

Source: The Gallup Organization, Assessing Americans' Mental Health, *December 2, 2004, Internet site http://www.gallup.com*

Women Are More Likely to Report Mental Health Problems

The prevalence of mental health conditions also varies by race and Hispanic origin.

Emotional extremes—either up or down—are a common manifestation of mental health problems. It's no surprise, then, that one of the most commonly reported mental problems is nervousness or restlessness, with 11 percent of adults saying they experience this feeling at least some of the time.

Women are more likely than men to report experiencing the mental states examined here. Thirteen percent of women say they feel sad at least some of the time compared with 8 percent of men, for example. Some of the differences between the sexes may be a result of women's greater willingness to admit having problems.

There are also differences by race and Hispanic origin in the likelihood of experiencing mental problems. Blacks and Hispanics are more likely than non-Hispanic whites to report feeling sad at least some of the time. Blacks are more likely than other groups to feel as though "everything is an effort." But non-Hispanic whites are more likely than other racial or ethnic groups to feel nervous or restless at least some of the time.

■ The lower socioeconomic status of blacks and Hispanics is probably behind their greater likelihood of experiencing certain mental problems.

Blacks are most likely to feel that "everything is an effort"

(percent of people aged 18 or older with selected mental health conditions during the past thirty days some, most, or all of the time, by race and Hispanic origin, 2002)

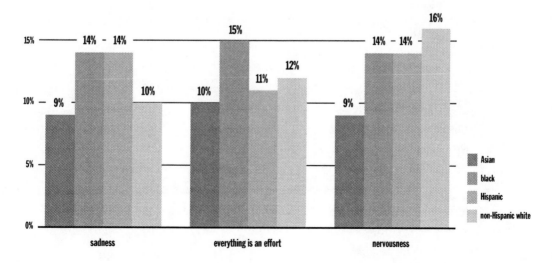

Table 12.5 Mental Health Conditions among Adults by Age, 2002

(number and percent of people aged 18 or older with selected mental health conditions during the past thirty days, by type of condition and age, 2002; numbers in thousands)

	total	18 to 44	45 to 64	65 to 74	75 or older
Total people	205,825	108,114	64,650	17,809	15,252
Sadness					
All or most of the time	5,838	2,903	2,083	463	388
Some of the time	15,746	7,775	5,269	1,420	1,281
Hopelessness					
All or most of the time	4,264	2,078	1,640	266	280
Some of the time	8,246	4,212	2,897	548	589
Worthlessness					
All or most of the time	3,981	1,752	1,632	265	332
Some of the time	6,606	3,355	2,236	496	519
Everything is an effort					
All or most of the time	9,678	5,086	3,186	693	714
Some of the time	15,135	8,014	4,872	1,196	1,052
Nervousness					
All or most of the time	8,251	3,834	3,142	646	629
Some of the time	22,577	12,414	7,062	1,738	1,363
Restlessness					
All or most of the time	9,879	5,166	3,533	613	567
Some of the time	22,543	12,145	7,217	1,797	1,384
PERCENT WITH CONDITION BY AGE					
Total people	100.0%	100.0%	100.0%	100.0%	100.0%
Sadness					
All or most of the time	2.9	2.7	3.3	2.7	2.6
Some of the time	7.8	7.3	8.3	8.1	8.7
Hopelessness					
All or most of the time	2.1	2.0	2.6	1.5	1.9
Some of the time	4.1	4.0	4.6	3.1	4.0
Worthlessness					
All or most of the time	2.0	1.6	2.6	1.5	2.3
Some of the time	3.3	3.2	3.5	2.8	3.5
Everything is an effort					
All or most of the time	4.8	4.8	5.0	4.0	4.9
Some of the time	7.5	7.5	7.7	6.9	7.2
Nervousness					
All or most of the time	4.1	3.6	4.9	3.7	4.3
Some of the time	11.2	11.7	11.1	10.0	9.3
Restlessness					
All or most of the time	4.9	4.9	5.6	3.5	3.9
Some of the time	11.2	11.4	11.4	10.3	9.4

(continued)

PERCENT DISTRIBUTION OF THOSE WITH CONDITION BY AGE	total	18 to 44	45 to 64	65 to 74	75 or older
Total people	**100.0%**	**52.5%**	**31.4%**	**8.7%**	**7.4%**
Sadness					
All or most of the time	100.0	49.7	35.7	7.9	6.6
Some of the time	100.0	49.4	33.5	9.0	8.1
Hopelessness					
All or most of the time	100.0	48.7	38.5	6.2	6.6
Some of the time	100.0	51.1	35.1	6.6	7.1
Worthlessness					
All or most of the time	100.0	44.0	41.0	6.7	8.3
Some of the time	100.0	50.8	33.8	7.5	7.9
Everything is an effort					
All or most of the time	100.0	52.6	32.9	7.2	7.4
Some of the time	100.0	53.0	32.2	7.9	7.0
Nervousness					
All or most of the time	100.0	46.5	38.1	7.8	7.6
Some of the time	100.0	55.0	31.3	7.7	6.0
Restlessness					
All or most of the time	100.0	52.3	35.8	6.2	5.7
Some of the time	100.0	53.9	32.0	8.0	6.1

Source: National Center for Health Statistics, Summary Health Statistics for U.S. Adults: National Health Interview Survey, 2002, *Series 10, No. 222, 2004; calculations by New Strategist*

Table 12.6 Mental Health Conditions among Adults by Sex, 2002

(number and percent of people aged 18 or older with selected mental health conditions during the past thirty days, by type of condition and sex, 2002; numbers in thousands)

	total	men	women
Total people	**205,825**	**98,749**	**107,076**
Sadness			
All or most of the time	5,838	2,001	3,836
Some of the time	15,746	6,133	9,612
Hopelessness			
All or most of the time	4,264	1,565	2,699
Some of the time	8,246	3,229	5,017
Worthlessness			
All or most of the time	3,981	1,407	2,574
Some of the time	6,606	2,920	3,686
Everything is an effort			
All or most of the time	9,678	4,090	5,588
Some of the time	15,135	5,958	9,177
Nervousness			
All or most of the time	8,251	3,034	5,217
Some of the time	22,577	8,801	13,776
Restlessness			
All or most of the time	9,879	4,161	5,717
Some of the time	22,543	9,778	12,765
PERCENT WITH CONDITION BY SEX			
Total people	**100.0%**	**100.0%**	**100.0%**
Sadness			
All or most of the time	2.9	2.1	3.6
Some of the time	7.8	6.3	9.1
Hopelessness			
All or most of the time	2.1	1.6	2.6
Some of the time	4.1	3.3	4.8
Worthlessness			
All or most of the time	2.0	1.4	2.4
Some of the time	3.3	3.0	3.5
Everything is an effort			
All or most of the time	4.8	4.2	5.3
Some of the time	7.5	6.1	8.7
Nervousness			
All or most of the time	4.1	3.1	4.9
Some of the time	11.2	9.0	13.1
Restlessness			
All or most of the time	4.9	4.2	5.4
Some of the time	11.2	10.1	12.1

(continued)

PERCENT DISTRIBUTION OF THOSE WITH CONDITION BY SEX	total	men	women
Total people	**100.0%**	**48.0%**	**52.0%**
Sadness			
All or most of the time	100.0	34.3	65.7
Some of the time	100.0	38.9	61.0
Hopelessness			
All or most of the time	100.0	36.7	63.3
Some of the time	100.0	39.2	60.8
Worthlessness			
All or most of the time	100.0	35.3	64.7
Some of the time	100.0	44.2	55.8
Everything is an effort			
All or most of the time	100.0	42.3	57.7
Some of the time	100.0	39.4	60.6
Nervousness			
All or most of the time	100.0	36.8	63.2
Some of the time	100.0	39.0	61.0
Restlessness			
All or most of the time	100.0	42.1	57.9
Some of the time	100.0	43.4	56.6

Source: National Center for Health Statistics, Summary Health Statistics for U.S. Adults: National Health Interview Survey, 2002, *Series 10, No. 222, 2004; calculations by New Strategist*

Table 12.7 Mental Health Conditions among Adults by Race and Hispanic Origin, 2002

(number and percent of people aged 18 or older with selected mental health conditions during the past thirty days, by type of condition, race, and Hispanic origin, 2002; numbers in thousands)

	total	Asian	black	Hispanic	non-Hispanic white
Total people	205,825	7,270	23,499	22,691	149,584
Sadness					
All or most of the time	5,838	129	882	831	3,875
Some of the time	15,746	456	2,271	2,064	10,610
Hopelessness					
All or most of the time	4,264	84	481	665	2,899
Some of the time	8,246	248	1,088	1,038	5,657
Worthlessness					
All or most of the time	3,981	80	490	490	2,799
Some of the time	6,606	203	781	849	4,613
Everything is an effort					
All or most of the time	9,678	202	1,613	1,040	6,546
Some of the time	15,135	475	1,835	1,338	11,144
Nervousness					
All or most of the time	8,251	110	822	988	6,114
Some of the time	22,577	477	2,341	2,103	17,213
Restlessness					
All or most of the time	9,879	119	1,099	1,052	7,389
Some of the time	22,543	450	2,486	1,959	17,209
PERCENT WITH CONDITION BY RACE AND HISPANIC ORIGIN					
Total people	100.0%	100.0%	100.0%	100.0%	100.0%
Sadness					
All or most of the time	2.9	1.9	3.7	4.1	2.6
Some of the time	7.8	6.6	10.0	9.5	7.2
Hopelessness					
All or most of the time	2.1	1.3	2.0	3.2	2.0
Some of the time	4.1	3.6	4.9	5.1	3.8
Worthlessness					
All or most of the time	2.0	1.2	2.1	2.5	1.9
Some of the time	3.3	2.9	3.4	4.1	3.1
Everything is an effort					
All or most of the time	4.8	3.3	6.8	5.1	4.4
Some of the time	7.5	6.7	8.1	6.0	7.6
Nervousness					
All or most of the time	4.1	1.8	3.5	4.8	4.1
Some of the time	11.2	6.7	10.2	9.6	11.8
Restlessness					
All or most of the time	4.9	2.1	4.7	5.0	5.0
Some of the time	11.2	6.6	10.8	9.1	11.8

(continued)

PERCENT DISTRIBUTION OF THOSE WITH CONDITION BY RACE AND HISPANIC ORIGIN	total	Asian	black	Hispanic	non-Hispanic white
Total people	**100.0%**	**3.5%**	**11.4%**	**11.0%**	**72.7%**
Sadness					
All or most of the time	100.0	2.2	15.1	14.2	66.4
Some of the time	100.0	2.9	14.4	13.1	67.4
Hopelessness					
All or most of the time	100.0	2.0	11.3	15.6	68.0
Some of the time	100.0	3.0	13.2	12.6	68.6
Worthlessness					
All or most of the time	100.0	2.0	12.3	12.3	70.3
Some of the time	100.0	3.1	11.8	12.9	69.8
Everything is an effort					
All or most of the time	100.0	2.1	16.7	10.7	67.6
Some of the time	100.0	3.1	12.1	8.8	73.6
Nervousness					
All or most of the time	100.0	1.3	10.0	12.0	74.1
Some of the time	100.0	2.1	10.4	9.3	76.2
Restlessness					
All or most of the time	100.0	1.2	11.1	10.6	74.8
Some of the time	100.0	2.0	11.0	8.7	76.3

Note: Numbers by race and Hispanic origin will not sum to total because not all races are shown and Hispanics may be of any race.
Source: National Center for Health Statistics, Summary Health Statistics for U.S. Adults: National Health Interview Survey, 2002, *Series 10, No. 222, 2004; calculations by New Strategist*

Income Is Linked to Mental Health Problems

The prevalence of mental health conditions also varies by education.

Adults with lower incomes are most likely to report having certain mental health problems, such as sadness or restlessness. Fully 24 percent of people with household incomes below $20,000 reported feeling restless at least some of the time during the past month, for example. The percentage reporting this problem declines steadily with income, to just 12 percent of those with incomes of $75,000 or more.

It's not hard to explain the greater mental health problems of those with low incomes, since they are more likely to experience difficulties such as not being able to pay their bills. Economic problems can lead to mental health problems, particularly among those predisposed to mental problems. But people with pre-existing mental conditions may also have more difficulty holding down a job, leading to lower incomes.

Education is also linked to certain mental health conditions. Those with lower levels of education are more likely to report having each of the conditions examined here. But determining what role, if any, education plays in mental health is complicated. People with higher levels of education also have higher incomes, for example.

■ The interaction between socioeconomic circumstances and mental health is complex, with interplay in both directions. Socioeconomics influence mental health, and mental health affects economic status.

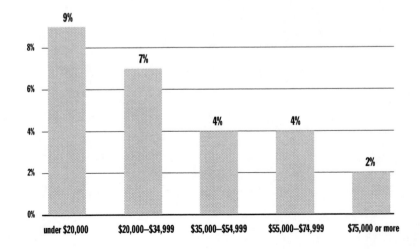

Many low-income people feel like "everything is an effort"

(percent of people aged 18 or older who felt like "everything is an effort" all or most of the time during the past 30 days, by household income, 2002)

Table 12.8 Mental Health Conditions among Adults by Household Income, 2002

(number and percent of people aged 18 or older with selected mental health conditions during the past thirty days, by type of condition, and household income, 2002; numbers in thousands)

	total	under $20,000	$20,000– $34,999	$35,000– $54,999	$55,000– $74,999	$75,000 or more
Total people	205,825	37,369	29,671	31,814	23,984	41,572
Sadness						
All or most of the time	5,838	2,167	1,095	810	456	352
Some of the time	15,746	4,727	2,800	2,551	1,288	1,802
Hopelessness						
All or most of the time	4,264	1,599	785	530	303	313
Some of the time	8,246	2,785	1,479	1,254	715	767
Worthlessness						
All or most of the time	3,981	1,528	820	442	273	281
Some of the time	6,606	2,145	1,231	1,055	493	712
Everything is an effort						
All or most of the time	9,678	3,238	2,009	1,366	899	706
Some of the time	15,135	4,043	2,371	2,479	1,459	2,538
Nervousness						
All or most of the time	8,251	2,978	1,689	1,068	662	726
Some of the time	22,577	5,316	3,356	3,826	2,314	4,189
Restlessness						
All or most of the time	9,879	3,106	1,879	1,493	814	1,231
Some of the time	22,543	5,390	3,570	3,704	2,574	3,948
PERCENT WITH CONDITION BY HOUSEHOLD INCOME						
Total people	100.0%	100.0%	100.0%	100.0%	100.0%	100.0%
Sadness						
All or most of the time	2.9	6.4	3.8	2.6	2.0	0.9
Some of the time	7.8	13.3	9.6	8.1	5.4	4.3
Hopelessness						
All or most of the time	2.1	4.8	2.7	1.6	1.3	0.8
Some of the time	4.1	8.2	5.2	3.9	3.2	1.8
Worthlessness						
All or most of the time	2.0	4.5	2.8	1.4	1.3	0.8
Some of the time	3.3	6.2	4.3	3.4	2.5	1.7
Everything is an effort						
All or most of the time	4.8	9.4	6.9	4.3	4.0	1.9
Some of the time	7.5	11.6	8.2	7.8	6.2	5.9
Nervousness						
All or most of the time	4.1	8.7	5.9	3.3	2.8	2.0
Some of the time	11.2	15.0	11.5	11.9	9.1	9.9
Restlessness						
All or most of the time	4.9	9.1	6.6	4.7	3.5	3.0
Some of the time	11.2	15.3	12.2	11.5	10.7	9.1

(continued)

PERCENT DISTRIBUTION OF THOSE WITH CONDITION BY HOUSEHOLD INCOME	total	under $20,000	$20,000–$34,999	$35,000–$54,999	$55,000–$74,999	$75,000 or more
Total people	**100.0%**	**18.2%**	**14.4%**	**15.5%**	**11.7%**	**20.2%**
Sadness						
All or most of the time	100.0	37.1	18.8	13.9	7.8	6.0
Some of the time	100.0	30.0	17.8	16.2	8.2	11.4
Hopelessness						
All or most of the time	100.0	37.5	18.4	12.4	7.1	7.3
Some of the time	100.0	33.8	17.9	15.2	8.7	9.3
Worthlessness						
All or most of the time	100.0	38.4	20.6	11.1	6.9	7.1
Some of the time	100.0	32.5	18.6	16.0	7.5	10.8
Everything is an effort						
All or most of the time	100.0	33.5	20.8	14.1	9.3	7.3
Some of the time	100.0	26.7	15.7	16.4	9.6	16.8
Nervousness						
All or most of the time	100.0	36.1	20.5	12.9	8.0	8.8
Some of the time	100.0	23.5	14.9	16.9	10.2	18.6
Restlessness						
All or most of the time	100.0	31.4	19.0	15.1	8.2	12.5
Some of the time	100.0	23.9	15.8	16.4	11.4	17.5

Source: National Center for Health Statistics, Summary Health Statistics for U.S. Adults: National Health Interview Survey, 2002, *Series 10, No. 222, 2004; calculations by New Strategist*

Table 12.9 Mental Health Conditions among Adults by Education, 2002

(number and percent of people aged 18 or older with selected mental health conditions during the past thirty days, by type of condition and educational attainment, 2002; numbers in thousands)

	total	not a high school graduate	high school graduate	some college	college graduate
Total people	**205,825**	**28,248**	**52,556**	**48,091**	**47,197**
Sadness					
All or most of the time	5,838	1,496	1,748	1,223	443
Some of the time	15,746	3,623	4,523	3,453	2,055
Hopelessness					
All or most of the time	4,264	1,130	1,231	876	416
Some of the time	8,246	1,743	2,396	1,870	1,032
Worthlessness					
All or most of the time	3,981	1,149	1,256	678	340
Some of the time	6,606	1,386	1,778	1,609	845
Everything is an effort					
All or most of the time	9,678	2,187	2,979	1,977	1,045
Some of the time	15,135	2,591	3,950	3,889	2,633
Nervousness					
All or most of the time	8,251	2,182	2,360	1,647	942
Some of the time	22,577	3,157	5,660	5,553	4,854
Restlessness					
All or most of the time	9,879	2,080	2,734	2,195	1,118
Some of the time	22,543	3,312	5,595	5,935	4,417
PERCENT WITH CONDITION BY EDUCATION					
Total people	**100.0%**	**100.0%**	**100.0%**	**100.0%**	**100.0%**
Sadness					
All or most of the time	2.9	5.6	3.4	2.5	1.0
Some of the time	7.8	13.4	8.7	7.2	4.6
Hopelessness					
All or most of the time	2.1	4.3	2.4	1.8	0.9
Some of the time	4.1	6.4	4.6	3.8	2.1
Worthlessness					
All or most of the time	2.0	4.3	2.4	1.4	0.7
Some of the time	3.3	5.1	3.4	3.4	1.8
Everything is an effort					
All or most of the time	4.8	8.2	5.8	4.1	2.3
Some of the time	7.5	9.3	7.7	8.0	5.6
Nervousness					
All or most of the time	4.1	7.9	4.6	3.4	2.0
Some of the time	11.2	11.4	11.0	11.5	10.2
Restlessness					
All or most of the time	4.9	7.8	5.3	4.5	2.4
Some of the time	11.2	11.9	10.9	12.4	9.4

(continued)

	total	not a high school graduate	high school graduate	some college	college graduate
PERCENT DISTRIBUTION OF THOSE WITH CONDITION BY EDUCATION					
Total people	**100.0%**	**13.7%**	**25.5%**	**23.4%**	**22.9%**
Sadness					
All or most of the time	100.0	25.6	29.9	20.9	7.6
Some of the time	100.0	23.0	28.7	21.9	13.1
Hopelessness					
All or most of the time	100.0	26.5	28.9	20.5	9.8
Some of the time	100.0	21.1	29.1	22.7	12.5
Worthlessness					
All or most of the time	100.0	28.9	31.5	17.0	8.5
Some of the time	100.0	21.0	26.9	24.4	12.8
Everything is an effort					
All or most of the time	100.0	22.6	30.8	20.4	10.8
Some of the time	100.0	17.1	26.1	25.7	17.4
Nervousness					
All or most of the time	100.0	26.4	28.6	20.0	11.4
Some of the time	100.0	14.0	25.1	24.6	21.5
Restlessness					
All or most of the time	100.0	21.1	27.7	22.2	11.3
Some of the time	100.0	14.7	24.8	26.3	19.6

Source: National Center for Health Statistics, Summary Health Statistics for U.S. Adults: National Health Interview Survey, 2002, *Series 10, No. 222, 2004; calculations by New Strategist*

One in Five High School Girls Has Considered Suicide

Serious attempts at suicide are relatively rare, however.

An alarmingly large number of high school students, particularly girls, say they have seriously considered committing suicide. Twenty-one percent of girls in grades 9 through 12
have considered suicide in the past year, as have 13 percent of boys. The percentage of girls
who thought about suicide is highest among tenth graders and declines with age. Among
boys, there is a slight rise after grade nine. Suicide attempts also decline among girls as they
move into the higher grades, but among boys there is little change.

Among black students, boys are more likely than girls to have made a serious suicide
attempt that required medical attention. Hispanic girls also have a relatively high rate of
serious suicide attempts. This finding suggests that cultural factors may influence the likelihood of carrying through on suicidal ideations.

■ Although few high school students actually attempt suicide, the relatively large share
who consider it indicates a need for more support services for teenagers.

Hispanic girls are most likely to seriously consider suicide

*(percent of students in grades 9 through 12 who seriously considered
suicide in the past year, by race, Hispanic origin, and sex, 2003)*

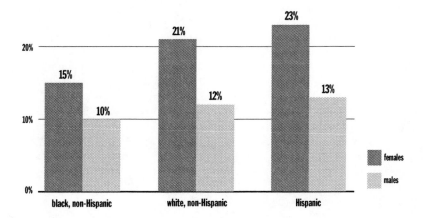

Table 12.10 Suicidal Ideation among High School Students, 2003

(percent of students in grades 9 through 12 who seriously considered or attempted suicide or made a suicide attempt that required medical attention in the past twelve months, by grade, race, Hispanic origin, and sex, 2003)

	considered suicide		attempted suicide		suicide attempt required medical attention	
	female	male	female	male	female	male
Total	**21.3%**	**12.8%**	**11.5%**	**5.4%**	**3.2%**	**2.4%**
Ninth grade	22.2	11.9	14.7	5.8	3.9	3.1
Tenth grade	23.8	13.2	12.7	5.5	3.2	2.1
Eleventh grade	20.0	12.9	10.0	4.6	2.9	2.0
Twelfth grade	18.0	13.2	6.9	5.2	2.2	1.8
Black, non-Hispanic	14.7	10.3	9.0	7.7	2.2	5.2
White, non-Hispanic	21.2	12.0	10.3	3.7	2.4	1.1
Hispanic	23.4	12.9	15.0	6.1	5.7	4.2

Source: National Center for Health Statistics, Health, United States, 2004; *Internet site http://www.cdc.gov/nchs/hus.htm*

Nine Percent of Adults Have Had a Serious Mental Illness

Most have not received treatment, however.

Nearly 20 million adults—9 percent of people aged 18 or older—experienced a bout of mental illness in the past year that was serious enough to substantially interfere with or limit one or more major life activities. Women are more likely than men to have (or admit having) a serious mental illness—12 percent of women versus a smaller 7 percent of men. Among both men and women, the percentage with a serious mental illness declines with age.

Only 47 percent of people with serious mental problems received mental health treatment or counseling for problems other than drug or alcohol use. Among women, 52 percent received treatment. Among men, only 38 percent were treated. The percentage of people receiving treatment rises with age. Non-Hispanic whites are more likely than other racial or ethnic groups to get treatment for mental problems.

■ One of the barriers to treatment of the seriously mentally ill is their own inability either to recognize their mental illness or to get treatment. It often falls on the people around them to make sure they get the help they need.

Women under age 50 are most likely to have serious mental problems

(percent of people aged 18 or older with serious mental illness in the past year, by age and sex, 2003)

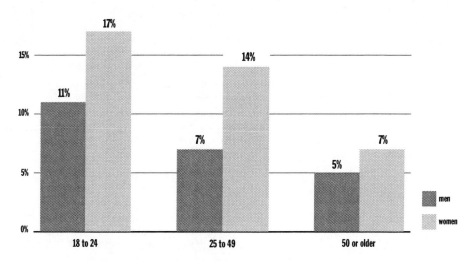

Table 12.11 Serious Mental Illness by Selected Characteristics and Age, 2003

(number and percent of people aged 18 or older with serious mental illness in the past year, by selected characteristics and age, 2003; numbers in thousands)

	number				percent			
	total	18 to 25	26 to 49	50 or older	total	18 to 25	26 to 49	50 or older
Total with illness	19,588	4,420	10,418	4,750	9.2%	13.9%	10.4%	5.9%
Sex								
Men	6,887	1,690	3,438	1,758	6.7	10.6	7.0	4.7
Women	12,702	2,730	6,980	2,992	11.5	17.3	13.8	6.8
Race and Hispanic origin								
Not Hispanic	17,257	3,735	9,186	4,336	9.2	14.3	10.7	5.8
American Indian	96	22	66	–	8.9	11.9	11.9	–
Asian	536	196	311	29	6.1	13.6	6.4	1.2
Black	1,992	532	1,108	351	8.4	12.4	9.4	4.6
White	14,308	2,877	7,575	3,856	9.5	14.6	11.3	6.0
Hispanic	2,331	686	1,231	414	9.0	12.1	8.5	7.3
Education								
Not a high school graduate	4,276	1,030	1,949	1,297	11.3	15.0	13.3	7.9
High school graduate	6,360	1,525	3,212	1,623	9.5	13.9	10.7	6.2
Some college	5,388	1,388	3,022	979	10.3	14.0	11.9	5.7
College graduate	3,564	478	2,235	851	6.5	12.0	7.5	4.0
Employment status								
Employed full-time	9,583	1,948	6,034	1,601	8.2	13.4	8.5	5.1
Employed part-time	2,861	1,061	1,366	435	10.0	13.0	12.1	4.7
Unemployed	1,230	445	540	–	15.2	16.5	13.3	–
Other	5,914	967	2,478	2,469	10.0	15.4	18.5	6.3

Note: Serious mental illness is defined as a diagnosable mental, behavioral, or emotional disorder that meets the criteria found in the fourth edition of the Diagnostic and Statistical Manual of Mental Disorders *and results in functional impairment that substantially interferes with or limits one or more major life activities. Other employment status includes retirees, the disabled, homemakers, students, and others not in the labor force. (–) means sample is too small to make a reliable estimate.*
Source: SAMHSA, Office of Applied Studies, National Survey on Drug Use and Health, 2003; Internet site http://oas.samhsa. gov/NHSDA/2k3NSDUH/appg.htm#tabg.1

Table 12.12 Treatment for Serious Mental Illness by Selected Characteristics, 2003

(number of people aged 18 or older with serious mental illness in the past year and percent receiving mental health treatment for problems other than drug or alcohol use, by selected characteristics, 2003; numbers in thousands)

	total with serious mental illness	received treatment number	received treatment percent of total
Total with illness	**19,588**	**9,253**	**47.3%**
Age			
Aged 18 to 25	4,420	1,551	35.2
Aged 26 to 49	10,418	5,144	49.4
Aged 50 or older	4,750	2,558	54.0
Sex			
Men	6,887	2,649	38.5
Women	12,702	6,604	52.1
Race and Hispanic origin			
Not Hispanic	17,257	8,571	49.7
American Indian	96	–	–
Asian	536	91	17.0
Black	1,992	725	36.6
White	14,308	7,548	52.8
Hispanic	2,331	682	29.3
Education			
Not a high school grad.	4,276	1,666	39.0
High school graduate	6,360	2,821	44.4
Some college	5,388	2,729	50.9
College graduate	3,564	2,036	57.1
Employment status			
Employed full-time	9,583	4,061	42.4
Employed part-time	2,861	1,368	47.9
Unemployed	1,230	444	36.4
Other	5,914	3,380	57.2

Note: Recipients of mental health treatment are defined as having received inpatient or outpatient care, or using prescription medication for problems with emotions, nerves, or mental health. Respondents were not to include treatment for drug or alcohol use. Serious mental illness is defined as a diagnosable mental, behavioral, or emotional disorder that meets the criteria found in the fourth edition of the Diagnostic and Statistical Manual of Mental Disorders *and results in functional impairment that substantially interferes with or limits one or more major life activities. Other employment status includes retirees, the disabled, homemakers, students, and others not in the labor force. (–) means sample is too small to make a reliable estimate.*
Source: SAMHSA, Office of Applied Studies, National Survey on Drug Use and Health, 2003; Internet site http://oas.samhsa.gov/NHSDA/2k3NSDUH/appg.htm#tabg.1

13

Sexual Attitudes and Behavior

■ **Americans have increasingly liberal attitudes toward sexual behavior.**

Most favor sex education in the public schools, 44 percent say premarital sex is not wrong at all, and 32 percent say homosexual sex is not wrong either.

■ **Nearly half of 15-to-19-year-olds have had sexual intercourse.**

The likelihood of being sexually active increases with age, from between 30 and 32 percent among 15-to-17-year-olds to 71 percent of girls and 65 percent of boys aged 18 to 19.

■ **Many teens do not use birth control when they first have sex.**

The younger teenagers are at first sexual intercourse, the less likely they are to use birth control.

■ **Most adults have had only one sex partner in the past year.**

Fifteen percent admit to having two or more sex partners, however.

■ **Among adults, the birth control pill is the most widely used contraceptive.**

Thirty-one percent of contracepting women use the pill, 27 percent are sterilized, and 18 percent have partners who use condoms.

Americans Have Increasingly "Liberal" Attitudes toward Sex

They are less likely to think homosexuality and premarital sex are wrong.

Americans have long favored sex education in public schools, worrying that it could lead to problems if children are not adequately informed about sex. In the late 1970s, as much as 21 percent of the public opposed sex education in public schools. Opposition bottomed out at 10 percent in 1990. Today, a slightly larger but still small 11 percent are against sex education in public schools.

Opinions about premarital sex have undergone a significant transformation since the 1970s. In 1972 only 26 percent of adults felt that premarital sex was "not wrong at all." By 2002, the share holding this view had grown to 44 percent. The proportion of Americans believing premarital sex is always wrong fell from 35 to 27 percent during those years.

Attitudes about homosexuality have also changed, although the shift has been more gradual. In 1973, only 11 percent of adults thought sex between two people of the same sex was not wrong at all. By 2002, this proportion had grown to 32 percent. At the same time, the proportion saying homosexual sex is always wrong fell from 70 to 53 percent.

■ Changing attitudes about sexual issues are largely the result of "generational replacement." As older generations die, they are replaced by younger generations with different attitudes.

Many people think premarital sex is OK

(percent of people aged 18 or older who think premarital sex is not wrong at all, 1972 and 2002)

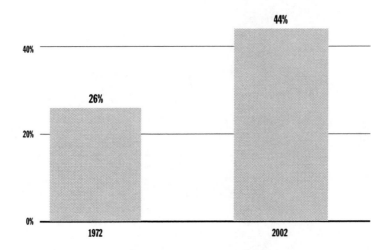

Table 13.1 Sex Education in Public Schools, 1974 to 2002

"Would you be for or against sex education in the public schools?"

(number of respondents aged 18 or older, and percent distribution by response, 1974–2002)

	number of respondents	total	favor	oppose	depends	don't know
2002	908	100.0%	86.7%	11.3%	0.0%	2.0%
2000	1,868	100.0	85.2	12.4	0.0	2.4
1998	1,863	100.0	85.1	12.7	0.0	2.3
1996	1,954	100.0	85.3	12.3	0.0	2.4
1994	1,965	100.0	85.0	12.1	0.0	2.9
1993	1,077	100.0	82.6	14.8	0.0	2.6
1991	1,022	100.0	85.1	11.8	0.0	3.0
1990	924	100.0	87.6	9.8	0.0	2.6
1989	1,003	100.0	84.4	12.2	0.0	3.4
1988	984	100.0	84.7	12.6	0.0	2.7
1986	1,468	100.0	81.7	15.5	0.0	2.8
1985	1,526	100.0	82.0	15.5	0.0	2.5
1983	1,595	100.0	83.6	13.6	0.0	2.8
1982	1,856	100.0	81.6	15.2	0.0	3.2
1977	1,524	100.0	77.0	20.9	0.0	2.1
1975	1,488	100.0	76.3	20.0	0.0	3.7
1974	1,481	100.0	78.9	17.1	0.6	3.4

Source: General Social Surveys, National Opinion Research Center, University of Chicago; calculations by New Strategist

Table 13.2 Premarital Sex, 1972 to 2002

"There's been a lot of discussion about the way morals and attitudes about sex are changing in this country. If a man and woman have sex relations before marriage, do you think it is always wrong, almost always wrong, wrong only sometimes, or not wrong at all?"

(number of respondents aged 18 or older, and percent distribution by response, 1972–2002)

	number of respondents	total	always wrong	almost always wrong	sometimes wrong	not wrong at all	don't know
2002	903	100.0%	26.8%	8.1%	19.5%	43.6%	2.0%
2000	1,867	100.0	26.9	8.4	20.6	40.1	4.0
1998	1,869	100.0	25.5	8.9	20.2	41.9	3.5
1996	1,954	100.0	23.1	9.4	22.0	42.6	3.0
1994	1,967	100.0	25.2	9.8	19.8	42.2	3.1
1993	1,077	100.0	26.3	9.8	20.2	41.1	2.5
1991	1,021	100.0	26.8	9.6	18.2	42.6	2.7
1990	925	100.0	24.8	11.1	22.2	38.5	3.5
1989	1,002	100.0	27.1	8.4	22.1	39.3	3.1
1988	982	100.0	25.6	10.4	21.8	39.5	2.7
1986	1,464	100.0	27.0	8.7	22.4	39.2	2.7
1985	1,530	100.0	27.6	8.0	19.2	42.0	3.1
1983	1,592	100.0	26.8	9.7	23.7	37.8	1.9
1982	1,851	100.0	28.0	9.0	20.4	39.5	3.1
1978	1,528	100.0	28.6	11.5	19.9	37.8	2.2
1977	1,520	100.0	30.2	9.3	22.4	35.6	2.6
1975	1,485	100.0	29.7	11.9	23.0	31.5	3.9
1974	1,477	100.0	32.0	12.3	22.8	29.7	3.2
1972	1,602	100.0	35.1	11.4	23.3	26.2	4.1

Source: General Social Surveys, National Opinion Research Center, University of Chicago; calculations by New Strategist

Table 13.3 Homosexual Sex Relations, 1973 to 2002

"What about sexual relations between two adults of the same sex—
do you think it is always wrong, almost always wrong,
wrong only sometimes, or not wrong at all?"

(number of respondents aged 18 or older, and percent distribution by response, 1973–2002)

	number of respondents	total	always wrong	almost always wrong	sometimes wrong	not wrong at all	other	don't know
2002	919	100.0%	52.9%	4.7%	6.9%	31.8%	0.0%	3.8%
2000	1,850	100.0	53.9	4.1	7.3	26.4	0.0	8.3
1998	1,874	100.0	54.3	5.3	6.5	27.5	0.0	6.5
1996	1,908	100.0	56.5	4.9	5.8	26.4	0.0	6.5
1994	1,991	100.0	62.9	3.8	5.8	22.0	0.0	5.4
1993	1,068	100.0	62.8	4.1	6.9	20.9	0.0	5.2
1991	986	100.0	70.9	3.9	4.2	15.0	0.0	6.1
1990	916	100.0	72.6	4.6	5.8	12.2	0.0	4.8
1989	1,029	100.0	70.7	3.9	5.7	15.0	0.0	4.8
1988	973	100.0	74.0	4.5	5.4	12.3	0.0	3.7
1987	1,801	100.0	74.4	4.2	6.7	12.0	0.0	2.7
1985	1,531	100.0	73.0	3.9	6.8	13.3	0.0	3.1
1984	1,466	100.0	70.6	4.8	7.2	13.8	0.0	3.7
1982	1,847	100.0	70.0	5.2	6.7	14.0	0.0	4.2
1980	1,465	100.0	69.9	5.7	5.8	13.9	0.0	4.6
1977	1,522	100.0	68.6	5.5	7.2	14.2	0.0	4.5
1976	1,488	100.0	67.1	5.9	7.5	15.3	0.0	4.2
1974	1,484	100.0	67.0	4.8	7.5	12.3	3.4	4.9
1973	1,497	100.0	70.3	6.3	7.3	10.6	2.1	3.3

Source: General Social Surveys, National Opinion Research Center, University of Chicago; calculations by New Strategist

Most Teenagers Think Anything Goes between Consenting Adults

But most do not think unmarried 16-year-olds should have sex.

Teenagers aged 15 to 19 have fairly liberal attitudes about many sexual issues. Nearly three-quarters agree or agree strongly that whatever consenting adults want to do in the bedroom is all right. Interestingly, teenagers make a distinction between 16-year-olds and 18-year-olds when it comes to premarital sex. The majority thinks it is all right for unmarried 18-year-olds to have sex, but most do not feel 16-year-olds should.

Teenaged boys and girls differ in their opinions on premarital childbearing, with girls considerably more likely to think it is OK for a woman to have a child out of wedlock (65 percent of girls versus 50 percent of boys). Surprisingly, boys are more likely than girls to think marriage is better than going through life single (69 percent of boys versus 55 percent of girls).

Having a child out of wedlock might be all right in theory, but teens would clearly prefer not to do so. Among never-married girls aged 15 to 19, fully 60 percent say they would be "very upset" if they got pregnant and another 27 percent would be "a little upset." Boys are more likely than girls to say they would be a little or very pleased to get a girl pregnant—although most (85 percent) say a pregnancy would make them a little or very upset.

■ Given the liberal sexual attitudes of teenagers, it is likely that American society will become even more tolerant of sexuality.

Teens' tolerance of premarital sex has limits

(percent of people aged 15 to 19 who agree or agree strongly with selected questions, by sex, 2002)

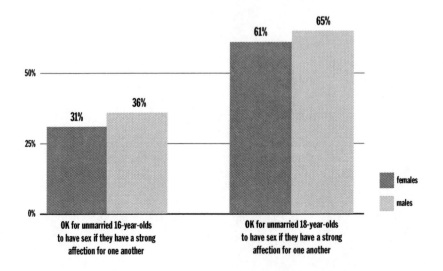

Table 13.4 Attitudes of People Aged 15 to 19 toward Sexual Activity, Childbearing, and Cohabitation, 2002

(percent distribution of people aged 15 to 19 by how much they agree with selected questions, by sex, 2002)

	total	strongly agree	agree	disagree	strongly disagree	neither agree nor disagree
Females						
Any sexual act between two consenting adults is all right	100.0%	12.4%	60.6%	20.8%	4.6%	1.6%
It is all right for unmarried 18-year-olds to have sexual relations if they have strong affection for one another	100.0	9.0	51.9	25.3	11.9	1.9
It is all right for unmarried 16-year-olds to have sexual relations if they have strong affection for one another	100.0	2.7	27.8	42.2	25.3	1.9
It is OK for an unmarried female to have a child	100.0	11.4	53.4	24.5	8.3	2.3
It is better for a person to get married than to go through life being single	100.0	10.3	44.2	32.7	10.0	3.0
A young couple should not live together unless they are married	100.0	8.2	27.9	51.6	11.2	1.2
Divorce is usually the best solution when a couple can't seem to work out their marriage problems	100.0	9.2	38.8	36.6	13.3	2.2
Males						
Any sexual act between two consenting adults is all right	100.0	12.4	61.3	21.3	2.8	2.3
It is all right for unmarried 18-year-olds to have sexual relations if they have strong affection for one another	100.0	10.3	54.7	25.8	8.3	0.9
It is all right for unmarried 16-year-olds to have sexual relations if they have strong affection for one another	100.0	3.1	32.6	42.3	20.3	1.9
It is OK for an unmarried female to have a child	100.0	5.2	44.7	38.3	9.5	2.2
It is better for a person to get married than to go through life being single	100.0	19.9	49.2	24.6	4.0	2.3
A young couple should not live together unless they are married	100.0	7.3	25.0	55.1	11.7	0.9
Divorce is usually the best solution when a couple can't seem to work out their marriage problems	100.0	6.5	35.2	40.1	15.7	2.5

Source: National Center for Health Statistics, Teenagers in the United States: Sexual Activity, Contraceptive Use, and Childbearing, 2002; *Vital and Health Statistics Series 23, No. 24, 2004; Internet site http://www.cdc.gov/nchs/nsfg.htm*

Table 13.5 Attitudes of People Aged 15 to 19 toward Pregnancy, 2002

(percent distribution of never-married people aged 15 to 19 by response to question, "If you got pregnant now/got a female pregnant now, how would you feel?" by sex, 2002)

	total	very upset	a little upset	a little pleased	very pleased
TOTAL NEVER-MARRIED FEMALES	**100.0%**	**60.2%**	**26.7%**	**8.0%**	**4.7%**
Age					
Aged 15 to 17	100.0	67.5	21.2	8.2	2.8
Aged 18 to 19	100.0	49.0	35.1	7.8	7.6
Race and Hispanic origin					
Black, non-Hispanic	100.0	50.5	32.5	11.7	5.0
Hispanic	100.0	46.4	29.0	14.9	9.8
White, non-Hispanic	100.0	65.8	24.2	5.5	3.8
TOTAL NEVER-MARRIED MALES	**100.0**	**51.4**	**33.4**	**11.0**	**3.7**
Age					
Aged 15 to 17	100.0	58.9	29.9	8.1	2.8
Aged 18 to 19	100.0	41.8	37.8	14.6	4.7
Race and Hispanic origin					
Black, non-Hispanic	100.0	35.9	43.1	14.0	6.3
Hispanic	100.0	38.2	35.1	17.0	9.7
White, non-Hispanic	100.0	59.0	30.6	8.5	1.3

Source: National Center for Health Statistics, Teenagers in the United States: Sexual Activity, Contraceptive Use, and Childbearing, 2002; Vital and Health Statistics Series 23, No. 24, 2004; Internet site http://www.cdc.gov/nchs/nsfg.htm

Some Teenagers Are More Likely than Others to Have Sex

Many have had multiple partners.

Among 15-to-19-year-olds, 47 percent of girls and 46 percent of boys admit to having had sex. Because many teenagers may decline to answer the question honestly, the proportions may be even higher than these statistics suggest.

Not surprisingly, the likelihood of being sexually active increases with age, from 30 to 32 percent among 15-to-17-year-olds to 71 percent of girls and 65 percent of boys aged 18 to 19. Teens living with both parents at age 14 are less likely than those in other family arrangements to have had sex. Among non-Hispanic blacks and Hispanics, boys are more likely than girls to have had sex, while among non-Hispanic whites the opposite is true.

Sexual activity increases as children move through high school. Only 21 percent of 9th graders say they are currently sexually active, for example, compared with 49 percent of 12th graders. The likelihood of having had multiple sexual partners also increases with age.

Boys become sexually active at a younger age than girls and they report having more sexual partners. But from 10th grade on, girls are more likely than boys to be currently sexually active.

■ Because sexual activity is the norm in high school, sex education in middle school is a must.

Most 11th and 12th graders have had sex

(percent of students in grades 9 through 12 who have ever had sexual intercourse, by grade, 2002)

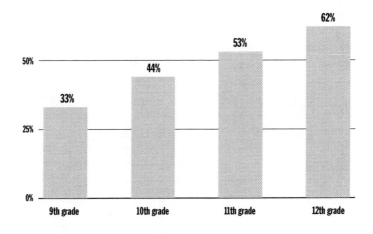

Table 13.6   People Aged 15 to 19 Who Have Had Sexual Intercourse by Selected Characteristics, 2002

(percent of people aged 15 to 19 who have ever had sexual intercourse, by selected characteristics and sex, 2002)

	females	males
Total people aged 15 to 19	**46.8%**	**46.0%**
Age		
Aged 15 to 17	30.3	31.6
Aged 18 to 19	70.6	64.7
Mother's age at first birth		
Under age 20	58.0	56.2
Aged 20 or older	41.6	42.5
Mother's education		
Not a high school graduate	47.2	48.7
High school graduate	51.6	52.0
Some college or more	43.3	41.9
Family structure at age 14		
Both biological/adoptive parents	40.2	40.8
Single parents, stepparents, no parents	58.1	57.5
Race and Hispanic origin		
Black, non-Hispanic	57.0	63.4
Hispanic	40.4	55.5
White, non-Hispanic	46.4	41.1

Source: National Center for Health Statistics, Teenagers in the United States: Sexual Activity, Contraceptive Use, and Childbearing, 2002; *Vital and Health Statistics Series 23, No. 24, 2004; Internet site http://www.cdc.gov/nchs/nsfg.htm*

Table 13.7 Sexual Behavior of 9th to 12th Graders by Sex, 2003

(percent of 9th to 12th graders engaging in selected sexual activities, by sex and grade, 2003)

	total	9th grade	10th grade	11th grade	12th grade
Total					
Ever had sexual intercourse	46.7%	32.8%	44.1%	53.2%	61.6%
First sexual intercourse before age 13	7.4	9.3	8.5	5.4	5.5
Four or more sex partners during lifetime	14.4	10.4	12.6	16.0	20.3
Currently sexually active*	34.3	21.2	30.6	41.1	48.9
Condom use during last sexual intercourse	63.0	69.0	69.0	60.8	57.4
Birth control pill use before last sexual intercourse	17.0	8.7	12.7	19.6	22.6
Females					
Ever had sexual intercourse	45.3	27.9	43.1	53.1	62.3
First sexual intercourse before age 13	4.2	5.3	5.7	3.2	1.9
Four or more sex partners during lifetime	11.2	6.4	8.8	13.4	17.9
Currently sexually active*	34.6	18.3	31.2	42.9	51.0
Condom use during last sexual intercourse	57.4	66.1	66.4	55.5	48.5
Birth control pill use before last sexual intercourse	20.6	11.6	13.5	24.1	27.2
Males					
Ever had sexual intercourse	48.0	37.3	45.1	53.4	60.7
First sexual intercourse before age 13	10.4	13.2	11.2	7.5	8.8
Four or more sex partners during lifetime	17.5	14.2	16.4	18.6	22.2
Currently sexually active*	33.8	24.0	30.0	39.2	46.5
Condom use during last sexual intercourse	68.8	71.2	71.8	66.7	67.0
Birth control pill use before last sexual intercourse	13.1	6.6	11.8	14.8	17.5

* Sexual intercourse during the three months preceding the survey.
Source: Centers for Disease Control and Prevention, Youth Risk Behavior Surveillance—United States, 2003, *Mortality and Morbidity Weekly Report, Surveillance Summaries, Vol. 53/SS02, May 21, 2004*

Younger Teens Are Less Likely to Use Contraception

Hispanic teenagers are least likely to use birth control.

Among teenaged girls, the younger they were when they first had sexual intercourse, the less likely they were to use a contraceptive. More than one-third of girls aged 15 to 19 who first had intercourse when they were 14 or younger did not use any type of contraception. The share who used a condom, which reduces the risk of pregnancy and sexually transmitted diseases, rose with age to a high of 71 percent among those first having intercourse at ages 17 to 19.

Boys show a different pattern of contraceptive use. As is true with girls, the boys who first had intercourse at age 14 or younger were least likely to use contraception. But unlike the pattern with girls, boys who first had intercourse at ages 15 to 16 were most likely to use birth control. Boys aged 17 to 19 when they first had sex were less likely than those aged 15 to 16 to use contraception. Among both boys and girls, Hispanics were least likely to use birth control when they first had sex.

Not all teens are having sex, of course. Among sexually inexperienced 15-to-19-year-olds, the reason most commonly given for avoiding sex is that it is against their religion or morals. Fear of pregnancy and fear of sexually transmitted disease are also compelling reasons to delay having sex. The most commonly cited reason for not having sex among non-Hispanic black teenage girls is to avoid sexually transmitted diseases. For non-Hispanic black and Hispanic teen boys, it is fear of getting a girl pregnant.

■ The relatively large percentage of teenagers who do not use birth control when they first have sex suggests more efforts are needed to either prevent teens from having sex or to convince them to use contraception.

Many teens have unprotected sex

(percent of 15-to-19-year-olds who did not use contraception at first sexual intercourse, by age and sex, 2002)

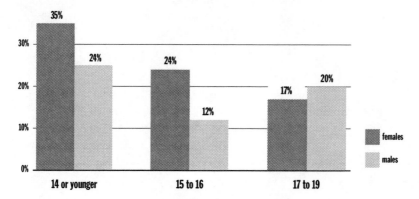

Table 13.8 Contraceptive Use among People Aged 15 to 19, 2002

(number of people aged 15 to 19 who have ever had sexual intercourse and percent distribution by method of contraception at first sexual intercourse, by sex, age, race, and Hispanic origin, 2002; numbers in thousands)

| | total | | | | | | |
	number	percent	no method	condom	pill	withdrawal	dual methods
TOTAL FEMALES	**4,598**	**100.0%**	**25.5%**	**66.4%**	**16.5%**	**7.5%**	**13.1%**
Age at first sexual intercourse							
Age 14 or younger	1,290	100.0	34.8	58.5	11.4	6.7	9.8
Aged 15 to 16	2,235	100.0	24.1	68.6	16.3	7.2	13.3
Aged 17 to 19	1,074	100.0	17.4	71.3	22.7	9.3	16.7
Race and Hispanic origin							
Black, non-Hispanic	854	100.0	29.0	61.2	13.3	5.6	8.7
Hispanic	615	100.0	33.8	55.5	8.6	8.2	9.0
White, non-Hispanic	2,905	100.0	22.0	71.8	18.4	8.2	15.3
TOTAL MALES	**4,697**	**100.0**	**18.0**	**70.9**	**14.9**	**9.8**	**10.4**
Age at first sexual intercourse							
Age 14 or younger	1,513	100.0	24.1	72.0	8.4	3.9	7.8
Aged 15 to 16	1,977	100.0	11.9	77.3	14.7	13.2	11.7
Aged 17 to 19	1,207	100.0	20.4	59.1	23.4	11.4	11.5
Race and Hispanic origin							
Black, non-Hispanic	934	100.0	14.4	84.9	11.4	–	11.5
Hispanic	903	100.0	26.6	67.4	5.8	4.0	5.5
White, non-Hispanic	2,672	100.0	15.2	68.2	19.3	13.4	11.5

Note: (–) means sample is too small to make a reliable estimate.
Source: National Center for Health Statistics, Teenagers in the United States: Sexual Activity, Contraceptive Use, and Childbearing, *2002; Vital and Health Statistics Series 23, No. 24, 2004; Internet site http://www.cdc.gov/nchs/nsfg.htm*

Table 13.9 Reason People Aged 15 to 19 Have Never Had Sexual Intercourse, 2002

(percent distribution of people aged 15 to 19 who have never had sexual intercourse by reason for not having intercourse, by sex, age, race, and Hispanic origin, 2002)

	age		race and Hispanic origin		
	15 to 17	18 to 19	black non-Hispanic	white non-Hispanic	Hispanic
FEMALES					
Total females without sexual experience	**100.0%**	**100.0%**	**100.0%**	**100.0%**	**100.0%**
Against religion or morals	37.5	38.7	19.2	42.1	29.8
Don't want to get pregnant	19.1	17.3	14.0	18.3	24.2
Don't want to get a sexually transmitted disease	9.1	–	25.9	3.7	8.6
Haven't found the right person yet	15.9	21.8	18.6	19.3	13.5
In a relationship, but waiting for the right time	6.1	8.0	5.1	4.9	11.4
Other reason	12.3	12.7	17.2	11.6	12.4
MALES					
Total males without sexual experience	**100.0**	**100.0**	**100.0**	**100.0**	**100.0**
Against religion or morals	29.3	36.9	21.4	35.9	18.9
Don't want to get a girl pregnant	27.4	19.5	28.1	23.1	42.1
Don't want to get a sexually transmitted disease	12.0	–	20.2	9.0	11.7
Haven't found the right person yet	17.9	28.2	13.6	19.4	19.0
In a relationship, but waiting for the right time	4.3	5.9	–	4.5	–
Other reason	9.2	4.7	9.9	8.2	5.6

Note: (–) means sample is too small to make a reliable estimate.
Source: National Center for Health Statistics, Teenagers in the United States: Sexual Activity, Contraceptive Use, and Childbearing, *2002; Vital and Health Statistics Series 23, No. 24, 2004; Internet site http://www.cdc.gov/nchs/nsfg.htm*

Most Adults Have Had Only One Sex Partner in the Past Year

But the percentage having multiple partners is up slightly from 1993.

From 1993 through 2002, the majority of respondents to the National Opinion Research Center's General Social Survey said they had had only one sex partner in the past year. The share fell slightly, however, from 66 to 61 percent between 1993 and 2002. The percentage of people having had no sex partners increased slightly during those years.

In 1993, only 11 percent of adults admitted to having two or more sex partners during the past year. By 2002, the figure had crept up to 15 percent.

■ The small increase in the percentage of people having two or more sex partners in the past year does not yet signify a trend. There is some evidence from other studies, however, that concern about sexually transmitted diseases has waned—which could lead to an increase in sexual activity.

Fifteen percent have had two or more sex partners in past year

(percent of people aged 18 or older who had two or more sexual partners in the past twelve months, 1993 to 2002)

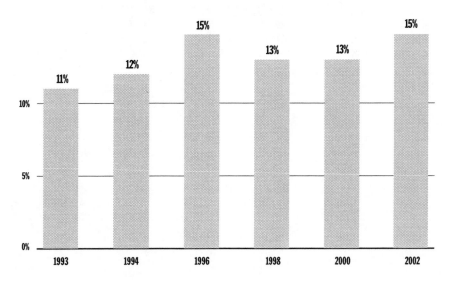

Table 13.10 People Aged 18 or Older by Number of Sex Partners in Past Year, 1993 to 2002

"How many sex partners have you had in the last 12 months?"

(number of respondents aged 18 or older and percent distribution by response, 1993 to 2002)

	number of respondents	total	no partners	one partner	two partners	three partners	four partners	five or more partners	more than one	don't know	no answer
2002	2,276	100.0%	22.5%	61.4%	7.0%	3.6%	1.7%	2.1%	0.2%	0.2%	1.3%
2000	2,400	100.0	21.7	62.6	6.3	3.3	1.8	1.9	0.1	–	2.4
1998	2,451	100.0	20.9	64.7	6.7	2.3	1.6	1.9	0.5	0.0	1.4
1996	2,657	100.0	18.7	64.9	7.2	3.4	1.7	1.7	0.9	0.1	1.4
1994	2,791	100.0	21.8	63.9	6.8	2.6	1.3	1.5	0.1	–	2.0
1993	1,492	100.0	21.0	65.9	5.8	2.2	1.7	1.7	–	–	1.7

Note: (–) means less than 0.05.
Source: General Social Surveys, National Opinion Research Center, University of Chicago

Birth Control Pill Is First Choice for Contraception

Sterilization is the second-most common birth control method.

Among women using contraception, the most popular is the pill, with 31 percent saying they use this method. Almost 7 percent use hormone-based contraceptives in other forms, including patches and injections. The second-most common form of contraception is female sterilization, used by 27 percent. The popularity of these methods has reduced reliance on other means of contraception. In 2002 fewer than 1 percent of women used a diaphragm, down from 9 percent in 1982. But condom use rose from 12 to 18 percent during those years in response to concerns about sexually transmitted disease.

The use of contraceptives varies by age. As would be expected, the share of women who have been sterilized, or whose partner has been sterilized, increases with age. Use of the pill declines with age, as does use of condoms.

Non-Hispanic white women are more likely than non-Hispanic black or Hispanic women to use some form of contraception. Non-Hispanic whites are less likely to have been sterilized, however. Forty-three percent of non-Hispanic white women have used family planning services compared with 40 percent of black and Hispanic women.

■ The percentage of women who are trying to get pregnant peaks at 7 percent among those aged 30 to 34.

Condom use has increased the most

(percent of women aged 15 to 44 using selected methods of contraception, 1982 and 2002)

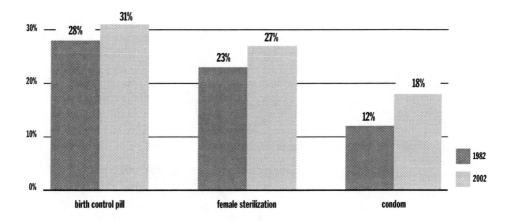

Table 13.11 Contraceptive Use by Type, 1982 and 2002

(number of women aged 15 to 44 using contraception and percent distribution by current method used, 1982 and 2002; numbers in thousands)

	2002	1982
Number using contraception	**38,109**	**30,142**
Total using contraception	**100.0%**	**100.0%**
Female sterilization	27.0	23.2
Male sterilization	9.2	10.9
Pill	30.6	28.0
Implant, Lunelle, or Patch	1.2	–
Three-month injectable (Depo-Provera)	5.3	–
Intrauterine device (IUD)	2.0	7.1
Diaphragm	0.3	8.1
Condom	18.0	12.0
Periodic abstinence—calendar rhythm method	1.2	3.3
Periodic abstinence—natural family planning	0.4	0.6
Withdrawal	4.0	2.0
Other methods	0.9	1.3

Note: Other methods includes Today sponge, cervical cap, female condom, and other methods.
Source: National Center for Health Statistics, Use of Contraception and Use of Family Planning Services in the United States: *1982–2002, Advance Data, No. 350, 2004; Internet site http://www.cdc.gov/nchs/nsfg.htm*

Table 13.12 Contraceptive Use by Age, 2002

(total number of women aged 15 to 44 and percent distribution by contraceptive status and age, 2002; numbers in thousands)

	total	15 to 19	20 to 24	25 to 29	30 to 34	35 to 39	40 to 44
TOTAL WOMEN AGED 15 TO 44							
Number	**61,561**	**9,834**	**9,840**	**9,249**	**10,272**	**10,853**	**11,512**
Percent	**100.0%**	**100.0%**	**100.0%**	**100.0%**	**100.0%**	**100.0%**	**100.0%**
Using contraception	**61.9**	**31.5**	**60.7**	**68.0**	**69.2**	**70.8**	**69.1**
Female sterilization	16.7	–	2.2	10.3	19.0	29.2	34.7
Male sterilization	5.7	–	0.5	2.8	6.4	10.0	12.7
Pill	18.9	16.7	31.9	25.6	21.8	13.2	7.6
Implant, Lunelle, or Patch	0.8	0.4	0.9	1.7	0.9	0.5	0.2
Three-month injectable (Depo-Provera)	3.3	4.4	6.1	4.4	2.9	1.5	1.1
Intrauterine device (IUD)	1.3	0.1	1.1	2.5	2.2	1.0	0.8
Diaphragm	0.2	–	0.1	0.3	0.1	–	0.4
Condom	11.1	8.5	14.0	14.0	11.8	11.1	8.0
Periodic abstinence							
Calendar rhythm method	0.7	–	0.8	0.3	0.9	1.1	1.2
Natural family planning	0.2	–	–	0.4	0.2	0.3	0.4
Withdrawal	2.5	0.8	3.1	5.3	2.6	2.4	1.0
Other methods	0.6	0.6	0.2	0.4	0.4	0.5	1.1
Not using contraception	**38.1**	**68.5**	**39.3**	**32.0**	**30.8**	**29.2**	**30.9**
Surgically sterile—female (noncontraceptive)	1.5	–	–	0.4	0.9	2.1	4.9
Nonsurgically sterile, male or female	1.6	0.7	0.7	0.9	1.4	1.2	4.4
Pregnant or postpartum	5.3	3.5	9.5	8.4	6.9	3.8	0.8
Seeking pregnancy	4.2	1.2	2.8	5.5	7.0	5.1	3.3
Other nonuse							
Never had intercourse or no intercourse in past 3 months	18.1	56.2	17.9	8.9	7.6	9.1	10.8
Had intercourse during past 3 months	7.4	6.9	8.4	8.0	7.0	7.7	6.7

Note: Other methods includes Today sponge, cervical cap, female condom, and other methods. (–) means percentage is less than 0.05.
Source: National Center for Health Statistics, Use of Contraception and Use of Family Planning Services in the United States: 1982–2002, *Advance Data, No. 350, 2004; Internet site http://www.cdc.gov/nchs/nsfg.htm*

Table 13.13　Contraceptive Use by Race and Hispanic Origin, 2002

(total number of women aged 15 to 44 and percent distribution by contraceptive status, race, and Hispanic origin, 2002; numbers in thousands)

	total	non-Hispanic black	non-Hispanic white	Hispanic
TOTAL WOMEN AGED 15 TO 44				
Number	**61,561**	**8,587**	**40,420**	**9,107**
Percent	**100.0%**	**100.0%**	**100.0%**	**100.0%**
Using contraception	**61.9**	**57.4**	**64.5**	**59.0**
Female sterilization	16.7	22.3	15.5	19.9
Male sterilization	5.7	1.4	7.5	2.6
Pill	18.9	12.9	22.2	13.0
Implant, Lunelle, or Patch	0.8	0.5	0.5	1.8
Three-month injectable (Depo-Provera)	3.3	5.6	2.7	4.3
Intrauterine device (IUD)	1.3	0.8	0.9	3.2
Diaphragm	0.2	0.1	0.2	–
Condom	11.1	11.4	10.7	10.9
Periodic abstinence				
Calendar rhythm method	0.7	0.3	0.8	0.6
Natural family planning	0.2	0.1	0.2	0.3
Withdrawal	2.5	1.5	2.5	2.2
Other methods	0.6	0.5	0.7	0.3
Not using contraception	**38.1**	**42.6**	**35.5**	**41.0**
Surgically sterile—female (noncontraceptive)	1.5	1.5	1.7	0.9
Nonsurgically sterile, male or female	1.6	1.5	1.7	1.7
Pregnant or postpartum	5.3	5.9	4.6	6.9
Seeking pregnancy	4.2	4.2	3.9	5.2
Other nonuse				
Never had intercourse or no intercourse in past three months	18.1	19.4	17.0	18.7
Had intercourse during past 3 months	7.4	10.2	6.7	7.7

Note: Other methods includes Today sponge, cervical cap, female condom, and other methods. (–) means percentage is less than 0.05.
Source: National Center for Health Statistics, Use of Contraception and Use of Family Planning Services in the United States: 1982–2002, *Advance Data, No. 350, 2004; Internet site http://www.cdc.gov/nchs/nsfg.htm*

Table 13.14 Use of Family Planning Services by Selected Characteristics, 2002

(number of women aged 15 to 44 and percent using family planning services, by selected characteristics and type of service, 2002; numbers in thousands)

			type of family planning service used				
	number	used at least one type of family planning service	birth control method	birth control counseling	birth control checkup or test	sterilization counseling	sterilization operation
TOTAL WOMEN AGED 15 TO 44	**61,561**	**41.7%**	**33.9%**	**18.6%**	**23.6%**	**4.4%**	**1.9%**
Age							
Aged 15 to 17	5,819	31.8	22.2	19.0	15.8	1.1	–
Aged 18 to 19	4,016	51.6	43.9	26.5	31.0	0.9	–
Aged 20 to 24	9,840	63.3	54.0	30.6	35.7	1.4	1.2
Aged 25 to 29	9,249	55.4	46.3	23.8	30.2	3.6	2.2
Aged 30 to 34	10,272	47.0	39.1	18.3	27.2	7.1	2.6
Aged 35 to 39	10,853	30.5	23.9	12.7	18.6	6.6	3.0
Aged 40 to 44	11,512	19.5	14.0	7.0	10.8	5.2	2.0
Race and Hispanic origin							
Black, non-Hispanic	8,587	39.6	30.6	20.7	21.5	5.0	2.2
Hispanic	9,107	39.7	28.9	22.6	20.6	7.0	2.3
White, non-Hispanic	40,420	43.2	36.4	17.4	25.4	3.7	1.7
Marital or cohabiting status							
Currently married	28,327	39.5	31.5	16.0	21.3	5.8	2.5
Currently cohabiting	5,570	50.4	43.2	21.5	30.2	4.6	1.8
Not cohabiting							
Never married	21,568	44.4	36.4	22.5	25.4	2.4	0.7
Formerly married	6,096	34.5	28.0	14.3	22.0	4.7	3.1
Parity							
No births	25,622	45.3	38.8	20.8	27.1	1.3	0.3
One birth	11,193	51.0	43.0	22.9	27.6	4.5	1.4
Two births	13,402	38.1	29.3	16.5	21.4	6.3	3.7
Three or more births	11,343	28.6	19.5	11.8	14.5	9.2	3.8
Ratio of income to poverty level							
0 to 149 percent	14,582	39.3	29.7	20.1	21.4	7.3	2.8
150 to 299 percent	14,502	39.3	31.9	16.5	22.2	5.3	2.3
300 percent or more	22,643	45.5	39.3	17.4	26.6	3.4	1.8

Note: (–) means not applicable or zero.

Source: National Center for Health Statistics, Use of Contraception and Use of Family Planning Services in the United States: 1982–2002, *Advance Data, No. 350, 2004; Internet site http://www.cdc.gov/nchs/nsfg.htm*

14

Weight and Exercise

■ **Only 39 percent of adults are at a healthy weight.**

Women are more likely than men to have a healthy weight.

■ **Men and women are at least 24 pounds heavier today than they were in the 1960s.**

The average man weighs 191 pounds. The average woman weighs 164.

■ **Most Americans are overweight.**

Sixty-nine percent of men and 62 percent of women are overweight.

■ **Only 9 percent of high school girls are overweight.**

Thirty-six percent of high school girls think they are overweight, however.

■ **Most adults want to lose weight.**

The percentage of women who want to lose weight climbed from 45 to 67 percent between 1954 and 2004.

■ **Most Americans do not get enough exercise.**

Fewer than half meet recommendations for moderate physical activity.

Shifts in Eating Habits Reflect Fads and Findings

Some positive changes are apparent, but other changes hint at relaxed habits.

Between 1990 and 2002, Americans changed some of their dietary habits. The popularity of low-carbohydrate diets may account for some of the changes in food intake—such as increased consumption of red meat, poultry, fish, shellfish, and eggs. Low-carb diets may also play a role in the greater consumption of cheese, yogurt, and cream.

Ongoing efforts by nutritionists and public health professionals to get Americans to eat a better diet have yet to result in big changes. But they may account for the greater consumption of fresh fruits and vegetables. Nutrition education may also be why people are drinking more skim milk and less whole and 2-percent milk. Overall milk consumption has declined, however.

The beverage of choice continues to be carbonated soft drinks. Not only do Americans consume more soft drinks than any other beverage, they drink more than they once did. Consumption of soft drinks rose from 46.2 gallons in 1990 to 49.3 gallons in 2000. Coffee consumption was down, however, as was consumption of alcoholic beverages. Bottled water, on the other hand, is increasingly popular.

■ The decline in the consumption of potatoes may be related to the low-carb craze. If so, potato consumption may increase as people become disillusioned with low-carb regimens.

Americans are consuming more fruits and vegetables—and more sugar

(number of pounds of selected foods consumed per person, 1990 and 2002)

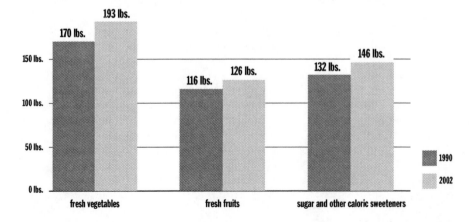

Table 14.1 Food and Beverage Consumption, 1990 and 2002

(number of pounds of selected foods and gallons of selected beverages consumed per person, 1990 and 2002; percent change in consumption, 1990–2002)

	2002	1990	percent change 1990–2002
Red meat	114.0	112.2	1.6%
Beef	64.5	63.9	0.9
Pork	48.2	46.4	3.9
Poultry	70.7	56.2	25.8
Chicken	56.8	42.4	34.0
Turkey	14.0	13.8	1.4
Fish and shellfish	15.6	14.9	4.7
Eggs	255.0	234.0	9.0
Shell	180.0	186.0	−3.2
Processed	75.0	48.0	56.3
Beverage milk	21.9	25.7	−14.8
Plain whole milk	7.3	10.2	−28.4
Plain 2% milk	7.0	9.1	−23.1
Plain skim milk	5.8	4.9	18.4
Flavored milk	1.6	1.1	45.5
Yogurt	13.7	7.4	85.1
Cream	12.1	8.7	39.1
Sour cream and dips	6.7	4.7	42.6
Cheese	30.5	24.6	24.0
American	12.8	11.1	15.3
Cheddar	9.6	9.0	6.7
Italian	12.4	9.0	37.8
Mozzarella	9.7	6.9	40.6
Other	5.3	4.5	17.8
Swiss	1.1	1.4	−21.4
Cream, Neufchatel	2.4	1.7	41.2
Cottage cheese	2.6	3.4	−23.5
Frozen dairy products	26.4	28.4	−7.0
Ice cream	16.7	15.8	5.7
Low-fat ice cream	6.5	7.7	−15.6
Sherbet	1.1	1.2	−8.3
Frozen yogurt	1.5	2.8	−46.4
Butter*	4.6	4.4	4.5
Margarine*	8.2	10.9	−24.8
Salad and cooking oils*	33.7	25.2	33.7
Flour and cereal products	191.3	180.9	5.7
Wheat flour products	136.7	135.9	0.6
Rice products	19.2	15.8	21.5
Corn products	29.7	21.4	38.8
Oat products	4.5	6.5	−30.8
Caloric sweeteners	146.1	132.4	10.3
Sugar	63.2	64.4	−1.9
Corn sweeteners	81.5	66.8	22.0
Peanuts (shelled)	5.8	6.0	−3.3
Tree nuts	3.1	2.4	29.2
Fresh fruits	125.6	116.2	8.1
Noncitrus	103.2	94.9	8.7
Apples	16.0	19.6	−18.4
Bananas	26.8	24.3	10.3

(continued)

	2002	1990	percent change 1990–2002
Cantaloupes	11.3	9.2	22.8%
Grapes	8.6	7.9	8.9
Peaches and nectarines	5.3	5.5	–3.6
Pears	2.9	3.2	–9.4
Pineapples	3.8	2.0	90.0
Plums and prunes	1.3	1.5	–13.3
Strawberries	4.7	3.2	46.9
Watermelons	13.9	13.3	4.5
Other nonctirus fruits	8.6	5.2	65.4
Citrus	22.4	21.4	4.7
Oranges	10.6	12.4	–14.5
Grapefruit	4.8	4.4	9.1
Other citrus fruit	7.0	4.6	52.2
Processed fruits	146.0	155.9	–6.4
Frozen fruits	4.6	3.8	21.1
Dried fruits	10.6	12.1	–12.4
Canned fruits	16.7	21.0	–20.5
Fresh vegetables	193.4	170.2	13.6
Asparagus	1.0	0.6	66.7
Broccoli	5.0	3.4	47.1
Cabbage	8.4	8.3	1.2
Carrots	9.5	8.3	14.5
Cauliflower	1.5	2.2	–31.8
Celery	6.5	7.2	–9.7
Corn	9.0	6.7	34.3
Cucumbers	6.7	4.7	42.6
Head lettuce	22.4	27.7	–19.1
Mushrooms	2.6	2.0	30.0
Onions	18.5	15.1	22.5
Snap beans	2.1	1.1	90.9
Bell peppers	7.0	4.5	55.6
Potatoes	45.0	46.7	–3.6
Sweet potatoes	3.7	4.4	–15.9
Tomatoes	18.4	15.5	18.7
Other fresh vegetables	26.1	11.8	121.2
Processed vegetables	218.6	215.5	1.4
Frozen vegetables	78.0	66.8	16.8
Canned vegetables	99.8	110.4	–9.6
Potato chips	17.0	16.4	3.7
Tea	7.8	6.9	13.0
Coffee	23.6	26.8	–11.9
Bottled water**	17.7	8.0	121.3
Carbonated soft drinks*	49.3	46.2	6.7
Diet*	11.6	10.7	8.4
Regular*	37.7	35.6	5.9
Fruit juices	8.0	8.0	0.0
Fruit drinks, cocktails, ades**	7.7	6.3	22.2
Alcoholic beverages	25.2	27.4	–8.0
Beer	21.8	23.9	–8.8
Wine	2.1	2.0	5.0
Distilled spirits	1.3	1.5	–13.3

* Latest data available are for 2000.
** Latest data available are for 1999.
Note: Alcoholic beverage consumption is per person aged 21 or older.
Source: Bureau of the Census, Statistical Abstract of the United States: 2004–2005, Internet site http://www.census.gov/prod/www/statistical–abstract–04.html; calculations by New Strategist

Few Americans Are at a Healthy Weight

Asians are most likely to be at a healthy weight.

The majority of people aged 18 or older are overweight. Only 39 percent are within a healthy weight range, and just 2 percent are underweight. Women are more likely than men to be at a healthy weight—47 versus 32 percent.

Sixty percent of Asians are at a healthy weight, the largest share among all racial and ethnic groups. Many Asians are immigrants who still adhere to a traditional diet. In general, Asian diets include less fat and carbohydrates than the American fast-food diet, and portions are smaller. Studies show, however, that second-generation immigrants are more likely to adopt an American diet. As they do, weight problems are likely to grow.

■ Americans love to sample foods from other cultures, but they often adapt those foods to suit their palate by adding fat and calories.

Blacks and Hispanics are least likely to be at a healthy weight

(percent of people aged 18 or older who are at a healthy weight, by race and Hispanic origin, 2002)

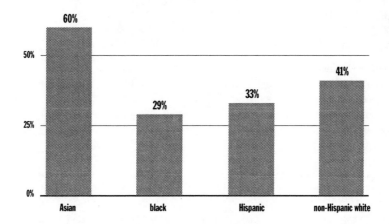

Table 14.2 Self-Reported Weight Status of People Aged 18 or Older by Selected Characteristics, 2002

(number of people aged 18 or older and percent distribution by weight status as measured by body mass index, by selected characteristics, 2002; numbers in thousands)

	total	underweight	healthy weight	overweight total	obese
Total	205,825	2.0%	39.4%	58.5%	23.5%
Sex					
Men	98,749	1.1	32.0	66.9	23.8
Women	107,076	3.0	46.9	50.0	22.9
Age					
Aged 18 to 44	108,114	2.5	44.2	53.3	21.4
Aged 45 to 64	64,650	1.1	32.1	66.9	27.8
Aged 65 to 74	17,809	1.7	31.7	66.6	27.3
Aged 75 or older	15,252	3.5	45.4	51.0	15.9
Race and Hispanic origin					
Asian	7,270	5.6	59.9	34.5	7.0
Black	23,499	1.7	29.4	68.9	34.8
Hispanic	22,691	1.4	33.4	65.2	25.4
Non-Hispanic white	149,584	2.1	41.4	56.6	21.9
Education					
Less than high school	28,248	1.5	32.1	66.4	29.7
High school graduate	52,556	2.0	34.6	63.4	27.5
Some college	48,091	1.7	36.1	62.2	25.8
College graduate	47,197	1.7	43.6	54.7	17.4
Household income					
Less than $20,000	37,369	2.9	40.4	56.7	26.4
$20,000 to $34,999	29,671	1.9	37.4	60.8	26.8
$35,000 to $54,999	31,814	1.9	37.9	60.2	24.0
$55,000 to $74,999	23,984	1.8	37.5	60.7	23.0
$75,000 or more	41,572	1.7	42.2	56.1	19.8

Note: Underweight is a body mass index (BMI) below 18.5; healthy weight is a BMI of 18.5 to 24.9; overweight is a BMI of 25.0 to 29.9; obese is a BMI of 30.0 or more. Body mass index is calculated by dividing weight in kilograms by height in meters squared. Respondents self-reported height and weight measurements. Numbers by race and Hispanic origin will not sum to total because not all races are shown and Hispanics may be of any race.
Source: National Center for Health Statistics, Summary Health Statistics for U.S. Adults: National Health Interview Survey, 2002, *Series 10, No. 222, 2004; Internet site http://www.cdc.gov/nchs/nhis.htm*

Four Decades of Overeating Tips the Scales

Both men and women grew by at least 24 pounds.

In 1960–62, the average weight of men aged 20 to 74 was 166 pounds. By 1999–02, the average man had packed on an additional 25 pounds, bringing his weight to 191 pounds. A similar change took place among women, whose average weight rose from 140 to 164 pounds.

For women, the biggest weight increase has occurred among those aged 20 to 34, a gain of 29 pounds between 1960–62 and 1999–02. Men aged 65 to 74 gained the most during those years, their average weight rising by almost 33 pounds.

Regardless of race or Hispanic origin, the 40-to-59 age group is packing the most pounds. Within the age group, non-Hispanic whites weigh the most among men, nearly 200 pounds on average. Among women in the age group, non-Hispanic blacks weigh the most, tipping the scales at an average of 189 pounds.

■ Because weight gain occurs slowly, many do not realize they are gaining weight until they no longer fit into their clothes.

The average man weighs almost 200 pounds

(average weight in pounds of people aged 20 to 74, by sex, 1960–62 and 1990–99)

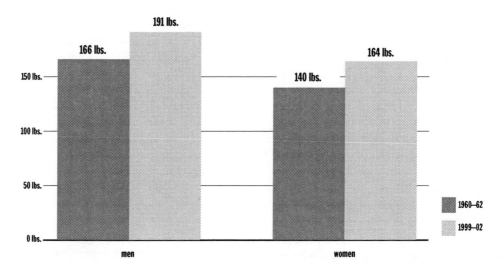

Table 14.3 Average Measured Weight by Sex and Age, 1960–62 and 1999–02

(average weight in pounds of people aged 20 to 74, by sex and age, 1960–62 and 1999–02; change in pounds 1960–62 to 1999–02)

	1999–02	1960–62	change in pounds
Men aged 20 to 74	**191.0**	**166.3**	**24.7**
Aged 20 to 29	183.4	163.9	19.5
Aged 30 to 39	189.1	169.9	19.2
Aged 40 to 49	196.0	169.1	26.9
Aged 50 to 59	195.4	167.7	27.7
Aged 60 to 74	191.5	158.9	32.6
Women aged 20 to 74	**164.3**	**140.2**	**24.1**
Aged 20 to 29	156.5	127.7	28.8
Aged 30 to 39	163.0	138.8	24.2
Aged 40 to 49	168.2	142.8	25.4
Aged 50 to 59	169.2	146.5	22.7
Aged 60 to 74	164.7	147.3	17.4

Note: Data are based on measured height and weight of a sample of the civilian noninstitutionalized population.
Source: National Center for Health Statistics, Mean Body Weight, Height, and Body Mass Index, United States 1960–2002, Advance Data, No. 347, 2004; Internet site http://www.cdc.gov/nchs/pressroom/04news/americans.htm; calculations by New Strategist

Table 14.4   Average Measured Weight by Sex, Age, Race, and Hispanic Origin, 1999–02

(average weight in pounds of people aged 20 or older, by sex, age, race, and Hispanic origin, 1999–02)

	men	women
Total people	**189.8**	**162.9**
BLACK, NON-HISPANIC		
Total aged 20 or older	**189.2**	**182.4**
Aged 20 to 39	189.1	179.2
Aged 40 to 59	191.1	189.3
Aged 60 or older	186.5	176.6
HISPANIC (MEXICAN)		
Total aged 20 or older	**177.3**	**157.1**
Aged 20 to 39	172.5	152.9
Aged 40 to 59	183.6	165.5
Aged 60 or older	175.7	150.7
WHITE, NON-HISPANIC		
Total aged 20 or older	**193.1**	**161.7**
Aged 20 to 39	189.7	158.4
Aged 40 to 59	199.5	167.6
Aged 60 or older	188.8	158.0

Note: Data are based on measured height and weight of a sample of the civilian noninstitutionalized population.
Source: National Center for Health Statistics, Mean Body Weight, Height, and Body Mass Index, United States 1960–2002, Advance Data, *No. 347, 2004; Internet site http://www.cdc.gov/nchs/pressroom/04news/americans.htm; calculations by New Strategist*

Most Americans Are Overweight

The ranks of the obese are growing.

The percentage of men who are overweight rose from 50 to 69 percent between 1960–62 and 1999-02. Among women, the figure rose from 40 to 62 percent during those years. Even more alarming is the increase in obesity. Among men, the obesity rate rose from 11 to 28 percent, while among women it increased from 16 to 34 percent.

The percentage of Americans who are overweight or obese rises with age, peaking in the 55-to-64 age group. Forty-two percent of women aged 55 to 64 are obese, as are 36 percent of men.

Among men by race and Hispanic origin, the percentage of the overweight ranges from a low of 62 percent among non-Hispanic blacks to a high of 70 percent among non-Hispanic whites and Hispanics. Among women, non-Hispanic whites are least likely to be overweight (58 percent), while non-Hispanic blacks are most likely to weigh too much (77 percent).

■ Obesity looms as a serious public health problem. Growing numbers of overweight and obese adults will lead to a growing number of people with serious health problems.

More than one-third of women are obese

(percent of people aged 20 to 74 who are obese, by sex, 1960–62 and 1999–02)

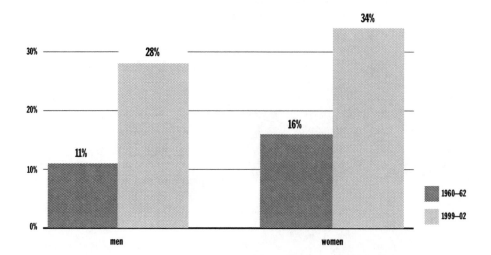

Table 14.5 Adults Measured as Overweight and Obese by Sex and Age, 1960–62 and 1999–02

(percent of people aged 20 to 74 who are overweight or obese, by sex and age, 1960–62 and 1999–02; percentage point change, 1960–62 to 1999–02)

	overweight			obese		
	1999–02	1960–62	percentage point change	1999–02	1960–62	percentage point change
Men aged 20 to 74	**68.8%**	**49.5%**	**19.3**	**28.1%**	**10.7%**	**17.4**
Aged 20 to 34	57.4	42.7	14.7	21.7	9.2	12.5
Aged 35 to 44	70.5	53.5	17.0	28.5	12.1	16.4
Aged 45 to 54	75.7	53.9	21.8	30.6	12.5	18.1
Aged 55 to 64	75.4	52.2	23.2	35.5	9.2	26.3
Aged 65 to 74	76.2	47.8	28.4	31.9	10.4	21.5
Women aged 20 to 74	**61.7**	**40.2**	**21.5**	**34.0**	**15.7**	**18.3**
Aged 20 to 34	52.8	21.2	31.6	28.4	7.2	21.2
Aged 35 to 44	60.6	37.2	23.4	32.1	14.7	17.4
Aged 45 to 54	65.1	49.3	15.8	36.9	20.3	16.6
Aged 55 to 64	72.2	59.9	12.3	42.1	24.4	17.7
Aged 65 to 74	70.9	60.9	10.0	39.3	23.2	16.1

Note: Overweight is defined as a body mass index of 25 or higher. Obesity is defined as a body mass index of 30 or higher. Body mass index is calculated by dividing weight in kilograms by height in meters squared. Data are based on measured height and weight of a sample of the civilian noninstitutionalized population.
Source: National Center for Health Statistics, Health, United States, 2004, Internet site http://www.cdc.gov/nchs/hus.htm

Table 14.6 Adults Measured as Overweight and Obese by Sex and Age, 1999—02

(percent of people aged 20 or older who are overweight or obese, by sex and age, 1999–02)

	overweight	obese
Total people	**65.2%**	**30.5%**
Total men	**68.6**	**27.5**
Aged 20 to 34	57.4	21.7
Aged 35 to 44	70.5	28.5
Aged 45 to 54	75.7	30.6
Aged 55 to 64	75.4	35.5
Aged 65 to 74	76.2	31.9
Aged 75 or older	67.4	18.0
Total women	**62.0**	**33.4**
Aged 20 to 34	52.8	28.4
Aged 35 to 44	60.6	32.1
Aged 45 to 54	65.1	36.9
Aged 55 to 64	72.2	42.1
Aged 65 to 74	70.9	39.3
Aged 75 or older	59.9	23.6

Note: Overweight is defined as a body mass index of 25 or higher. Obesity is defined as a body mass index of 30 or higher. Body mass index is calculated by dividing weight in kilograms by height in meters squared. Data are based on measured height and weight of a sample of the civilian noninstitutionalized population.
Source: National Center for Health Statistics, Health, United States, 2004, *Internet site http://www.cdc.gov/nchs/hus.htm*

Table 14.7 Adults Measured as Overweight and Obese by Sex, Race, and Hispanic Origin, 1999–02

(percent of people aged 20 or older who are overweight or obese, by sex, race, and Hispanic origin, 1999–02)

	overweight	obese
Total people	**65.2%**	**30.5%**
Female	**62.0**	**33.4**
Black, non-Hispanic	76.8	48.8
Hispanic (Mexican)	69.3	37.0
White, non-Hispanic	58.2	31.3
Male	**68.6**	**27.5**
Black, non-Hispanic	61.7	27.5
Hispanic (Mexican)	70.1	26.0
White, non-Hispanic	69.9	28.4

Note: Overweight is defined as a body mass index of 25 or higher. Obesity is defined as a body mass index of 30 or higher. Body mass index is calculated by dividing weight in kilograms by height in meters squared. Data are based on measured height and weight of a sample of the civilian noninstitutionalized population.
Source: National Center for Health Statistics, Health, United States, 2004, *Internet site http://www.cdc.gov/nchs/hus.htm*

Boys Are More Likely than Girls to Be Overweight

But the majority of children and teenagers are not overweight.

Given that most adults are overweight, it is not surprising that some children and teenagers also need to lose weight. Among people aged 6 to 19, 16 percent are overweight.

The likelihood of being overweight varies by race and Hispanic origin. Among boys, Hispanics of Mexican heritage are most likely to be overweight, with more than one-quarter classified as weighing too much. Among girls, non-Hispanic blacks are most likely to be overweight, with 24 percent of those aged 12 to 19 weighing more than they should.

A survey of high school students shows ninth graders to be more likely than older students to be overweight, at 15 percent. High school girls are more likely than boys to think they are overweight (36 versus 23 percent), although boys are more likely than girls to actually be overweight (17 versus 9 percent).

■ Overweight children nearly always become overweight adults, with resulting health problems.

Among boys, Hispanics are most likely to be overweight

(percent of children aged 6 to 11 who are overweight, by sex, race, and Hispanic origin, 1999–02)

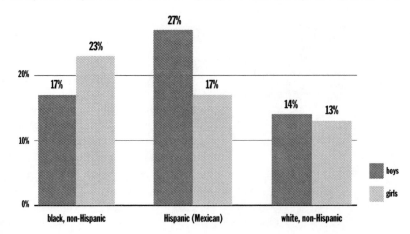

Table 14.8 Children Measured as Overweight by Age, Sex, Race, and Hispanic Origin, 1999–02

(percent of people aged 6 to 19 who are overweight, by age, sex, race, and Hispanic origin, 1999–02)

	6 to 11	12 to 19
Total overweight	**15.8%**	**16.1%**
Boys	**16.9**	**16.7**
Black, non-Hispanic	17.0	18.7
Hispanic (Mexican)	26.5	24.7
White, non-Hispanic	14.0	14.6
Girls	**14.7**	**15.4**
Black, non-Hispanic	22.8	23.6
Hispanic (Mexican)	17.1	19.6
White, non-Hispanic	13.1	12.7

Note: Overweight is defined as a body mass index of 25 or higher. Obesity is defined as a body mass index of 30 or higher. Body mass index is calculated by dividing weight in kilograms by height in meters squared. Data are based on measured height and weight of a sample of the civilian noninstitutionalized population.
Source: National Center for Health Statistics, Health, United States, 2004, *Internet site http://www.cdc.gov/nchs/hus.htm*

(percent of ninth to twelfth graders by weight status and dieting behavior, by sex and grade, 2003)

	total	9th grade	10th grade	11th grade	12th grade
Total					
At risk for becoming overweight*	15.4%	15.4%	15.0%	16.8%	14.4%
Overweight**	13.5	15.3	13.7	12.9	11.4
Described themselves as overweight	29.6	27.7	29.6	30.5	31.4
Were trying to lose weight	43.8	42.2	45.1	44.1	44.6
Ate less food, fewer calories, or foods low in fat to lose weight or to avoid gaining weight in past 30 days	42.2	40.4	42.7	42.8	43.7
Exercised to lose weight or to avoid gaining weight in past 30 days	57.1	57.6	59.2	56.8	54.6
Went without eating for at least 24 hours to lose weight or to avoid gaining weight in past 30 days	13.3	14.6	12.7	13.8	11.2
Took diet pills, powders, or liquids without a doctor's advice to lose weight or avoid gaining weight in past 30 days	9.2	8.0	8.3	10.1	10.8
Vomited or took a laxative to lose weight or to avoid gaining weight in past 30 days	6.0	6.2	6.4	5.7	5.5
Females					
At risk for becoming overweight*	15.3	15.6	15.3	16.9	13.2
Overweight**	9.4	11.2	9.3	8.6	8.0
Described themselves as overweight	36.1	33.1	36.1	36.9	38.7
Were trying to lose weight	59.3	54.1	62.2	60.4	61.7
Ate less food, fewer calories, or foods low in fat to lose weight or to avoid gaining weight in past 30 days	56.2	53.0	58.1	56.4	57.9
Exercised to lose weight or to avoid gaining weight in past 30 days	65.7	65.7	68.9	64.5	63.2
Went without eating for at least 24 hours to lose weight or to avoid gaining weight in past 30 days	18.3	18.8	18.5	19.6	15.7
Took diet pills, powders, or liquids without a doctor's advice to lose weight or avoid gaining weight in past 30 days	11.3	9.2	10.9	12.6	13.0
Vomited or took a laxative to lose weight or to avoid gaining weight in past 30 days	8.4	7.9	9.3	8.8	7.3

(continued)

	total	9th grade	10th grade	11th grade	12th grade
Males					
At risk for becoming overweight*	15.5%	15.3%	14.7%	16.6%	15.6%
Overweight**	17.4	19.0	17.9	17.0	14.7
Described themselves as overweight	23.5	22.6	23.2	24.3	24.1
Were trying to lose weight	29.1	31.2	28.3	28.3	28.0
Ate less food, fewer calories, or foods low in fat to lose weight or to avoid gaining weight in past 30 days	28.9	28.8	27.8	29.4	29.8
Exercised to lose weight or to avoid gaining weight in past 30 days	49.0	50.2	49.8	49.4	46.4
Went without eating for at least 24 hours to lose weight or to avoid gaining weight in past 30 days	8.5	10.7	7.0	8.2	6.9
Took diet pills, powders, or liquids without a doctor's advice to lose weight or avoid gaining weight in past 30 days	7.1	7.0	5.8	7.7	8.5
Vomited or took a laxative to lose weight or to avoid gaining weight in past 30 days	3.7	4.6	3.5	2.6	3.8

Students at risk of becoming overweight were between the 85th and 95th percentile for body mass index, by age and sex, based on reference data.

*** Students who were overweight were at or above the 95th percentile for body mass index, by age and sex, based on reference data.*

Source: Centers for Disease Control and Prevention, Youth Risk Behavior Surveillance–United States, 2003, Mortality and Morbidity Weekly Report, Surveillance Summaries, Vol. 53/SS02, May 21, 2004

Most Adults Want to Lose Weight

But strategies for doing so vary widely.

Given that most adults need to lose weight, it is not surprising that the majority of respondents to a 2004 Gallup poll say they want to lose weight. The percentage of men and women who want to lose weight has been rising since 1954, more or less in tandem with increases in the percentage of people who are overweight.

The share of people who want to lose weight is larger than the percentage making an effort to do so. Among adults aged 18 or older, only 38 percent say they are trying to lose weight. People aged 45 to 54 are most likely to be trying to drop pounds, with 45 percent making the attempt.

Among people trying to lose or maintain their current weight, exercise is the most popular strategy. Sixty-one percent say they are using exercise or physical activity for weight control. Thirty percent have cut both calories and fat in an attempt to become slimmer or at least maintain their weight, while 27 percent have reduced their fat intake only. A relatively small 14 percent say they are simply eating fewer calories.

■ Although exercise is considered an important component of a weight loss program, dietary changes are almost always necessary as well.

Two-thirds of women want to lose weight

(percent of people aged 18 or older who want to lose weight, by sex, 1954 and 2004)

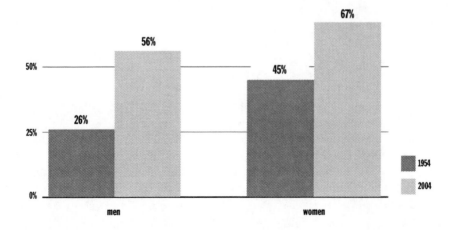

Table 14.10 People Who Want to Lose Weight, 1954 to 2004

(percent of people aged 18 or older who want to lose weight, by sex, selected years, 1954 to 2004)

	men	women
2004	56%	67%
2003	51	68
2002	49	66
2001	49	68
1999	44	58
1996	45	63
1990	42	61
1957	25	45
1955	24	49
1954	26	45

Source: The Gallup Organization, **Personal Weight Situation***; Internet site http://www.gallup.com/*

Table 14.11 Weight Loss Behavior by Age, 2000

(percent of people aged 18 or older engaging in selected weight loss behaviors, by age, 2000)

	total	18 to 24	25 to 34	35 to 44	45 to 54	55 to 64	65 or older
Trying to lose weight	38.0%	30.2%	38.0%	40.4%	44.7%	42.6%	30.6%
Trying to maintain weight	58.9	51.9	56.9	59.8	63.1	60.8	58.4
Eating fewer calories to lose/ maintain weight*	13.5	11.4	12.1	13.9	15.2	13.2	12.0
Eating less fat to lose/maintain weight*	27.4	25.3	25.8	27.7	28.3	29.1	29.4
Eating fewer calories and less fat to lose/maintain weight*	29.6	25.5	27.0	30.1	32.6	33.0	29.0
Using physical activity or exercise to lose/maintain weight*	60.7	74.7	67.7	64.0	60.5	55.4	43.3
Advised by health professional to lose weight	11.7	4.0	8.4	11.3	16.0	17.7	11.2

* Among those trying to lose or maintain weight.
Source: Centers for Disease Control and Prevention, Behavioral Risk Factor Surveillance System Prevalence Data, 2000; Internet site http://apps.nccd.cdc.gov/brfss/index.asp

Americans Do Not Get Enough Exercise

Fewer than half meet the recommendation for moderate physical activity.

The increase in the percentage of overweight and obese adults is the result of a simple formula: calories in minus calories out. Americans are consuming more calories, but most are not getting enough exercise to burn off their increased caloric intake.

Fewer than half (46 percent) of adults meet the recommendation for physical activity. The 54 percent majority do not meet recommended activity levels and 24 percent are physically inactive. Men are more likely than women to meet recommended activity levels.

The share of people who get enough exercise is highest among young adults aged 18 to 29 (50 percent), then steadily falls with age. Among people aged 75 or older, only 28 percent get enough exercise. There are also differences by race and Hispanic origin, with non-Hispanic whites more likely than blacks or Hispanics to meet exercise recommendations.

■ Physical activity increases with education, in part because the educated are more aware of what they need to do to be healthy.

The majority of college graduates get enough exercise

(percent of people aged 18 or older who participated in the recommended level of physical activity in the past month, by educational attainment, 2003)

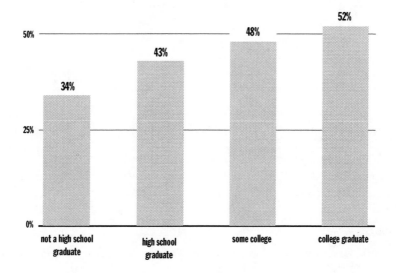

Table 14.12 Participation in Leisure-Time Physical Activity, 2003

(percent of people aged 18 or older engaging in leisure-time physical activity, by selected demographic characteristics and level of activity, 2003)

	people who meet recommended activity	people with insufficient activity	
		total	physically inactive
Total people	**46.0%**	**54.0%**	**24.3%**
Men	**48.2**	**51.8**	**22.0**
Aged 18 to 29	57.8	42.2	17.1
Aged 30 to 44	48.7	51.3	20.7
Aged 45 to 64	43.2	56.8	24.4
Aged 65 to 74	45.7	54.3	24.9
Aged 75 or older	36.7	63.3	31.0
Women	**44.0**	**56.0**	**26.3**
Aged 18 to 29	50.1	49.9	21.9
Aged 30 to 44	47.7	52.3	23.4
Aged 45 to 64	42.6	57.4	26.7
Aged 65 to 74	37.1	62.9	31.2
Aged 75 or older	27.6	72.4	42.0
Race and Hispanic origin			
Black, non-Hispanic	36.3	63.7	32.7
Hispanic	37.5	62.5	36.0
White, non-Hispanic	49.0	51.0	20.9
Other	43.5	56.5	25.2
Education			
Less than 12 years	33.8	66.2	45.7
12 years	43.1	56.9	30.5
Some college (13–15 years)	47.5	52.5	21.0
College (16+ years)	51.9	48.1	13.1
Household income			
Less than $10,000	34.7	65.3	42.2
$10,000 to $19,999	37.0	63.0	38.9
$20,000 to $34,999	43.6	56.4	29.4
$35,000 to $49,999	47.3	52.7	21.9
$50,000 or more	53.6	46.4	13.6

Note: Recommended activity is physical activity at least five times per week for thirty minutes each time or vigorous physical activity for twenty minutes each time at least three times per week. Insufficient activity is physical activity that does not meet the recommended level. The physically inactive are people with no reported physical activity.
Source: Bureau of the Census, Statistical Abstract of the United States: 2004–2005; Internet site http://www.census.gov/prod/www/statistical-abstract-04.html; calculations by New Strategist

Table 14.13 Frequency of Vigorous Physical Activity among People Aged 18 or Older, 2002

(number of people aged 18 or older and percent distribution by number of leisure-time periods per week of vigorous physical activity lasting ten minutes or more, by selected characteristics, 2002; numbers in thousands)

	total	frequency of vigorous physical activity per week				
		never	less than one	one to two	three to four	five or more
Total	205,825	59.2%	3.0%	12.3%	13.2%	12.3%
Sex						
Men	98,749	53.1	3.4	14.3	14.1	15.0
Women	107,076	65.0	2.5	10.4	12.3	9.8
Age						
Aged 18 to 44	108,114	49.7	3.7	15.6	16.2	14.8
Aged 45 to 64	64,650	63.2	2.7	11.0	12.2	10.9
Aged 65 to 74	17,809	77.1	1.4	5.9	6.7	8.9
Aged 75 or older	15,252	88.1	0.9	2.2	3.8	4.9
Race and Hispanic origin						
Asian	7,270	64.7	3.6	11.5	11.1	9.0
Black	23,499	67.4	2.4	10.3	10.6	9.3
Hispanic	22,691	71.1	1.7	9.6	8.4	9.2
Non-Hispanic white	149,584	55.7	3.2	13.2	14.4	13.4
Education						
Less than high school	28,248	80.7	1.5	6.1	4.7	7.1
High school graduate	52,556	68.0	2.5	10.0	8.9	10.6
Some college	48,091	58.3	3.2	12.5	14.2	11.8
College graduate	47,197	46.0	3.8	16.3	19.3	14.6
Household income						
Less than $20,000	37,369	72.1	1.8	8.3	8.0	9.9
$20,000 to $34,999	29,671	65.9	2.5	10.2	10.2	11.2
$35,000 to $54,999	31,814	57.3	3.0	13.6	13.2	13.0
$55,000 to $74,999	23,984	54.2	3.9	14.3	14.5	13.1
$75,000 or more	41,572	45.4	4.2	15.9	19.4	15.1

Note: Vigorous physical activity is defined as activity that causes heavy sweating and large increases in breathing or heart rate. Numbers by race and Hispanic origin will not sum to total because not all races are shown and Hispanics may be of any race.
Source: National Center for Health Statistics, Summary Health Statistics for U.S. Adults: National Health Interview Survey, 2002, *Series 10, No. 222, 2004; Internet site http://www.cdc.gov/nchs/nhis.htm*

Sports Participation Is Declining

Fewer Americans are engaging in a variety of sports.

Americans lead increasingly sedentary lives. A survey of sports participation by the National Sporting Goods Association shows that participation in many sports is declining.

Exercise walking is one of the most popular forms of physical activity. But among people aged 7 or older, the percentage engaging in exercise walking more than once during the past twelve months fell slightly between 1998 and 2003, from 32 to 31 percent. In fact, participation in most of the sports considered here declined during the five-year period.

Children aged 7 to 11 are also less likely to participate in many sports long popular with the age set. They were less likely to ride a bicycle or to play baseball or softball in 2003 than in 1998. But their participation in skateboarding increased. Among teenagers, participation in many popular sports fell during those years. Even basketball participation declined, with only 32 percent of 12-to-17-year-olds participating in basketball more than once in 2003, down from 44 percent in 1998.

■ Children's declining participation in sports makes it less likely that they will be physically active as adults.

Playing basketball fell 12 percentage points among teens

(percentage point change in percent of people aged 7 to 17 participating in selected sports more than once during the past year, by age, 2003)

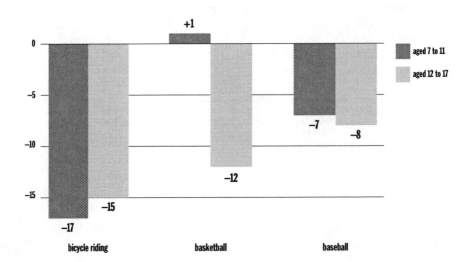

Table 14.14 Sports Participation of People Aged 7 or Older, 1998 and 2003

(number and percent of people aged 7 or older participating in selected sports more than once during past year, 1998 and 2003; percent change in number and percentage point change in share, 1998–2003; numbers in millions)

	number participating		percent change	percent participating		percentage point change
	2003	1998		2003	1998	
Total people	**256.2**	**242.9**	**5.5%**	–	–	–
Archery (target)	3.9	4.8	–19.1	1.5%	2.0%	–0.5
Backpacking/wilderness camping	13.7	14.6	–6.2	5.3	6.0	–0.7
Baseball	14.6	15.9	–7.7	5.7	6.5	–0.8
Basketball	27.9	29.4	–5.2	10.9	12.1	–1.2
Bicycle riding	36.3	43.5	–16.7	14.2	17.9	–3.7
Billiards/pool	30.5	32.3	–5.7	11.9	13.3	–1.4
Boating (motor)	24.2	25.7	–5.9	9.4	10.6	–1.1
Bowling	39.4	40.1	–1.6	15.4	16.5	–1.1
Camping (vacation/overnight)	51.4	46.5	10.7	20.1	19.1	0.9
Exercise walking	79.5	77.6	2.4	31.0	31.9	–0.9
Exercising (aerobic)	28.0	25.8	8.8	10.9	10.6	0.3
Exercising with equipment	48.6	46.1	5.4	19.0	19.0	0.0
Fishing	38.2	43.6	–12.4	14.9	17.9	–3.0
Football (tackle)	8.7	8.1	6.1	3.4	3.3	0.1
Football (touch)	9.3	10.8	–14.0	3.6	4.4	–0.8
Golf	25.7	27.5	–6.7	10.0	11.3	–1.3
Hiking	25.0	27.2	–7.9	9.8	11.2	–1.4
Hockey (ice)	1.8	2.1	–14.2	0.7	0.9	–0.2
Hunting with bow and arrow	5.0	5.6	–11.4	2.0	2.3	–0.4
Hunting with firearms	17.9	17.3	3.6	7.0	7.1	–0.1
Ice/figure skating	5.1	7.8	–34.6	2.0	3.2	–1.2
Kayaking/rafting	4.7	3.2	47.1	1.8	1.3	0.5
Kick boxing	3.0	2.3	31.7	1.2	0.9	0.2
Martial arts	4.8	4.6	5.7	1.9	1.9	0.0
Mountain biking (off road)	8.2	8.6	–4.7	3.2	3.5	–0.3
Muzzleloading	3.1	3.1	0.0	1.2	1.3	–0.1
Running/jogging	22.9	22.5	1.8	8.9	9.3	–0.3
Sailing	2.6	3.6	–26.2	1.0	1.5	–0.5
Skateboarding	9.0	5.8	55.3	3.5	2.4	1.1
Skating (in-line)	16.0	27.0	–40.9	6.2	11.1	–4.9
Skiing (alpine)	6.8	7.7	–11.8	2.7	3.2	–0.5
Skiing (cross country)	1.9	2.6	–26.8	0.7	1.1	–0.3
Snowboarding	6.3	3.6	73.5	2.5	1.5	1.0
Soccer	11.1	13.2	–15.8	4.3	5.4	–1.1
Softball	11.8	15.6	–24.1	4.6	6.4	–1.8
Swimming	47.0	58.2	–19.3	18.3	24.0	–5.6
Target shooting	17.0	18.9	–9.9	6.6	7.8	–1.1
Tennis	9.6	11.2	–14.7	3.7	4.6	–0.9
Volleyball	10.4	14.8	–29.4	4.1	6.1	–2.0
Water skiing	5.5	7.2	–24.4	2.1	3.0	–0.8
Workout at club	29.5	26.5	11.0	11.5	10.9	0.6

Note: (–) means not applicable.
Source: National Sporting Goods Association, Internet site http://www.nsga.org

Table 14.15 Sports Participation of Children Aged 7 to 17, 1993 and 2003

(number and percent of people aged 7 to 17 participating in selected sports more than once during past year, 1993 and 2003; percent change in number and percentage point change in share, 1993–2003; numbers in thousands)

	number participating		percent change	percent participating		percentage point change
	2003	1993		2003	1993	
AGE 7 TO 11						
Total children	**19,859**	**18,561**	**7.0%**	–	–	–
Baseball	4,514	5,422	–16.7	22.7%	29.2%	–6.5
Basketball	6,299	5,751	9.5	31.7	31.0	0.7
Bicycle riding	8,591	11,204	–23.3	43.3	60.4	–17.1
Fishing	3,684	4,623	–20.3	18.6	24.9	–6.4
Golf	1,293	840	53.9	6.5	4.5	2.0
Ice hockey	388	243	59.7	2.0	1.3	0.6
In-line skating	5,949	4,558	30.5	30.0	24.6	5.4
Skateboarding	3,484	2,284	52.5	17.5	12.3	5.2
Skiing (alpine)	778	453	71.7	3.9	2.4	1.5
Snowboarding	1,146	290	295.2	5.8	1.6	4.2
Soccer	4,715	4,543	3.8	23.7	24.5	–0.7
Softball	1,919	2,886	–33.5	9.7	15.5	–5.9
Tennis	997	1,003	–0.6	5.0	5.4	–0.4
Volleyball	1,274	1,333	–4.4	6.4	7.2	–0.8
AGE 12 TO 17						
Total children	**24,654**	**21,304**	**15.7**	–	–	–
Baseball	4,079	5,283	–22.8	16.5	24.8	–8.3
Basketball	7,871	9,361	–15.9	31.9	43.9	–12.0
Bicycle riding	6,537	8,794	–25.7	26.5	41.3	–14.8
Fishing	4,062	4,945	–17.9	16.5	23.2	–6.7
Golf	2,300	1,692	35.9	9.3	7.9	1.4
Ice hockey	410	433	–5.3	1.7	2.0	–0.4
In-line skating	3,693	3,627	1.8	15.0	17.0	–2.0
Skateboarding	3,568	2,110	69.1	14.5	9.9	4.6
Skiing (alpine)	868	1,549	–44.0	3.5	7.3	–3.8
Snowboarding	2,029	713	184.6	8.2	3.3	4.9
Soccer	3,552	3,063	16.0	14.4	14.4	0.0
Softball	2,890	3,817	–24.3	11.7	17.9	–6.2
Tennis	2,054	2,464	–16.6	8.3	11.6	–3.2
Volleyball	3,359	5,443	–38.3	13.6	25.5	–11.9

Note: (–) means not applicable.
Source: National Sporting Goods Association, Internet site http://www.nsga.org

Most Children Engage in Free-Time Physical Activities

A smaller proportion take part in organized activities.

Among children aged 9 to 13, nearly 40 percent participated in some type of organized physical activity in the past week. An even larger 77 percent took part in free-time physical activities.

Reliance on organized activities for children's physical recreation creates problems for some families. Participation often has a cost, for example, and this can effectively exclude families who cannot afford the fee. In fact, nearly half of parents (47 percent) say expense is a barrier to their children's participation in physical activities.

The demand by many organizations that parents help out also is a barrier to children's participation. Twenty-one percent of parents say a lack of parental time is a barrier to their child's participation in physical activities. Transportation is another problem, mentioned by 26 percent of parents. Sixteen percent of parents say a lack of neighborhood safety is a barrier.

■ Although most children engage in some kind of physical activity during an average week, few are getting enough exercise.

Cost is the number-one barrier to children's participation

(percent of parents reporting barriers to children's participation in physical activities, 2002)

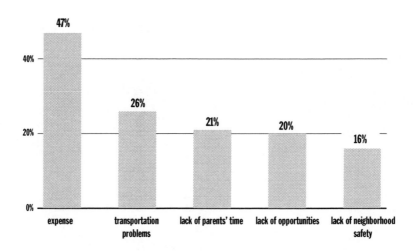

Table 14.16 Participation of Children Aged 9 to 13 in Physical Activities, 2002

(percent of children aged 9 to 13 participating in physical activities during past seven days and percent of parents reporting barriers to children's participation, by selected demographic characteristics, 2002)

	participated in organized physical activity during past seven days	participated in free-time physical activity during past seven days	barriers to children's participation in physical activities				
			transportation problems	lack of opportunities	expense	lack of parents' time	lack of neighborhood safety
Total children	**39.5%**	**77.4%**	**25.6%**	**20.1%**	**46.6%**	**21.0%**	**16.1%**
Sex							
Female	38.6	74.1	26.9	20.8	47.5	22.8	17.6
Male	38.3	80.5	24.4	19.5	45.8	19.2	14.6
Age							
Aged 9	36.1	75.8	25.6	20.5	46.3	20.3	16.9
Aged 10	37.5	77.0	26.2	19.2	46.4	21.6	18.0
Aged 11	43.1	78.0	26.1	21.1	46.0	20.7	16.9
Aged 12	37.7	77.5	24.9	20.0	49.0	20.8	15.9
Aged 13	38.1	78.0	25.2	19.8	45.4	21.5	12.4
Race and Hispanic origin							
Black, non-Hispanic	24.1	74.7	32.6	30.6	54.9	23.3	13.3
Hispanic	25.9	74.6	36.9	30.8	62.3	23.3	41.2
White, non-Hispanic	46.6	79.3	18.9	13.4	39.5	19.1	8.5
Parental education							
Not a high school graduate	19.4	75.3	42.7	36.7	65.9	27.3	42.9
High school graduate	28.3	75.4	32.3	23.8	54.8	20.5	18.2
Some college or more	46.8	78.7	19.3	15.4	39.2	20.0	10.2
Household income							
Less than $25,000	23.5	74.1	44.5	35.6	70.6	25.6	29.4
$25,000 to $50,000	32.8	78.6	28.9	21.9	53.6	20.4	17.8
$50,000 or more	49.1	78.3	14.4	11.5	30.8	19.0	8.6

Source: Centers for Disease Control and Prevention, Physical Activity Levels among Children Aged 9–13 Years—United States, 2002, *MMWR, Vol. 52, No. 33, August 22, 2003*

Glossary

Abortion Includes legal abortions only; defined as a procedure performed by a licensed physician or someone acting under the supervision of a licensed physician to induce the termination of a pregnancy.

Acquired immunodeficiency syndrome (AIDS) All 50 states and the District of Columbia report AIDS cases to the Centers for Disease Control and Prevention (CDC) using a uniform case definition and case report form.

Acute condition. *See* Condition.

Adjusted for inflation Income or a change in income that has been adjusted for the rise in the cost of living, or the consumer price index (CPI-U-RS).

Age of householder. *See* Householder, age of.

AIDS. *See* Acquired immunodeficiency syndrome.

Alternative medicine. *See* Complementary and alternative medicine.

Ambulatory care Medical care provided at a health care facility or provider's office to persons who are not currently admitted to the health care institution on the premises.

Ambulatory patient Person seeking care from a health care facility or provider's office who is not currently admitted to the health care institution on the premises. *See* Ambulatory care.

American Indians In this book, American Indians include Alaska Natives.

Asians In this book, Asians include Native Hawaiians and other Pacific Islanders unless those groups are shown separately.

Assisted living The National Center for assisted Living defines assisted living as a congregate residential setting that provides and coordinates personal care services, 24-hour supervision, assistance, activities, and health-related services.

Average length of stay In the National Health Interview Survey, average length of stay per discharged patient is computed by dividing the total number of hospital days for a specified group by the total number of discharges for that group. In the National Hospital Discharge Survey, average length of stay is computed by dividing the total number of days of care, counting the date of admission but not the date of discharge, by the number of patients discharged.

Baby-boom generation Americans born between 1946 and 1964.

Behavioral Risk Factor Surveillance System (BRFSS) The BRFSS is a collaborative project of the Centers for Disease Control and Prevention and U.S. states and territories. It is an ongoing data collection program designed to measure behavioral risk factors in the adult population aged 18 or older. All 50 states, three territories, and the District of Columbia take part in the survey, making the BRFSS the primary source of information on the health-related behaviors of Americans.

Birth rate. *See* Rate: Birth and related rates.

Birth weight The first weight of the newborn obtained after birth. Low birthweight is defined as less than 2,500 grams, or 5 pounds 8 ounces.

Blacks Blacks include those who identified themselves as "black" or "African American."

Body Mass Index (BMI) BMI is calculated by dividing weight in kilograms by height in meters squared. It is used to determine who is overweight and obese.

Cause of death For the purpose of national mortality statistics, every death is attributed to one underlying condition based on information reported on the death certificate and using the international rules for selecting the underlying cause of death from the reported conditions.

Central cities The largest city in a metropolitan area is called the central city. The balance of the metropolitan area outside the central city is regarded as the "suburbs."

Chronic condition. *See* Condition.

Complementary and alternative medicine (CAM) Complementary and alternative medicine is defined as a group of diverse medical and health care systems, practices, and products that are not presently considered to be part of conventional medicine.

Condition A health condition is a departure from a state of physical or mental well-being. An impairment is a health condition that includes chronic or permanent health defects resulting from disease, injury, or congenital malformations. Based on duration, there are two categories of conditions, acute and chronic. An acute condition is a condition that has lasted less than three months and has involved either a physician visit (medical attention) or restricted activity. A chronic condition is a condition lasting three months or more or one that is classified as chronic regardless of its time of onset (for example, diabetes, heart conditions, emphysema, and arthritis).

Consumer Expenditure Survey The Consumer Expenditure Survey (CEX) is an ongoing study of the day-to-day spending of American households administered by the Bureau of Labor Statistics. The CEX includes an interview survey and a diary survey. The average spending figures shown in this book are the integrated data from both the diary and interview components of the survey. Two separate, nationally representative samples are used for the interview and diary surveys. For the interview survey, about 7,500 consumer units are interviewed on a rotating panel basis each quarter for five consecutive quarters. For the diary survey, 7,500 consumer units keep weekly diaries of spending for two consecutive weeks.

Consumer price index (CPI) The CPI is prepared by the Bureau of Labor Statistics. It is a monthly measure of the average change in prices paid by urban consumers for a fixed basket of goods and services. The medical care component of the CPI shows trends in medical care prices based on specific indicators of hospital, medical, dental, and drug prices.

Consumer unit *(on selected spending tables only)* The term consumer unit is used by the Bureau of Labor Statistics in the annual Consumer Expenditure Survey. For convenience, the terms consumer unit and household are used interchangeably in the spending tables of this book, although consumer units are somewhat different from households. A consumer unit comprises all related members of a household or a financially independent member of a household. Thus, a household may include more than one consumer unit. *See also* Household.

Current Population Survey The CPS is a nationally representative survey of the civilian noninstitutional population aged 15 or older. It is taken monthly by the Census Bureau for the Bureau of Labor Statistics, collecting information from more than 50,000 households on employment and unemployment. In March of each year, the survey includes the Annual Social and Economic Supplement, which is the source of most national data on the characteristics of Americans, such as their incomes, living arrangements, and health insurance status.

Current smoker Current smokers are defined as those who answer "everyday" or "some days" to the question: "Do you smoke everyday, some days, or not at all?"

Death rate. *See* Rate: Death and related rates.

Diagnosis. *See* First-listed diagnosis.

Disability (2000 Census data) The 2000 Census defined the disabled as those who were blind, deaf, or had severe vision or hearing impairments, and/or had a condition that substantially limited one or more

basic physical activities such as walking, climbing stairs, reaching, lifting, or carrying. It also included people who, because of a physical, mental, or emotional condition lasting six months or more, have difficulty learning, remembering, concentrating, dressing, bathing, getting around inside the home, going outside the home alone to shop or visit a doctor's office, or working at a job or business.

Disability (National Health Interview Survey) The NHIS estimates the number of people aged 18 or older who have difficulty in physical functioning, probing whether respondents could perform nine activities by themselves without using special equipment. The categories are walking a quarter mile; standing for two hours; sitting for two hours; walking up 10 steps without resting; stooping, bending, kneeling; reaching over one's head; grasping or handling small objects; carrying a 10-pound object; and pushing/pulling a large object. Adults who reported that any of these activities was very difficult or they could not do it at all were defined as having physical difficulties.

Disability, work (Current Population Survey) The CPS considers a person to have a work disability if one or more of the following conditions are met: 1) Answered "yes" to the March supplement question, "Does anyone in this household have a health problem or disability which prevents them from working or which limits the kind or amount of work they can do?" 2) Answered "yes" to the March supplement question, "Is there anyone in this household who ever retired or left a job for health reasons?" 3) Identified by the core questionnaire as currently not in the labor force because of a disability. 4) Identified by the March supplement as a person who did not work at all in the previous year because of illness or disability. 5) Under age 65 and covered by Medicare in previous year. 6) Under age 65 and received Supplemental Security Income (SSI) in previous year. 7) Received VA disability income in previous year.

Discharge The National Health Interview Survey defines a hospital discharge as the completion of any continuous period of stay of one or more nights in a hospital by an inpatient, not including well newborn infants. According to the National Hospital Discharge Survey, discharge is the formal release of an inpatient (excluding newborn infants) by a hospital, that is, the termination of a period of hospitalization (including stays of zero nights) by death or by disposition to a place of residence, nursing home, or another hospital.

Earnings A type of income, earnings is the amount of money a person receives from his or her job. *See also* Income.

Emergency department An emergency department is a hospital facility staffed 24-hours a day for the provision of unscheduled outpatient services to patients whose conditions require immediate care. Off-site emergency departments open less than 24 hours are included if staffed by the hospital's emergency department. An emergency department visit is a direct personal exchange between a patient and a physician or other health care provider working under the physician's supervision for the purpose of seeking care and receiving personal health services.

Employed All civilians who did any work as a paid employee or farmer/self-employed worker, or who worked 15 hours or more as an unpaid farm worker or in a family-owned business, during the reference period. All those who have jobs but who are temporarily absent from their jobs due to illness, bad weather, vacation, labor management dispute, or personal reasons are considered employed.

Expenditures. *See* Health expenditures, consumer; Health expenditures, national.

Family A group of two or more people (one of whom is the householder) related by birth, marriage, or adoption and living in the same household.

Family household A household maintained by a householder who lives with one or more people related to him or her by blood, marriage, or adoption.

Federal hospital. *See* Hospital.

Female/male householder A woman or man who maintains a household without a spouse present. May head family or nonfamily households.

Fertility rate. *See* Rate: Birth and related rates.

First-listed diagnosis In the National Hospital Discharge Survey, this is the first recorded final diagnosis on the medical record face sheet.

Foreign-born population People who are not U.S. citizens at birth.

Full-time employment Full-time is 35 or more hours of work per week during a majority of the weeks worked.

Full-time, year-round employment Indicates 50 or more weeks of full-time employment during the previous calendar year.

General Social Survey The General Social Survey (GSS) is a biennial survey of the attitudes of Americans taken by the University of Chicago's National Opinion Research Center (NORC). NORC conducts the GSS through face-to-face interviews with an independently drawn, representative sample of 1,500 to 3,000 noninsti-

tutionalized English-speaking people aged 18 or older who live in the United States.

Generation X Americans born between 1965 and 1976.

Gestation The period of gestation is defined as beginning with the first day of the last normal menstrual period and ending with the day of birth or day of termination of pregnancy.

Gross domestic product (GDP) GDP is the market value of the goods and services produced by labor and property located in the United States. The suppliers (that is, the workers and, for property, the owners) may be either U.S. residents or residents of the rest of the world.

Group quarters population The group quarters population includes all people not living in households. Two general categories of people in group quarters are recognized: 1) the institutionalized population, which includes people under formally authorized, supervised care or custody in institutions at the time of enumeration such as correctional institutions, nursing homes, and juvenile institutions; and 2) the noninstitutionalized population, which includes all people who live in group quarters other than institutions such as college dormitories, military quarters, and group homes.

Health expenditures, consumer Consumer spending statistics show the amounts spent out-of-pocket on health care products and services by individual consumer units during a 12-month period, including the amount spent on sales tax. The full cost of each purchase is recorded even though full payment may not have been made at the date of purchase. Average expenditure figures may be artificially low for infrequently purchased items such as eyeglasses because figures are calculated using all consumer units within a demographic segment rather than just purchasers.

Health expenditures, Medical Expenditure Panel Survey (MEPS) The sum of direct payments for health care provided during the year, including out-of-pocket payments and payments by private insurance, Medicaid, Medicare, and other sources. Payments for over-the-counter drugs, alternative care services, and phone contacts with medical providers are not included in MEPS total expenditure estimates. Indirect payments not related to specific medical events, such as Medicaid Disproportionate Share and Medicare Direct Medical Education subsidies, also are not included. MEPS expenditures are classified into eight categories:

—*Hospital inpatient services* Room and board and all hospital diagnostic and laboratory expenses associated with the basic facility charge and payments for separately billed physician inpatient services.

—*Emergency Room services* Hospital diagnostic and laboratory expenses associated with ER facility charge and payments for separately billed inpatient services.
—*Outpatient services* Outpatient diagnostic and laboratory expenses associated with the basic facility charge and payments for separately billed inpatient services.
—*Medical provider visits* Visits to a medical provider seen in an office-based setting.
—*Prescribed medicines* All prescribed medications that were initially purchased or otherwise obtained during the calendar year, as well as any refills.
—*Dental services* Any type of dental care provider, including general dentists, dental hygienists, dental technicians, dental surgeons, orthodontists, endodontists, and periodontists.
—*Home health services* Care provided by home health agencies and independent home health providers. Agency providers accounted for most of the expenses in this category.

Health expenditures, national The total amount spent for all health services and supplies and health-related research and construction activities in the United States during a calendar year. Detailed estimates are available by source of expenditure (for example, out-of-pocket payments, private health insurance, and government programs) and by type of expenditure (for example, hospital care, physician services, and drugs). They are in current dollars for the year of report.
—*Personal health care expenditures* National outlays for goods and services relating directly to patient care. Expenditures in this category are total national health expenditures minus expenditures for research and construction, expenses for administering health insurance programs, and government public health activities.
—*Private expenditures* Outlays for services provided or paid for by nongovernmental sources—consumers, insurance companies, private industry, and philanthropic and other nonpatient care sources.
—*Public expenditures* Outlays for services provided or paid for by federal, state, and local government agencies or expenditures required by governmental mandate (such as workmen's compensation insurance payments).

Health maintenance organization (HMO) A prepaid health plan delivering comprehensive care to members through designated providers, having a fixed monthly payment for health care services, and requiring beneficiaries to be plan members for a specified period of time (usually one year).

Hispanic origin Of Mexican, Puerto Rican, Cuban, Central and South American, and other or unknown Spanish origins. Because Hispanic is an ethnic origin rather than a race, Hispanics may be of any race. While most Hispanics are white, there are black, Asian, American Indian, and even Native Hawaiian Hispanics.

HIV. *See* Human immunodeficiency virus infection.

Home health care Care provided to individuals and families in their place of residence for promoting, maintaining, or restoring health or for minimizing the effects of disability and illness including terminal illness.

Hospice care A program of palliative and supportive care services providing physical, psychological, social, and spiritual care for dying persons, their families, and other loved ones. Hospice care is available in home and inpatient settings.

Hospital In the National Hospital Ambulatory Medical Care Survey, hospitals include all those with an average length of stay for all patients of less than 30 days (short-stay) and hospitals whose specialty is general (medical or surgical) or children's general. Federal hospitals, hospital units of institutions, and hospitals with fewer than six beds staffed for patient use are excluded.

Household All the persons who occupy a housing unit. A household includes the related family members and all the unrelated persons, if any, such as lodgers, foster children, wards, and employees who share the housing unit. A person living alone is counted as a household. A group of unrelated people who share a housing unit as roommates or unmarried partners is also counted as a household, but group quarters such as college dormitories, prisons, and nursing homes are not.

Household, race/ethnicity of Households are categorized according to the race or ethnicity of the householder only.

Householder The householder is the person (or one of the persons) in whose name the housing unit is owned or rented or, if there is no such person, any adult member. With married couples, the householder may be either the husband or wife. The householder is the reference person for the household.

Householder, age of The age of the householder is used to categorize households into age groups. Married couples, for example, are classified according to the age of either husband or wife depending on which one identified him- or herself as the householder.

Human immunodeficiency virus (HIV) infection In 1987, the National Center for Health Statistics introduced a specific category for classifying HIV infection as a cause of death. Prior to that time, HIV deaths were classified under a variety of codes depending on the specific course taken by the disease. Therefore, beginning with 1987, death statistics for HIV infection are not strictly comparable with data for earlier years.

Incidence The number of cases of disease having their onset during a prescribed period of time. It is often expressed as a rate, for example, the incidence of measles per 1,000 children aged 5 to 15 during a specified year. Incidence is a measure of morbidity or other events that occur within a specified period of time. *See* Prevalence.

Income Money received in the preceding calendar year by each person aged 15 or older from each of the following sources: (1) earnings from longest job (or self-employment); (2) earnings from jobs other than longest job; (3) unemployment compensation; (4) workers' compensation; (5) Social Security; (6) Supplemental Security income; (7) public assistance; (8) veterans' payments; (9) survivor benefits; (10) disability benefits; (11) retirement pensions; (12) interest; (13) dividends; (14) rents and royalties or estates and trusts; (15) educational assistance; (16) alimony; (17) child support; (18) financial assistance from outside the household, and (19) other periodic income. Income is reported in several ways in this book. Household income is the combined income of all household members. Income of persons is all income accruing to a person from all sources. Earnings are the money a person receives from his or her job.

Institutionalized population. *See* Group Quarters Population.

Labor force The labor force includes both the employed and the unemployed (people who are looking for work). People are counted as in the labor force if they were working or looking for work during the reference week in which the Census Bureau fields the Current Population Survey.

Labor force participation rate The percent of the civilian noninstitutional population that is in the civilian labor force, which includes both the employed and the unemployed.

Length of stay. *See* Average length of stay.

Life expectancy The average number of years of life remaining to a person at a particular age and is based on a given set of age-specific death rates, generally the mortality conditions existing in the period mentioned. Life expectancy may be determined by race, sex, or other characteristics using age-specific death rates for the population with that characteristic.

Limitation of activity A long-term reduction in a person's capacity to perform the usual kind or amount of activities associated with his or her age group. Each

person is classified according to the extent to which his or her activities are limited, as follows: unable to carry on major activity, limited in the amount or kind of major activity performed, not limited in major activity but otherwise limited, and not limited in activity.

Live birth The complete expulsion or extraction from its mother of a product of conception, irrespective of the duration of the pregnancy, which, after such separation, breathes or shows any other evidence of life such as heartbeat, umbilical cord pulsation, or definite movement of voluntary muscles, whether the umbilical cord has been cut or the placenta is attached. Each product of such a birth is considered live born.

Live-birth order The total number of live births the mother has had, including the present birth, as recorded on the birth certificate. Fetal deaths are excluded.

Low birth weight. *See* Birth weight.

Major (or usual) activity The principal activity of a person or of his or her age-sex group. For children aged 1 to 5, major activity refers to ordinary play with other children; for children aged 5 to 17, major activity refers to school attendance; for adults aged 18 to 69, major activity usually refers to a job, housework, or school attendance; for persons aged 70 or older, major activity refers to the capacity for independent living (bathing, shopping, dressing, and eating without needing the help of another person).

Marital status The term married encompasses all married people including those separated from their spouses. Unmarried includes those who are single (never married), divorced, or widowed.

Married couples with or without children under age 18 Refers to married couples with or without own children under age 18 living in the same household. Couples without children under age 18 may be parents of grown children who live elsewhere, or they could be childless couples.

Median The median is the amount that divides the population or households into two equal portions: one below and one above the median. Medians can be calculated for income, age, and many other characteristics.

Median income The amount that divides the income distribution into two equal groups, half having incomes above the median, half having incomes below the median. The medians for households or families are based on all households or families. The median for persons are based on all persons aged 15 or older with income.

Medicaid This program provides health care services for certain low-income persons. It is state operated and administered but has federal financial participation. Within certain broad federally determined guidelines, states decide on eligibility; the amount, duration, and scope of services covered; rates of payment for providers; and methods of administering the program. Medicaid does not provide health services to all poor people in every state. The program was authorized in 1965 by Title XIX of the Social Security Act.

Medical Expenditure Panel Survey (MEPS) MEPS is a nationally representative survey that collects detailed information on the health status, access to care, health care use and expenses and health insurance coverage of the civilian noninstitutionalized population of the U.S. and nursing home residents. MEPS comprises four component surveys: the Household Component, the Medical Provider Component, the Insurance Component, and the Nursing Home Component. The Household Component is the core survey and is conducted each year, and includes 15,000 households and 37,000 people.

Medicare This nationwide health insurance program provides health insurance protection to people aged 65 or older, people entitled to Social Security disability payments for two or more years, and people with end-stage renal disease, regardless of income. The program was enacted July 30, 1965, as Title XVIII, Health Insurance for the Aged of the Social Security Act, and became effective on July 1, 1966. It consists of two separate but coordinated programs, hospital insurance (Part A) and supplementary medical insurance (Part B).

Mental illness The National Survey on Drug Use and Health defines serious mental illness as having a diagnosable mental, behavioral, or emotional disorder that met the criteria found in the 4th edition of the *Statistical Manual of Mental Disorders* and that resulted in functional impairment that substantially limited one or more major life activities.

Metropolitan area A county or group of counties that includes at least one city having a population of 50,000 or more plus adjacent counties that are metropolitan in character and are economically and socially integrated with the central city. In New England, towns and cities rather than counties are the units used in defining metropolitan areas. There is no limit to the number of adjacent counties included in the metropolitan area as long as they are integrated with the central city. A metropolitan area's boundaries may cross state lines.

Millennial generation Americans born between 1977 and 1994.

Monitoring the Future Project (MTF) The MTF survey is conducted by the University of Michigan Survey Research Center. The survey is administered to approximately 50,000 students in 420 public and private secondary schools every year. High school seniors have been surveyed annually since 1975. Students in 8th and 10th grade have been surveyed annually since 1991.

National Ambulatory Medical Care Survey (NAMCS) The NAMCS is an annual survey of visits to nonfederally employed office-based physicians who are primarily engaged in direct patient care. Data are collected from physicians rather than patients, with each physician assigned a one-week reporting period. During that week, a systematic random sample of visit characteristics are recorded by the physician or office staff.

National Compensation Survey (NCS) The Bureau of Labor Statistics' National Compensation Survey examines the incidence and detailed provisions of selected employee benefit plans in small, medium, and large private establishments, and state and local governments. Each year BLS economists visit a representative sample of establishments across the country, asking questions about the establishment, its employees, and their benefits.

National Health and Nutrition Examination Survey (NHANES) The NHANES is a continuous survey of a representative sample of the U.S. civilian noninstitutionalized population. Respondents are interviewed at home about their health and nutrition, and this interview is followed up by a physical examination that measures height and weight, among other things, in mobile examination centers.

National Health Interview Survey (NHIS) The NHIS is a continuing nationwide sample survey of the civilian noninstitutional population of the U.S. conducted by the Census Bureau for the National Center for Health Statistics. Each year, data are collected from more than 100,000 people about their illnesses, injuries, impairments, chronic and acute conditions, activity limitations, and the use of health services.

National Home and Hospice Care Survey These are a series of surveys of a nationally representative sample of home and hospice care agencies in the U.S., sponsored by the National Center for Health Statistics. Data on the characteristics of patients and services provided are collected through personal interviews with administrators and staff.

National Hospital Ambulatory Medical Care Survey (NHAMCS) The NHAMCS is an annual national probability sample survey of visits to emergency departments and outpatient departments at non-Federal, short stay and general hospitals. Data are collected by hospital staff from patient record forms.

National Hospital Discharge Survey This survey has been conducted annually since 1965, sponsored by the National Center for Health Statistics, to collect nationally representative information on the characteristics of inpatients discharged from nonfederal, short-stay hospitals in the U.S. The survey collects data from a sample of approximately 270,000 inpatient records acquired from a national sample of about 500 hospitals.

National Nursing Home Survey This is a series of national sample surveys of nursing homes, their residents, and staff conducted at various intervals since 1973-74 and sponsored by the National Center for Health Statistics. The latest survey was taken in 1999. data for the survey are obtained through personal interviews with administrators and staff, and occasionally with self-administered questionnaires, in a sample of about 1,500 facilities.

National Survey of Family Growth (NSFG) The 2002 NSFG, sponsored by the National Center for Health Statistics, is a nationally representative survey of the civilian noninstitutional population aged 15 to 44. In-person interviews were completed with 12,571 men and women, collecting data on marriage, divorce, contraception, and infertility. The 2002 survey updates previous NSFG surveys taken in 1973, 1976, 1988, and 1995.

National Survey on Drug Use and Health *(formerly called the National Household Survey on Drug Abuse)* This survey, sponsored by the Substance Abuse and Mental Health Services Administration, has been conducted since 1971. It is the primary source of information on the use of illegal drugs by the U.S. population. Each year, a nationally representative sample of about 70,000 individuals aged 12 or older are surveyed in the 50 states and the District of Columbia.

Native Hawaiian and other Pacific Islander The 2000 census identified this group for the first time as a separate racial category from Asians. In most survey data, however, the population is included with Asians.

Nonfamily household A household maintained by a householder who lives alone or who lives with people to whom he or she is not related.

Nonfamily householder A householder who lives alone or with nonrelatives.

Non-Hispanic People who do not identify themselves as Hispanic are classified as non-Hispanic. Non-Hispanics may be of any race.

Non-Hispanic white People who identify their race as white and who do not indicate a Hispanic origin.

Noninstitutionalized population. *See* Group Quarters Population.

Nonmetropolitan area Counties that are not classified as metropolitan. *See* Metropolitan area.

Nursing home An establishment with three or more beds that provides nursing or personal care services to the aged, infirm, or chronically ill.

Obese Having a body mass index (BMI) of 30 or higher. BMI is calculated by dividing weight in kilograms by height in meters squared.

Office In the National Health Interview Survey, the term office refers to the office of any physician in private practice not located in a hospital. In the National Ambulatory Medical Care Survey, an office is any location for a physician's ambulatory practice other than a hospital, nursing home, other extended care facility, patient home, industrial clinic, college clinic, and family planning clinic. Private offices in hospitals, however, are included.

Office visit In the National Ambulatory Medical Care Survey, an office visit is any direct personal exchange between an ambulatory patient and a physician or member of his or her staff for the purposes of seeking care and rendering health services.

Operation. *See* Procedure.

Outpatient department According to the National Hospital Ambulatory Medical Care Survey, an outpatient department is a hospital facility where nonurgent ambulatory medical care is provided, excluding ambulatory surgical centers, employee health services, and facilities providing chemotherapy, renal dialysis, methadone maintenance, and radiology. An outpatient department visit is a direct personal exchange between a patient and a physician or other health care provider working under the physician's supervision for the purpose of seeking care and receiving personal health services.

Outpatient visit The American Hospital Association defines outpatient visits as visits for receipt of medical, dental, or other services by patients who are not lodged in the hospital. Each appearance by an outpatient to each unit of the hospital is counted individually as an outpatient visit.

Outside central city The portion of a metropolitan county or counties that falls outside of the central city or cities; generally regarded as the suburbs.

Overweight Having a body mass index (BMI) of 25 or higher. BMI is calculated by dividing weight in kilograms by height in meters squared.

Part-time employment Part-time is less than 35 hours of work per week in a majority of the weeks worked during the year.

Patient A person who is formally admitted to the inpatient service of a hospital for observation, care, diagnosis, or treatment.

Percent change The change (either positive or negative) in a measure expressed as a proportion of the starting measure.

Percentage point change The change (either positive or negative) in a value which is already expressed as a percentage.

Personal health care expenditures. *See* Health expenditures, national.

Physical activity, recommended amount Physical activity at least five times a week for 30 minutes each time or vigorous physical activity at least three times a week for 20 minutes each time.

Physician Physicians are classified by the American Medical Association and others as licensed doctors of medicine or osteopathy, as follows:
—*Active (or professionally active) physician* Physician currently practicing medicine for a minimum of 20 hours per week. Excluded are physicians who are inactive, practicing medicine less than 20 hours per week, have unknown addresses, or practice specialties not classified (when specialty information is presented).
—*Federal physician* Physician employed by the federal government.
—*Hospital-based physician* Physician who spends plurality of time as salaried physician in a hospital.
—*Office-based physician* Physician who spends plurality of time working in a practice based in a private office. *See* Office; Physician contact; Physician specialty.

Physician specialty Any specific branch of medicine in which a physician may concentrate. Data are based on physician self-reports of their primary area of specialty. Physician data are broadly categorized into two general areas of practice: generalists and specialists.
—*Generalist physician* Synonymous with primary care generalist. Includes physicians practicing in the general fields of family and general practice, general internal medicine, and general pediatrics. Specifically excludes primary care specialists.
—*Primary care specialist* Physician practicing in the subspecialties of general and family practice, internal medicine, and pediatrics. The primary care subspe-

cialties for family practice include such specialties as geriatric medicine and sports medicine. For internal medicine they include such specialties as infectious diseases, medical oncology, and rheumatology. For pediatrics they include such specialties as critical care pediatrics, and pediatric cardiology.
—*Specialist physician* Those practicing in primary care subspecialties and all other specialist fields not included in the generalist definition. Specialist fields include allergy and immunology, anesthesiology, child and adolescent psychiatry, dermatology, general surgery, obstetrics and gynecology, and psychiatry.

Poverty level The official income threshold below which families and people are classified as living in poverty. The threshold rises each year with inflation and varies depending on family size and age of householder.

Prevalence The number of cases of a disease, infected persons, or persons with some other problem during a particular interval of time. It is often expressed as a rate, for example, the prevalence of diabetes per 1,000 persons during one year. *See* Incidence.

Primary admission diagnosis In the National Home and Hospice Care Survey, the primary admission diagnosis is the first-listed diagnosis at admission on the patient's medical record as provided by the agency staff member most familiar with the care provided to the patient.

Primary care specialties. *See* Physician specialty.

Private expenditures. *See* Health expenditures, national.

Procedure The National Hospital Discharge Survey defines procedure as a surgical or nonsurgical operation, diagnostic procedure, or special treatment assigned by the physician and recorded on the medical record of patients discharged from the inpatient service of short-stay hospitals. A maximum of four operations or diagnostic procedures are permitted per discharge. Procedures are subdivided into diagnostic and other nonsurgical procedures and surgical operations.
—*Diagnostic and other nonsurgical procedures* Procedures generally not considered to be surgery, including diagnostic endoscopy, radiography, and other tests as well as physical medicine and rehabilitation.
—*Surgical operations* Surgery is defined as a major or minor surgical episode performed in the operating room. During a single episode, multiple surgical procedures may be performed, and the National Hospital Discharge Survey codes up to four surgical procedures per surgical episode.

Proportion or share The value of a part expressed as a percentage of the whole. If there are 4 million people aged 25 and 3 million of them are white, then the white proportion is 75 percent.

Public expenditures. *See* Health expenditures, national.

Race Race is self-reported and can be defined in three ways. The "race alone" population is people who identify themselves as only one race. The "race in combination" population is people who identify themselves as more than one race, such as white and black. The "race, alone or in combination" population includes both those who identify themselves as one race and those who identify themselves as more than one race.

Rate The measure of some event, disease, or condition in relation to a unit of population, along with some specification of time.

Birth and related rates
—Birth rate: Calculated by dividing the number of live births in a population in one year by the midyear resident population. Birth rate is expressed as the number of live births per 1,000 population. The rate may be restricted to births to women of specific age, race, marital status, or geographic location.
—Fertility rate: The number of live births per 1,000 women of reproductive age, 15 to 44.

Death and related rates
—Death rate: Calculated by dividing the number of deaths in a population in one year by the midyear resident population. Death rate is expressed as the number of deaths per 100,000 population. The rate may be restricted to deaths in specific age, race, sex, or geographic groups or from specific causes of death.
—Infant mortality rate: Calculated by dividing the number of infant deaths during one year by the number of live births reported in the same year.

Regions The four regions and nine census divisions of the United States are composed as follows:

Northeast
—New England: Connecticut, Maine, Massachusetts, New Hampshire, Rhode Island, and Vermont
—Middle Atlantic: New Jersey, New York, and Pennsylvania

Midwest
—East North Central: Illinois, Indiana, Michigan, Ohio, and Wisconsin
—West North Central: Iowa, Kansas, Minnesota, Missouri, Nebraska, North Dakota, and South Dakota

South
—South Atlantic: Delaware, District of Columbia, Florida, Georgia, Maryland, North Carolina, South Carolina, Virginia, and West Virginia
—East South Central: Alabama, Kentucky, Mississippi, and Tennessee
—West South Central: Arkansas, Louisiana, Oklahoma, and Texas

West
—Mountain: Arizona, Colorado, Idaho, Montana, Nevada, New Mexico, Utah, and Wyoming
—Pacific: Alaska, California, Hawaii, Oregon, and Washington

Rounding Percentages are rounded to the nearest tenth of a percent; therefore, the percentages in a distribution do not always add exactly to 100.0 percent. The totals, however, are always shown as 100.0. Moreover, individual figures are rounded to the nearest thousand without being adjusted to group totals, which are independently rounded; percentages are based on the unrounded numbers.

Short-stay hospital. *See* Hospital.

Smoker. *See* Current smoker.

Suburbs. *See* Outside Central City.

Surgical operations. *See* Procedure.

Unemployed Unemployed people are those who, during the survey period, had no employment but were available and looking for work. Those who were laid off from their jobs and were waiting to be recalled are also classified as unemployed.

Unrelated individuals Persons who live alone or with others to whom they are not related by blood, marriage, or adoption.

White The "white" racial category includes many Hispanics (who may be of any race) unless the term "non-Hispanic white" is used. *See also* Non-Hispanic white.

Youth Risk Behavior Surveillance System (YRBSS) The YRBSS was created by the Centers for Disease Control to monitor health risks being taken by young people at the national, state, and local level. The national survey is taken every two years based on a nationally representative sample of 16,000 students in 9th through 12th grade in public and private schools.

Bibliography

Agency for Healthcare Research and Quality
  Internet site http://www.ahrq.gov/
  —2001 and 2002 Medical Expenditure Panel Surveys, Internet site http://www.meps .ahrq.gov/CompendiumTables/TC_TOC.htm

American Society for Aesthetic Plastic Surgery
  Internet site http://www.surgery.org/
  —Statistics, Internet site http://www.surgery.org/press/statistics.php

Bureau of Labor Statistics
  Internet site http://www.bls.gov/
  —2003 Consumer Expenditure Survey, Internet site http://www.bls.gov/cex/home.htm
  —*Employee Benefits in Private Industry in the United States: March 2004*, Internet site http://www.bls.gov/ncs/ebs/home.htm

Bureau of the Census
  Internet site http://www.census.gov/
  —2004 Current Population Survey Annual Social and Economic Supplement, Internet site http://www.census.gov/hhes/income/dinctabs.html
  —*Disability Status: 2000*, Census 2000 Brief, C2KBR-17, 2003, Internet site http://www .census.gov/population/www/cen2000/briefs.html
  —*Fertility of American Women: June 2002*, detailed tables, Internet site http://www .census.gov/population/www/socdemo/fertility/cps2002.html
  —*Income, Poverty, and Health Insurance Coverage in the United States: 2003*, Current Population Report, P60-226, 2004, Internet site http://www.census.gov/hhes/www/income03.html
  —*Statistical Abstract of the United States: 2004–2005*, Internet site http://www.census.gov/ prod/www/statistical-abstract-04.html

Centers for Disease Control and Prevention
  Internet site http://www.cdc.gov/
  —Behavioral Risk Factor Surveillance System, Prevalence Data, Internet site http://www .apps.nccd.cdc.gov/brfss/
  —"Physical Activity Levels among Children Aged 9–13 Years—United States, 2002," *Morbidity and Mortality Weekly Report*, Vol. 52, No. 33, August 22, 2003, Internet site http://www .cdc.gov/mmwr/
  —"Youth Risk Behavior Surveillance—United States, 2003," *Morbidity and Mortality Weekly Report*, Surveillance Summaries, Vol. 53/SS02, May 21, 2004, Internet site http://www. cdc.gov/mmwr/

Centers for Medicare and Medicaid Services
  Internet site http://www.cms.hhs.gov/
  —*2003 Data Compendium*, Internet site http://www.cms.hhs.gov/researchers/pubs/ datacompendium/current/

The Gallup Organization
  Internet site http://www.gallup.com/
  —Assessing Americans' Mental Health, Internet site http://www.gallup.com/poll/content/ login.aspx?ci=14218

—Personal Weight Situation, Internet site http://www.gallup.com/poll/content/login.aspx?ci=7264

—Public: Healthcare Costs and Availability Are Major Concerns, Internet site http://www.gallup.com/poll/content/login.aspx?ci=14098

Inter-University Consortium for Political and Social Research, University of Michigan
Internet site http://www.icpsr.umich.edu/org/index.html
—2003 Monitoring the Future Survey, Internet site http://monitoringthefuture.org/data/03data.html

The Kaiser Family Foundation
Internet site http://www.kff.org/
—*2003 Health Insurance Survey*, November 2004, Internet site http://www.kff.org/kaiser-polls/pomr110104pkg.cfm

National Alliance for Caregiving and AARP
Internet sites http://www.caregiving.org/ and http://www.aarp.org/
—*Caregiving in the U.S., 2004*, Internet site http://www.aarp.org/research/reference/publicopinions/aresearch-import-853.html

National Center for Assisted Living
Internet site http://www.ahca.org/
—*The Assisted Living Sourcebook*, Internet site http://www.ahca.org/research/index.html

National Center for Health Statistics
Internet site http://www.cdc.gov/nchs /
—1999 National Nursing Home Survey, http://www.cdc.gov/nchs/about/major/nnhsd/nnhsd.htm
—"2002 National Hospital Discharge Survey," *Advance Data*, No. 342, 2004, Internet site http://www.cdc.gov/nchs/about/major/hdasd/listpubs.htm
— "Births: Final Data for 2002," *National Vital Statistics Reports*, Vol. 52, No. 1, 2003, Internet site http://www.cdc.gov/nchs/births.htm
— "Births: Preliminary Data for 2003," *National Vital Statistics Reports*, Vol. 53, No. 9, 2004, Internet site http://www.cdc.gov/nchs/births.htm
—"Characteristics of Hospice Care Discharges and Their Length of Service: United States, 2000," *Vital and Health Statistics Report*, Series 13, No. 154, 2003, Internet site http://www.cdc.gov/nchs/pressroom/03facts/hospicecare.htm
—"Complementary and Alternative Medicine Use Among Adults: United States, 2002," *Advance Data No. 343*, 2004, Internet site http://www.cdc.gov/nchs/pressroom/04news/adultsmedicine.htm
— "Deaths: Final Data for 2002," *National Vital Statistics Reports*, Vol. 53, No. 5, 2004, Internet site http://www.cdc.gov/nchs/about/major/dvs/mortdata.htm
—"Estimated Pregnancy Rates for the United States, 1990–2000: An Update," *National Vital Statistics Report*, Vol. 52, No. 23, 2004, Internet site http://www.cdc.gov/nchs/births/htm
—*Health, United States, 2004*, Internet site http://www.cdc.gov/nchs/hus.htm
—"Mean Age of Mother, 1970–2000," *National Vital Statistics Report*, Vol. 51, No. 1, 2002, Internet site http://www.cdc.gov/nchs/births.htm
—"Mean Body Weight, Height, and Body Mass Index, United States 1960–2002," *Advance Data No. 347*, 2004, Internet site http://www.cdc.gov/nchs/pressroom/04news/americans.htm

—"National Ambulatory Medical Care Survey: 2002 Summary," *Advance Data No. 346*, 2004, Internet site http://www.cdc.gov/nchs/about/major/ahcd/adata.htm

—"National Hospital Ambulatory Medical Care Survey: 2002 Emergency Department Summary," *Advance Data No. 340*, 2004, Internet site http://www.cdc.gov/nchs/about/major/ahcd/adata.htm

—"National Hospital Ambulatory Medical Care Survey: 2002 Outpatient Department Summary," *Advance Data No. 345*, 2004, Internet site http://www.cdc.gov/nchs/about/major/ahcd/adata.htm

—*Summary Health Statistics for the U.S. Population: National Health Interview Survey, 2002*, Series 10, No. 220, 2004, Internet site http://www.cdc.gov/nchs/nhis.htm

—*Summary Health Statistics for U.S. Adults: National Health Interview Survey, 2002*, Series 10, No. 222, 2004, Internet site http://www.cdc.gov/nchs/nhis.htm

—*Summary Health Statistics for U.S. Children: National Health Interview Survey, 2002*, Series 10, No. 221, 2004, Internet site http://www.cdc.gov/nchs/nhis.htm

—"Teenagers in the United States: Sexual Activity, Contraceptive Use, and Childbearing, 2002," *Vital and Health Statistics*, Series 23, No. 24, 2004, Internet site http://www.cdc.gov/nchs/nsfg.htm

—"Use of Contraception and Use of Family Planning Services in the United States: 1982–2002," *Advance Data No. 350*, 2004, Internet site http://www.cdc.gov/nchs/nsfg.htm

National Institute of Mental Health
Internet site http://www.nimh.nih.gov/
—*The Numbers Count: Mental Disorders in America, 2001*, Internet site http://www.nimh.nih.gov/publicat/numbers.cfm

National Opinion Research Center, University of Chicago
Internet site http://www.norc.uchicago.edu/
—1972 to 2002 General Social Surveys

National Sporting Goods Association
Internet site http://www.nsga.org/
—Sports Participation, Internet site http://www.nsga.org/public/pages/index.cfm?pageid=864

Pew Internet & American Life Project
Internet site http://www.pewinternet.org/
—*Internet Health Resources, 2003*, Internet site http://www.pewinternet.org/PPF/r/95/report_display.asp
—*Prescription Drugs Online, 2004*, Internet site http://www.pewinternet.org/PPF/r/139/report_display.asp

Substance Abuse and Mental Health Services Administration
Internet site http://www.samhsa.gov/
—National Survey on Drug Use and Health, 2003, Internet site http://oas.samhsa.gov/nsduh.htm

Index

disabled, 250–252, 254, 259–261, 263
drug and alcohol abuse treatment, 33
drug use, 28
exercise, frequency of, 475–477
health care visits, 323–324, 326–330
health conditions 270–273
health insurance coverage, 166, 168, 171, 213
health status, 76
home health care patients, 364–365
hospital discharges of, 389, 391
hospital emergency room visits, 381, 384
hospital outpatient visits, 370–371, 374
in assisted living facilities, 47
in hospice care, 217
in nursing homes, 49–51
life expectancy, 246, 248
mental health problems, 415, 418–419, 429–431
overnight hospitals stays, 389–390
physician office visits, 339–340, 343–344
prescription drug use, 306–308
problems receiving health care, 80
spending on health care, 190–210
using Internet to get health information, 96–97
weight status, 459–467, 472–473
with AIDS, 297–299
with diabetes, 295–296
with high cholesterol, 290–293
with hypertension, 270–273, 286–289
Mental health problems
as cause of disability, 251
as diagnosis during hospital emergency room
visit, 386
as diagnosis during hospital inpatient care, 392–393,
395, 398
as diagnosis during hospital outpatient visit, 376
as diagnosis during physician office visit, 346
as reason for needing care, 45
attitude toward, 410, 412–413
average length of hospital stay for, 400
by age, 410, 414–417, 429–431
by education, 422, 425–426, 429–431
by income, 422–424
by labor force status, 429–431
by race and Hispanic origin, 415, 420–421, 429–431
by sex, 415, 418–419, 429–431
by type of problem, 410–411, 415–426
health insurance coverage of, 99, 101
in past 30 days, 74, 78, 415–426
number of events, 310–311
number of people experiencing event, 312–313,
410–411
spending on, 214, 314–319
therapy ordered or provided during hospital
outpatient visit, 379
therapy ordered or provided during physician office
visit, 356–357
treatment for, 429, 431
Mental health status, 414
Metropolitan status, childless women by, 130
Migraines, as health condition, 266–285
Military health insurance, 163, 167–169, 173–174
Miscarriage, 116–118

Mobility problems
as reason for needing care, 45
in nursing home residents, 49, 51
of patients in hospice care, 218

Native Hawaiians
health care visits, 323–324
hospital emergency room visits, 382
hospital outpatient visits, 372
physician office visits, 341
Nativity status
births by, 136, 148–150
childless women by, 130
health insurance coverage of children by, 173–175
Natural products as alternative medicine, 68
Nurses
in hospice care, 216, 219
seen during hospital emergency room visit, 383, 387
seen during hospital outpatient visit, 373, 377
seen during physician office visits, 354–355
spending on, 205, 207
Nursing homes
residents, 49–51
spending on, 154, 156, 159, 182, 184, 186, 188,
212, 214

Obesity. See Weight.
Occupation, health insurance coverage by, 176–178
Online. See Internet.
Operations. See Surgery.
Outdoor activities. See Recreational activities.
Outpatient services. See Hospital outpatient departments.
Overweight. See Weight.

Physical health, poor in past 30 days, 74, 78
Physical therapists, spending on, 205, 210
Physician assistants
seen during hospital emergency room visit, 387
seen during hospital outpatient visit, 373, 377
seen during physician office visits, 354–355
spending on, 205, 208
Physician office visits. See also Physicians.
by age, 323–324, 339–341
by continuity of care, 351–352
by diagnosis, 342, 346
by health condition, 310–319
by medications prescribed, 356–360
by physician's specialty, 347, 349, 353, 356, 358
by practice characteristics, 347, 350
by race, 323–324, 339, 341
by reason for visit, 342–345
by services provided, 347–348, 356–357
by sex, 323–324, 339–340
by source of payment, 322, 325, 343, 354–355
by type of provider seen, 354–355
for preventive care, 342–344
Physicians. See also Physician office visits.
attitude towards, 81–95, 336–338
in hospice care, 219
seen during hospital emergency room visit, 383, 387
seen during hospital outpatient visit, 373, 377
spending on, 154, 156, 159, 182, 184, 186, 188,
191–192, 212, 214
time spent with patient, 81, 84–85, 351, 353

physician office visits, 339, 341, 343–344
problems receiving health care, 80
using Internet for prescription drug information, 98
Whites, non-Hispanic. *See also* Whites.
alternative medicine use, 57
average age at giving birth, 133
births to, 136–138, 140–141, 147–148
childless, 130
cigarette smoking, 5–6, 10
contraceptive use, 449, 452
deaths of, 222, 228
dental visits, 365–368
disabled, 252, 255
drinking, 15–16
exercise, frequency of, 475–477
family planning services, use by, 449, 453
health care visits, 326–330, 334–335
health conditions, 274–277, 302–305
health insurance coverage, 166, 169, 171–175,
    211, 213
health status, 76–77
mental health problems, 415, 420–421, 429–431
overnight hospitals stays, 390
pregnancy, attitude toward, 440
pregnancy outcomes, 116, 118
prescription drug use, 306, 308
recreational activities, participation in, 482
spending on health care, 190–210
teenage sexual behavior, 441–442, 444–446
vaccinations of children, 300–301
weight status, 459–461, 463–464, 467–469
with AIDS, 297, 299
with diabetes, 294–296
with high cholesterol, 290, 292–293
with hypertension, 274–277, 286, 288–289
with problems receiving health care 332–333
Women *See also* Children and Teenagers.
abortion rate, 119–120
alternative medicine use, 55
attitudes toward health care, 82–85, 87–92, 94–95
average length of hospital stay, 389, 391
births to, 132–146
caregivers, 41–42
childless, 128–131
cigarette smoking, 4–7, 9–12
contraceptive use, 450–452
cosmetic surgery, 38–39
deaths of, 222, 224
dental visits, 363–366
disabled, 250–252, 254, 259–261, 263
drinking, 15–17, 19–20
drug and alcohol abuse treatment, 33
drug use, 28
exercise, frequency of, 475–477
family planning services, use of, 449, 453
health care visits, 323–324, 326–330
health conditions 270–273
health insurance coverage, 166, 168, 171, 213
health status, 76
home health care patients, 364–365
hospital discharges, 389, 391
hospital emergency room visits, 381, 384
hospital outpatient visits, 370–371, 374

in assisted living facilities, 47
in hospice care, 217
in nursing homes, 49–51
life expectancy, 246, 248
mental health problems, 415, 418–419, 429–431
overnight hospitals stays, 389–390
physician office visits, 339–340, 343–344
pregnancy outcomes, 116–118
prescription drug use, 306–308
problems receiving health care, 80
spending on health care, 190–210
using Internet to get health information, 96–97
weight status, 459–467, 472–473
with AIDS, 297–299
with diabetes, 295–296
with high cholesterol, 290–293
with hypertension, 270–273, 286–289